Neurology and Psychiatry: A Meeting of Minds

Les Métamorphoses du Jour. N.°59.

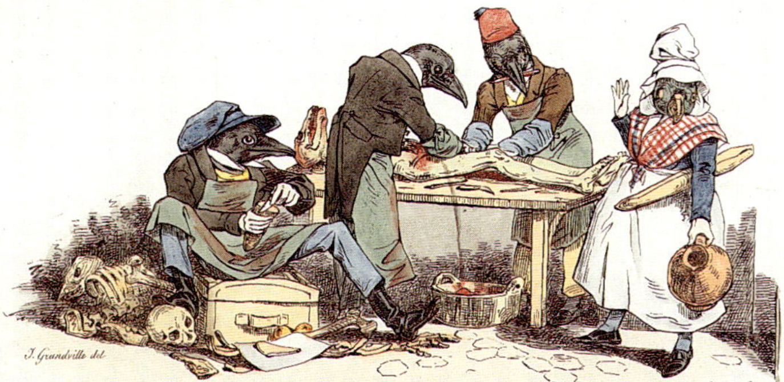

J. Grandville del. Lith. de Langlumé

Voulez vous déjeuner avec nous, la mère Piton?

chez Bulla rue S.t Jacques N.°38
et chez Martinet rue du Coq.

Neurology and Psychiatry
A Meeting of Minds

Editor
Jonathan Mueller, San Francisco, Calif.

Associate Editors
Charles D. Yingling, Leonard S. Zegans, San Francisco, Calif.

71 figures, 4 color plates and 14 tables, 1989

KARGER

Basel · München · Paris · London · New York · New Delhi · Singapore · Tokyo · Sydney

The editor thanks William E. Tate for the title of this book.

Library of Congress Cataloging-in-Publication Data
Neurology and psychiatry: a meeting of minds / editor, Jonathan Mueller; associate editors, Charles D. Yingling, Leonard S. Zegans.
Includes index.
1. Neuropsychiatry – Philosophy. 2. Neuropsychology – Philosophy.
I. Mueller, Jonathan, 1947–. II. Yingling, Charles D. III. Zegans, Leonard S.
[DNLM: 1. Neurology. 2. Neuropsychology. 3. Psychiatry. WL 103 N49335]
RC341.N435 1989 88–8276
152 – dc19
ISBN 3–8055–4712–9

Drug Dosage

The authors and the publisher have exerted every effort to ensure that drug selection and dosage set forth in this text are in accord with current recommendations and practice at the time of publication. However, in view of ongoing research, changes in government regulations, and the constant flow of information relating to drug therapy and drug reactions, the reader is urged to check the package insert for each drug for any change in indications and dosage and for added warnings and precautions. This is particularly important when the recommended agent is a new and/or infrequently employed drug.

Printed in Switzerland by Merkur Druck AG, Langenthal
ISBN 3–8055–4712–9

For Craig Van Dyke, MD

friend, boss, mentor and
perspicacious psychomaieutician.

J. M.

Contents

Neurobehavioral Syndromes

Neuropsychologic Approaches

Preface

Psychosomatics, biological psychiatry, organic psychiatry and neuropsychiatry are all terms that reflect psychiatry's growing recognition of structural and physiologic substrates for alterations in behavior, mood and thought. J. Mueller argues in the first chapter that without a framework for the integration of neuroscientific information, psychiatry runs the risk of being fragmented and destroyed, rather than invigorated by the neurosciences. He suggests that since neuroanatomy is unique in providing a conceptual framework for the assimilation of neurobiologic information, it needs to once again become psychiatry's core basic science. He then presents a rationale for the adoption of behavioral neurology and neuropsychology as two other key building blocks in the development of a modern neuropsychiatry that would return psychiatry to mainstream medicine.

M. R. Trimble compares the historical relationship of neurology to psychiatry in England and in the USA. He documents the continuous nature of British neuropsychiatry by considering the contributions of such figures as Willis, Ferrier, Jackson, Maudsley and Slater. Turning to North America, he offers several suggestions as to how neurology and psychiatry managed to drift so far asunder on this continent. After considering the important differences between neurobehavioral approaches, M. R. Trimble concludes by identifying those elements that tie neurology and psychiatry together.

Psychiatrists employ language to assess the inner world of patients' thoughts, as well as to gauge patients' awareness of their behavior and insight into their condition. Disruptions of the ability to 'propositionalize' occur in the aphasias, while impairment in melodic, intonational or 'prosodic' aspects of speech constitute a second area of great interest to neuropsychiatrists. As a neuroanatomist, A. B. Scheibel approaches language by utilizing Golgi techniques to elucidate the unfolding and maturation of the neural architecture that subserves language itself. His delineation of the evolving architecture of the dendritic arbor in Broca's area provides an elegant neuromorphologic correlate of Piaget's functional approach to the cognitive development of the child.

Psychomotor retardation and acceleration occur in a wide range of neurologic and psychiatric conditions. The anatomic underpinnings of brady- and tachyphrenia, of hypo- and hyperkinesia are now considerably less obscure than they were even five years ago. Long considered exclusively a motor domain, the basal ganglia now appear to play a crucial role in both motor and psychic spheres. W. J. H. Nauta's elegant chapter demonstrates how the anatomic connectivity of 'limbic' and 'nonlimbic' striatal regions may enable portions of the basal ganglia to play a central role in affect and cognition.

The fact that schizophrenic symptoms may be ameliorated with medications that block dopamine receptors has led neuroscientists to consider anatomic regions of the brain that receive strong dopaminergic inputs as likely suspects in the pathophysiology of schizophrenia. J. R. Stevens traces the history of attempts to implicate limbic regions such as the hippocampus, cingulate gyrus, ventral striatum, and striatal outflow pathways in the etiology of schizophrenia. Her masterful tour through these strategic limbic regions will be rewarding reading for all students of psychiatry, since it places modern efforts to understand the pathophysiology of schizophrenia in both an historic and anatomic context.

Since the advent of computed tomography (CT) in 1972, imaging of the brain has made extraordinary progress. Magnetic resonance imaging (MRI) now appears to be on the verge of superseding CT as the modality of choice for assessing the central nervous system. C. D. Yingling provides an analysis of the strengths and weaknesses of the major static and dynamic imaging techniques, assessing each of these in terms of their spatial and temporal resolution, invasiveness, and cost. This chapter is of particular value to psychiatric clinicians, since a growing literature employs single photon emission computed tomography (SPECT), positron emission tomography (PET), brain electrical activation mapping (BEAM) and various cerebral blood flow (CBF) measures to understand the physicochemical substrates of major psychiatric illnesses.

J. C. Mazziotta's chapter acquaints the reader with some of the most productive applications of PET, which has opened an era of dynamic in vivo neuropathology. In terms of stroke, PET has made two particularly striking contributions: (1) it demonstrates metabolic fluctuations in what has been termed the 'ischemic penumbra' adjacent to infarcted tissue, and (2) it characterizes the physiologic aftermath of strokes in terms of metabolic changes in regions remote from, but connected to, the site of injury ('diaschisis'). In vivo quantification of receptor density promises to have special relevance to the elucidation of psychiatric pathology. Although PET is still not available to clinicians who work outside major research centers, familiarity with PET is important to practicing neurologists and psychiatrists because a growing number of studies employ PET to study disorders ranging from stroke and epilepsy to schizophrenia and panic disorder.

Gilles de la Tourette's syndrome is well-known as a neurologic disorder characterized by multiple, chronic motor and vocal tics. Less appreciated is the range of intrapsychic phenomena that may also occur in the disorder. O. W. Sacks brings his skills as a phenomenological microscopist to bear on the subjective mental experiences of patients with Tourette's. In doing this he demonstrates, among other things, how this illness raises questions of the deepest nature regarding the authorship of mental as well as motor acts that are commonly, but simplistically, considered voluntary. Dr. Sacks' chapter argues forcibly and eloquently that without a strong psychodynamic orientation the data gathered by behavioral neurologists will be inadequate to afford any true understanding of the patient's experience of his illness.

Closed head injury is very common and personality change is one of its most frequent morbid consequences. Alterations in emotionality and behavior following head injury appears to reflect the frequency with which head trauma disrupts either limbic structures themselves or limbico-neocortical connections. The neuropathologic sequelae of head trauma may be either extensive and conspicuous or so subtle as to elude detection by most or all of our current neurodiagnostic armamentarium. Nevertheless, as event-related potential (ERP) technology continues to evolve, there is reason to hope that we will be increasingly able to characterize and quantify the extent of neural damage following closed-head injury. In his chapter M. P. Alexander challenges the widespread notion that the neuropathology of closed-head injury is so diffuse or 'messy' as to preclude meaningful correlations between lesion site and neurobehavioral symptoms. Instead, he schematizes the major types of resultant neuropathology and demonstrates how the behavioral sequelae of head injury can be understood on the basis of their pathoanatomy.

The lay public is aware that stroke may cause impairments in strength, sensation and speech. However, it tends to view emotional changes post-stroke as an understandable reaction to loss of function. From a neuropsychiatric perspective, however, stroke can be seen to produce direct, brain-based alterations in: (1) attention and perception, (2) cognition (language, constructions, memory, calculations and reasoning), (3) behavior, and (4) mood. Rehabilitation of the stroke patient depends on a clear delineation of the patient's acquired deficits, followed (against the backdrop of familiarity with the patient's premorbid goals, personality, and defensive style) by consideration of which areas are most likely to respond to psychosocial and pharmacologic interventions. Since depression may impede cooperation with rehabilitation efforts in many areas, recognition and treatment of post-stroke mood disorders may be a particularly strategic place to begin work with these patients. Depression following stroke is common and treatable, yet relatively few psychiatrists evaluate or treat the patients whom S. E. Starkstein and R. G. Robinson describe in their chapter.

Like syphilis in the last century, AIDS appears to be the prototype of a neuropsychiatric disorder. Because the clinical manifestations of AIDS are protean, physicians who work with these patients must (1) be able to integrate knowledge of neuropathology and neuroradiology, (2) develop sophistication in cognitive assessment, and (3) be aware of both psychodynamic and psychosocial factors. The chapter by Levy et al. begins with a review of the epidemiology of AIDS. Next it examines the remarkable range of AIDS-associated CNS pathologies and offers a lucid algorhythmic approach to the neurologic workup of patients suspected of having AIDS. The chapter concludes by considering the implications of AIDS for the daily practice of psychiatrists, neurologists and neurosurgeons.

R. J. Kiernan traces a history of great clinical neuropsychiatric interest, namely the evolution of bedside cognitive status testing. Practitioners of neurology and psychiatry test cognition informally on a frequent basis, yet few clinicians give much thought to the sensitivity or specificity of the questions they put to patients. Moreover, bedside assessment of cognition may vary greatly not only between clinicians, but also at different points in any one clinician's assessment of a particular patient. Dr. Kiernan's thoughtful chapter teases apart the particular contributions of neurologists, psychiatrists and psychologists to modern cognitive assessment. He describes limitations of current bedside cognitive testing and concludes by presenting a screening examination that falls midway between very brief tools for impressionistic assessment of cognition and more formal neuropsychologic batteries. It utilizes a structured format for testing and provides the examiner with a differentiated profile of the patient's cognitive deficits and strengths. He suggests that such a profile may serve as a starting place for clinicians who wish to formulate more sophisticated questions and hypotheses for neuropsychologists to answer.

In the 1940s and early 1950s neuropsychologists struggled to detect intellectual changes in patients who had undergone frontal lobotomy. Despite the important contributions of Luria and others since then, there exists today no simple bedside test that is pathognomonic for frontal lobe disease. Nevertheless, when impairment on such tasks as the Wisconsin Card Sorting Test and various maze learning tasks exists against the backdrop of preserved language, memory, calculations and ability, frontal lobe dysfunction is suggested. The chapter by D. F. Benson and D. T. Stuss will be of great help to those clinicians who have found it difficult to cull clinically relevant information from the profusion of theories on frontal lobe function. It first reviews frontal anatomy and connectivity, then reviews in a masterfully succinct fashion the most important theories of frontal lobe function. The authors conclude their chapter by proposing a hierarchical model of frontal lobe function that integrates their personal insights with previous theories.

A word, finally, on the allegoric significance of the frontispiece:

The nineteenth century French printmaker J. Grandville satirized the baser aspects of human nature by caricaturizing individuals as birds, insects and other 'lower' life forms. In this hand-colored pen lithograph from 1829 three somewhat roguish magpies are seen preparing the noontime repast. Their medical credentials are somewhat unclear, but they resemble surgeons or pathologists. Most importantly, they clearly enjoy their work and look forward to tasting the fruits of their labor. Madame Piton, demurely clad in a pristine smock, carries a baguette under her arm and is shown declining their invitation to lunch. Her gesture, and perhaps the green shading of her face, suggest horror at the indelicacy of their proposition.

Neurobiologists are currently preparing a feast for psychiatrists. The capacity of psychiatrists to be invigorated by this offering depends on their willingness to assimilate an organic psychiatry, whose chief organ will be the brain. Psychiatrists are being invited to dirty their hands and smocks by performing physical examinations and once again studying neuroanatomy and neuropathology. It is hoped that this volume will encourage psychiatric physicians in training to entertain such prospects with relish.

J. Mueller

Overview and History

Mueller (ed.): Neurology and Psychiatry: A Meeting of Minds,
pp. 2–13 (Karger, Basel 1989)

Internists of the Mind?

Jonathan Mueller[1]

Departments of Psychiatry and Neurology, UCSF School of Medicine and the San Francisco VA Medical Center, San Francisco, Calif., USA

> 'We must completely give up the idea of the psyche's being somehow connected with the brain . . .' C. G. Jung [1960]

Confusion as to what skills or knowledge distinguish psychiatrists from other 'mental health professionals' is not limited to the public sector. Psychiatric training programs continue to offer trainees a bewildering array of nonbiologic approaches to mental illness. These include sociology, medical anthropology, behavioral psychology, community mental health, hypnosis, numerous individual psychotherapeutic models, and group psychotherapy. The range and complexity of these alternative approaches do not compensate trainees for psychiatry's lack of a truly central basic science. Excessively pluralistic training approaches have produced psychiatrists whose professional identity is understandably confused and a profession whose relation to the medical community is problematic at best. Psychiatry must decide how it wishes to define itself.

Behavior reflects the interaction of environmental stimuli and contingencies with brain-based dispositions. Organic constraints on the range of possible behavior exist along a continuum. Patients with traditional psychiatric illness, together with brained-damaged individuals, differ from healthy 'normals' in the ease with which their neural mechanisms maintain-

[1] The author wishes to thank Drs. Craig Van Dyke, Joseph B. Martin, Walle J. H. Nauta, Marcel Kinsbourne, Roger Williams and Alan H. Ropper for their support and helpful suggestions.

ing homeostasis may be overwhelmed. The brain sciences offer increasingly broad opportunities for examining physiologic thresholds for disruption in behavioral and cognitive domains.

Until now biological psychiatry has been equated narrowly with chemotherapeutic approaches to psychiatric illness. Psychopharmacology, however, represents only one of the neurosciences relevant to modern psychiatry. The last two decades have witnessed tremendous strides in neuroanatomy, neuroimaging, neuroendocrinology, neuroimmunology, molecular genetics, and neuropsychology. Each of these areas harvests information that continues to revise our knowledge of the brain's structure and function. *Current Contents* recently listed 89 'core' neuroscience journals [Garfield, 1982]. As the functions of the brain become known in profoundly different ways, psychiatrists must take responsibility for understanding the structure, physiology, and pathology of the organ that subserves behavior.

Most psychiatrists' knowledge of neuroanatomy reflects what they recall from the first year of medical school. While an immense technology attains to ever greater sophistication in psychopharmacology, a largely unstructured view of the brain persists in the minds of most psychiatrists. Although psychiatrists may be able to discuss with sophistication mechanisms for the reuptake of neurotransmitters, they often have little idea as to where in the brain the relevant populations of receptors are located or what pathways lead to them. Many, for instance, have no clear idea of the location of, or connections to and from, such important forebrain regions as the nucleus accumbens septi [Stevens, 1973], the nucleus basalis of Meynert or the hippocampus [Price et al., 1982; Hyman et al., 1984] – structures of great relevance to the psychoses and Alzheimer-type dementia, respectively. Psychiatrists who regard knowledge of neuroanatomy as essentially irrelevant to their future fail to see that lack of familiarity with neuroanatomy effectively limits both the type of patients they will be able to treat and the type of information they will be able to learn. Psychopharmacology, for instance, will be understood increasingly with reference to specific neuroanatomic pathways and receptor populations. Elegant studies of neural circuits involved in the modulation of pain [Basbaum and Fields, 1978] foreshadow the inseparability of neurochemistry and neuroanatomy.

Without a working knowledge of neuroanatomy, psychiatrists will be unable to grasp important lessons from neighboring disciplines such as behavioral neurology and neuropsychology. Diseases that directly alter the neurophysiologic mechanisms underlying motivation, emotion and cognition constrain the types of psychiatric interventions from which a patient is likely to benefit. Without awareness of these syndromes clinicians run the risk of applying a narrow psychological model to the study of all behavior, or are obliged to restrict their practice to the care of patients in whom there is no evidence or suspicion of 'organicity'. This restriction becomes more and more problematic as an increasing percentage of the population faces senescence, as the AIDS epidemic progresses [Levy, 1989] and as organic factors are implicated in a growing range of psychiatric disorders. Unless psychiatrists begin to treat patients with structural brain pathology they will lose touch both with neuroanatomy and with the clinical neurosciences that are built on neuroanatomy.

Examples of a few lessons learned from stroke patients may clarify the types of practical insights regarding language and emotion that all psychiatrists should have when working with organically impaired patients.

Two patients in adjacent beds have sustained middle cerebral artery infarctions. The first patient has a lesion in the left or language-dominant hemisphere. His right hemiplegia is accompanied by a Broca (motor) aphasia and he is emotionally labile, given to bursts of irritability and tearfulness. The other patient with a right cerebral infarction has a left hemiplegia, but appears unconcerned about his motor deficit. Although his voice is colorless and uninflected, he has no problem with propositional speech and his mood is one of insouciance.

A consulting psychiatrist with no knowledge of the neural substrates of behavior might see the first patient as understandably depressed, given not only his motor deficit but also his loss of expressive language. Thus, his affective swings might be seen to reflect an 'appropriate' reaction to ego losses or damage to his 'self system'. If asked to consult on the second patient, the same psychiatrist might conclude that this patient is using massive or even 'psychotic' denial to avoid confronting his motor deficit.

Both of these interpretations reflect common sense approaches, but miss the mark entirely. Patients with left middle cerebral infarctions are more likely to manifest depressive phenomenology [Ross and Rush, 1981; Robinson et al., 1984; Starkstein and Robinson, 1989] and to demonstrate 'catastrophic reactions' when confronted with behavioral tasks that they previously could have performed. If their lesion is close to the left frontal pole, they are particularly likely to be depressed and have abnormal dexamethasone suppression tests [Finkelstein et al., 1982]. The language deficit of left hemisphere lesion patients complicates the physician's task in understanding to what degree they possess insight into their condition or are able to contemplate their future. Most importantly, tricyclic antidepressants may reverse the patient's mood disorder, thereby hastening departure from the hospital and improving participation in therapy of speech and physical impairments.

Acquired disorders of the ability to inflect and impart emotional color to spoken language were described as early as 1947 [Monrad-Krohn, 1947]. More recently, Ross [1981] has reported that individuals who sustain right hemisphere strokes may lose either the ability to express emotion in their voice or to perceive affective coloring in the speech of others. These alterations in prosody complicate the assessment of possible depression and can lead to either false-positive or false-negative diagnoses. Moreover, patients with right parietal damage often neglect (fail to report, attend, or orient to) deficits contralateral to their cerebral lesion [Heilman et al., 1985; Mesulam, 1979]. In 1914, Babinski [1914] used the term 'anosognosia' (a = without, noso = illness, gnosis = knowledge) to describe patients' neglect of left hemiplegia. He also observed patients with right hemisphere strokes who, although aware of a left hemiplegia, appeared indifferent to their deficit and never mentioned it to either physicians or friends over periods as long as several years. Regrettably, the term 'anasognosia', which stresses agnosia for (i. e. ignorance of) motor deficits, is often translated as 'denial of illness' [Weinstein and Kahn, 1955]. Distinguishing attentional and perceptual from psychodynamic reasons for ignoring or minimizing deficits is obviously important, since it may lead to different attitudes toward the patient and may suggest quite different treatment strategies.

Patients with fluent aphasia secondary to infarction of the dominant temporoparietal region may be misdiagnosed as schizophrenic since their bizarre speech is fluent and often unaccompanied by motor deficits [Benson, 1973]. Psychiatrists should also be aware of other aphasic disorders. Patients with dominant hemisphere infarction in the borderzone region between the middle and posterior cerebral arteries may develop a language disorder (i. e. transcortical sensory aphasia) characterized by severely impaired comprehension despite preservation of the ability to produce fluent spontaneous speech and to repeat words and phrases [Benson, 1979]. Preservation of repetition is commonly construed as evidence of intact comprehension and the patient's failure to cooperate with staff is assumed mistakenly to arise from negativism or a memory disorder.

Only to the degree that awareness of psychodynamics complements and strengthens the psychiatrist's understanding of cognitive, affective and behavioral changes that result *directly* from CNS damage will psychiatry enjoy the respect of other medical specialties. If differential diagnosis of neuropsychiatric illness were to become a cornerstone of training efforts, residents would quickly come to consider knowledge of neuroanatomy as more than preclinical esoterica. In the attempt to understand brain-behavior relationships, neuroanatomy would soon become as compelling to psychiatrists as nautical maps are to mariners. Confronted by patients with structural brain damage, the practical need to correlate localized neuropathology with altered emotion, motivation, cognition and motor behavior would fuel interest not only in neuroanatomy, but also in behavioral neurology and clinical neuropsychology.

The remainder of this chapter presents a rationale for the adoption of three building blocks that could form the foundation for a robust neuropsychiatry.

Neuroanatomy

Neuroanatomy must become the core basic science for psychiatric trainees. Study of the brain's actual structure would provide psychiatrists with an elegant and highly structured 3-dimensional matrix or 'cognitive map' [Tolman, 1948; O'Keefe and Nadel, 1978]. Onto this anatomic framework knowledge of neurochemistry [Valzelli, 1980], neuroendocrinology [Guilleman et al., 1985], neuroimmunology [Ader, 1981], neurobehavioral disorders [Pinkus and Tucker, 1985], and neuropsychology [Heilman and Valenstein, 1985] could be mapped with increasing sophistication.

Anterograde and retrograde tracing techniques, immunocytochemistry, enzyme histochemistry, and fluorescent dyes have created a renaissance in neuroanatomy [Heimer and RoBards, 1981; Chan-Palay and Palay, 1982; Emson, 1983]. Neuroanatomists, for instance, are beginning to map limbic inputs to the striatum [Nauta, 1982, 1989] that promise to have great relevance to the understanding of both 'psychomotor' slowing and acceleration. New techniques may allow neuropathologists to identify transmitter 'lesions' in neurological disorders such as Gilles de la Tourette disease and dystonia musculorum deformans where no structural pathology has previously been identified. Such techniques can also be expected to shed light on neuropsychiatric as well as traditional psychiatric disorders.

New tools offer powerful means of correlating changes in brain structure and physiology with neuropsychiatric symptomatology. X-ray computed axial tomography (CT) and magnetic resonance imaging (MRI) techniques identify with increasing sensitivity and precision structural abnormalities of the brain. Positron emission tomography (PET) is beginning to demonstrate functional correlates of altered metabolism and blood flow [Henry et al., 1983; Phelps and Mazziotta, 1985]. For instance, a pattern of bilateral temporoparietal glucose hypometabolism on PET has been suggested as unique to senile dementia of the Alzheimer type [Friedland et al., 1983]. Nuclear magnetic resonance (NMR) spectroscopy [Epstein, 1981; Shulman, 1983] may soon extend our ability to monitor in vivo brain metabolism in neuropsychiatric disorders to the molecular level.

Current concepts of brain-behavior relationships are still evolving, but already are too far advanced for psychiatrists to ignore. Previous notions of 'centers' for behavior have been replaced by the concept of chemically coded neuronal circuits subject to dynamic regulation by hormones and other neuromodulators. The rapidly shifting contributions of neural networks to a kinetic or cognitive 'melody' may be orchestrated by multiple neurotransmitters. Characterization of numerous peptidergic neuromodulators represents a major thrust of current neuroscience research [Krieger and Martin, 1981].

The boundaries between anatomy and physiology, between form and function, break down at an ultrastructural level. Anatomy is not static. Pharmacotherapy may alter structure as well as function. Neuroleptic drugs, for instance, appear to cause supersensitivity via sprouting of postsynaptic dopaminergic receptor sites in the neostriatum [Burt et al., 1977] and may also induce similar structural changes in the mesolimbic and mesocortical systems [Stevens and Livermore, 1978]. Whether we use words [Kandel, 1979] or drugs, as psychiatrists we may be facilitating or blocking specific neural pathways.

Behavioral Neurology

Psychiatrists can no longer afford to neglect the challenges and rewards of working with patients who have neurobehavioral disorders. The diagnosis, management, and study of schizophrenia, major affective disorders, character disorders, and the neuroses have been central to the training of psychiatrists. However, the aphasias, the amnesias, dementia syndromes, epileptic disorders, and traumatic brain injuries are uniquely instructive for the understanding of brain-behavior relationships. Remarkably, psychiatrists have managed to all but cede these important clinical areas to neurologists under the rubric of 'behavioral neurology'. In fact, each of these disorders could be considered a neuropsychiatric syndrome as appropriately as a neurobehavioral, or neurologic, disorder.

Heavy psychotherapy caseloads with patients who have character pathology, suffer from social maladjustment, marital discord or reactive depressions are interspersed with only an occasional 'token' brain-damaged patient in many psychiatric residencies. This situation leads understandably to disuse atrophy of whatever 'synaptic space' the psychiatric trainee once devoted to knowledge of the brain. Psychiatric residents continue to pay a high price for the profession's traditional fascination with neurotic or 'functional' psychopathology to the relative neglect of patients with brain damage.

Knowledge of neuroanatomy and neuropathology will mature, bear fruit, and nourish psychiatrists only to the extent that they directly experience their relevance to clinical neuropsychiatric phenomenology. Patients with neurobehavioral disorders therefore constitute a largely untapped resource for psychiatric training programs [Benson and Blumer, 1980; Mueller, 1983; Cummings, 1985; Mesulam, 1985].

Neuropsychology

Psychiatrists cannot hope to interact meaningfully with organically impaired patients until they are able to characterize these individuals' cognitive dysfunction. Recent advances in cognitive assessment [Kiernan et al., 1987; Schwamm et al., 1987; Kiernan, 1989] now enable clinicians to assess higher cortical functions in a brief but differentiated fashion. This in turn allows psychiatrists to expand the range of 'organic' disorders they can diagnose and treat. Psychiatrists who are unaware of the cognitive deficits associated with major psychiatric illness (e.g., alcoholic amnestic and dementia syndromes, depressive pseudodementia, or schizophrenia) [Taylor and Abrams, 1984] often fail to monitor either the course of illness or psychotherapeutic and/or pharmacologic interventions in terms of cognitive improvement or deterioration. Clinicians who document cognitive capacities that improve pari passu with treatment not only monitor an important parameter in their patients' illness, they also provide firm evidence of treatment efficacy. Specification of patient's cognitive and functional limitations helps to demystify both psychiatric illness and brain damage for family members. It also is of great practical importance for those involved in rehabilitation efforts [Erickson and Binder, 1986; Van Dyke et al., 1987].

At both clinical and research levels neuropsychology offers an objective methodology for consideration of mind-body and body-mind interactions. Rather than administering batteries simply to detect 'organicity' or localize pathology, neuropsychologists now attempt to characterize the behavioral consequences and functional deficits associated with brain lesions [Satz and Fletcher, 1981; Erickson and Binder, 1986]. Performance is no longer assessed exclusively in terms of the simple end product of complex cognitive processes. Instead, the level of analysis is shifting to delineation of individual differences in elementary stages of information processing [Butters and Cermak, 1980]. The convergence of information processing approaches and sophisticated electrophysiological probes of brain function suggest the possibility of examining cognitive processes in a way that respects and reflects the uniqueness of individual 'cognitive strategies' [Gevins et al., 1981; Ritter et al., 1981; Hunt, 1983]. These tools have major implications for the study of altered cognition following brain damage and perhaps even for the analysis of what psychiatrists term 'defensive styles'.

Apart from the writings of Goldstein, Luria and more recently Sacks, it has not been sufficiently stressed that acquired cognitive deficits impose enormous limitations on patients' capacities to sustain meaningful modes of what existentialists have termed 'being-in-the-world'. The manner in which cognitive deficits shape the range of affective experiences in interpersonal situations is still largely unexplored. Right hemisphere damage, however, appears to impose special restrictions on patients' ability to decode or perceive affective coloring in the speech of others [Ross, 1981]. It also may limit the richness and complexity of affective interactions by disrupting spatial analysis of visual display [Ekman et al., 1972; Benowitz et al., 1983]. By defining the raw materials or cognitive equipment available to the patient who attempts to negotiate reentry into the world following brain damage, neuropsychological assessment constitutes a practical cornerstone of psychosocial rehabilitation and specifies the ground of informed empathy.

Conclusion

The above suggestions in no way disparage traditional psychiatric skills. The author does suggest, however, that psychiatric training programs reconsider the mix of patients seen by residents who seek to treat mental disorders and yet wish to maintain their identity as physicians. As students of the brain and psyche, psychiatric residents should be taught to diagnose and treat both 'functional' and organic mental disorders [Caine and Joynt, 1986]. Psychiatric residents are too often made to feel they must choose *between* neurobiologic and psychodynamic approaches to mental illness. Divisiveness between biologically and dynamically oriented faculty imposes special strains on trainees. The integration of neurologic and psychodynamic perspectives will be a task of the greatest delicacy and importance [Sacks, 1989].

This chapter has attempted to underscore the timeliness and value of incorporating neuroanatomy, behavioral neurology and neuropsychology into the training of psychiatric residents. Neuropsychiatrists trained in these areas could be envisaged as doing the following: (1) performing initial neuropsychiatric evaluations; (2) assessing and triaging patients to appropriate caregivers (some or many of whom may be non-medical); (3) providing consultation regarding cognitive, emotional and behavioral disturbances, especially in the context of medical illness, and (4) bringing special skills to bear on the complex issues of managing and rehabilitating victims of brain disease. In these roles psychiatrists would render physicianly services both to their patients and to their medical colleagues. They would also begin to connect the psyche and the brain.

Summary

Psychiatry is at a crucial point in its evolution. Without a framework for the integration of neuroscientific knowledge it runs the risk of being fragmented and destroyed, rather than strengthened, by the neurosciences. The author has suggested that: (1) neuroanatomy provides a largely neglected but logical framework for the assimilation of neurobiologic as well as neuropsychiatric knowledge and as such should become psychiatry's central basic science; (2) behavioral neurology and neuropsychology represent two critical areas, training in which would allow psychiatrists to supplement their knowledge of psychopharmacology and psychotherapy with skill in the differential diagnosis and management of neuropsychiatric disorders.

References

Ader, R. (ed.): Psychoneuroimmunology (Academic Press, New York 1981).
Babinsky, M.J.: Contribution à l'étude des troubles mentaux dans l'hémiplégie organique (anosognosie). Revue neurol. *27:* 175–185 (1914).
Basbaum, A.I.; Fields, H.L.: Endogenous pain control mechanisms: review and hypothesis. Ann. Neurol. *4:* 451–462 (1978).
Benowitz, L.I.; Bear, D.M.; Rosenthal, R.; Mesulam, M.M.; Zaidel, E.; Sperry, R.W.: Hemispheric specialization in nonverbal communication. Cortex *19:* 5–11 (1983).
Benson, D.F.: Psychiatric aspects of aphasia. Br. J. Psychiat. *23:* 555–566 (1973).
Benson, D.F.: Aphasia, alexia, and agraphia (Churchill-Livingstone, New York 1979).
Benson, D.F.; Blumer, D. (eds): Psychiatric aspects of neurologic disorders, vol. 1, 2 (Grune & Stratton, New York 1975, 1980).
Burt, D.R.; Creese, I.; Snyder, S.H.: Antischizophrenic drugs: chronic treatment elevates receptor binding in the brain. Science *196:* 326–328 (1977).
Butters, N.; Cermak, L.S.: Alcoholic Korsakoff's syndrome: an information-processing approach to amnesia (Academic Press, New York 1980).
Caine, E.D.; Joynt, R.J.: Neuropsychiatry again. Archs Neurol., Chicago *43:* 325–327 (1986).
Chan-Palay, V.; Palay, S. (eds): Cytochemical methods in neuroanatomy (Liss, New York 1982).
Cummings, J.L.: Clinical neuropsychiatry (Grune & Stratton, Orlando 1985).
Ekman, P.V.; Friesen, W.V.; Ellsworth, P.: Emotion in the human face (Pergamon Press, New York 1972).
Emson, P.C.: Chemical neuroanatomy (Raven Press, New York 1983).
Epstein, F.H.: Nuclear magnetic resonance: a new tool in clinical medicine. New Engl. J. Med. *304:* 1360–1361 (1981).
Erickson, R.C.; Binder, I.M.: Cognitive deficits among functionally psychotic patients: a rehabilitative perspective. J. clin. exp. Neuropsychol. *8:* 257–274 (1986).
Finkelstein, S.J.; Benowitz, L.I.; Baldessarini, R.J.; Arana, G.W.; Levine, D.; Woo, E.; Bear, D.; Moya, K.; Stoll, A.L.: Mood, vegetative disturbance, and dexamethasone suppression test after stroke. Ann. Neurol. *12:* 463–478 (1982).
Friedland, R.P.; Budinger, T.F.; Ganz, E.; Yano, Y.; Mathis, C.A.; Koss, B.; Oben, B.A.; Guesman, R.H.; Derenzo, S.E.: Regional cerebral metabolic alterations in dementia of the Alzheimer type: positron emission tomography with flurodexoxyglucose. J. Comput. assist. Tomogr. *7:* 590–598 (1983).
Garfield, E.: Citation analysis of neuroscience journals: what they cite and who cites them. Current Contents *41:* 7–14 (1982).
Gevins, A.S.; Doyle, J.C.; Cutillo, B.A.; Schaffer, R.E.; Tannehill, R.S.; Ghannain, J.H.; Gilcrease, V.A.; Yeager, C.L.: Electrical potentials in human brain during cognition: new method reveals dynamic patterns of correlation. Science *213:* 918–922 (1981).
Guilleman, R.; Cohn, M.; Melnechuk, T.: Neural modulation of immunity (Raven Press, New York 1985).
Heilman, K.M.; Watson, R.T.; Valenstein, E.: Neglect and related disorders; in Heilman, Valenstein, Clinical neurology; 2nd ed., pp. 243–293 (Oxford University Press, New York 1985).

Heilman, K.M.; Valenstein, E. (eds): Clinical neuropsychology; 2nd ed. (Oxford University Press, New York 1985).
Heimer, L.; RoBards, M.J.: Neuroanatomical tract tracing methods (Plenum Press, New York 1981).
Henry, N.; Wagner, H., Jr.; Burns, D.; Dannals, R.F.; Wong, D.F.; Langstrom, B.; Duelfer, T.; Frost, J.J.; Ravert, H.T.; Links, J.M.; Rosenbloom, S.F.; Lukas, S.E.; Kramer, A.V.; Kuhar, M.J.: Imaging dopamine receptors in the human brain by positron tomography. Science *221:* 1264–1266 (1983).
Hunt, E.: On the nature of intelligence. Science *19:* 141–146 (1983).
Hyman, B.T.; Van Hoesen, G.W.; Damasio, A.R.; Barnes, C.L.: Alzheimer disease: cell specific pathology isolates the hippocampal formation. Science *225:* 1168–1170 (1984).
Jung, C.G.: Synchronicity: an acausal connecting principle. Collected works of C.G. Jung, vol. 8 (Princeton University Press, Princeton 1960).
Kandel, E.R.: Psychotherapy and the synapse. New Engl. J. Med. *301:* 1028–1037 (1979).
Kiernan, R.J.: Cognitive status testing: history, present status and future directions; in Mueller, Neurology and psychiatry, pp. 248–265 (Karger, Basel 1989).
Kiernan, R.J.; Mueller, J.; Langston, J.W.; Van Dyke, C.: The neurobehavioral cognitive status examination: a brief but differentiated approach to cognitive assessment. Ann. intern. Med. *107:* 481–485 (1987).
Krieger, D.T.; Martin, J.B.: Brain peptides. New Engl. J. Med. *304:* 876–895, 944–951 (1981).
Levy, R.M.: AIDS and the central nervous system: a challenge for the new neuropsychiatry; in Mueller, Neurology and psychiatry, pp. 210–245 (Karger, Basel 1989).
Mesulam, M.-M.: A cortical network for directed attention and unilateral neglect. Ann. Neurol. *10:* 309–325 (1979).
Mesulam, M.-M.: Principles of behavioral neurology (Davis, Philadelphia 1985).
Monrad-Krohn, G.H.: 'Dysprosody' or altered 'melody of language', Brain *70:* 405–415 (1947).
Mueller, J.: Neuroanatomic correlates of emotion; in Temoshok, Van Dyke, Zegans, Emotions in health and illness, pp. 95–121 (Grune & Stratton, New York 1983).
Nauta. W.J.H.: Limbic innervation of the striatum; in Friedhoff, Chase, Advances in neurology, pp. 41–46 (Raven Press, New York 1982).
Nauta, W.J.H.: Reciprocal links of the corpus striatum with the cerebral cortex and limbic system: a common substrate for movement and thought? in Mueller, Neurology and psychiatry, pp. 43–63 (Karger, Basel 1989).
O'Keefe, J.; Nadel, L.: The hippocampus as a cognitive map (Oxford University Press, New York 1978).
Phelps, E.P.; Mazziotta, J.C.: Positron emission tomography: human brain function and biochemistry. Science *228:* 799–809 (1985).
Pincus, J.H.; Tucker, G.T.: Behavioral neurology; 3rd ed. (Oxford University Press, New York 1985).
Price, D.L.; Whitehouse, P.J.; Struble, R.G.; Clark, A.W.; Coyle, J.T.; DeLong, M.R.; Hedreen, J.C.: Basal forebrain cholinergic systems in Alzheimer's disease and related dementias. Neurosci. Comment. *1:* 84–92 (1982).
Ritter, W.; Simpson, R.; Vaughan, H.G., Jr.; Macht, M.: Manipulation of even-related potential manifestations of information processing stages. Science *218:* 909–911 (1981).
Robinson, R.G.; Kubos, K.L.; Starr, L.B.; Rao, K.; Price, T.R.: Mood disturbances in stroke patients. Brain *107:* 81–93 (1984).

Ross, E.D.: The aprosodias: functional anatomic localization of the affective components of language in the right hemisphere. Archs Neurol. *38:* 561–569 (1981).
Ross, E.D.; Rush, J.: Diagnosis and neuroanatomic correlates of depression in brain-damaged patients. Archs gen. Psychiat. *38:* 1344–1354 (1981).
Sacks, O.W.: Neuropsychiatry and Tourette's; in Mueller, Neurology and psychiatry, pp. 156–174 (Karger, Basel 1989).
Satz, P.; Fletcher, J.M.: Emergent trends in neuropsychology: an overview. J. consult. clin. Psychol. *49:* 851–865 (1981).
Schwamm, L.H.; Van Dyke,C.; Kiernan, R.J.; Mervin, E.; Mueller, J.: The neurobehavioral cognitive status examination: comparison with the CCSE and MMSE in a neurosurgical population. Ann. intern. Med. *107:* 486–491 (1987).
Shulman, R.G.: NMR spectroscopy of living cells. Sci. Am. *248:* 86–93 (1983).
Starkstein, S.E.; Robinson, R.G.: Post-stroke mood disorders; in Mueller, Neurology and psychiatry, pp. 192–211 (Karger, Basel 1989).
Stevens, J.R.: An anatomy of schizophrenia? Archs gen. Psychiat. *29:* 117–189 (1973).
Stevens, J.R.; Livermore, A.: Kindling of the mesolimbic dopamine system: animal model of psychosis. Neurology *28:* 36–46 (1978).
Taylor, M.A.; Abrams, R.: Cognitive impairment in schizophrenia. Am. J. Psychiat. *141:* 196–201 (1984).
Tolman, E.C.: Cognitive maps in rats and men. Psychol. Rev. *55:*189–208 (1948).
Valzelli, L.: An approach to neuroanatomical and neurochemical psychophysiology (Wright, Littleton 1980).
Van Dyke, C.; Mueller, J.; Kiernan, R.J.: The case for psychiatrists as authorities on cognition. Psychosomatics *28 (2):* 87–89 (1987).
Weinstein, E.A.; Kahn, R.L.: Denial of illness (Thomas, Springfield 1955).

Jonathan Mueller, MD, San Francisco VA Medical Center (116 N),
4150 Clement Street, San Francisco, CA 94121 (USA)

Mueller (ed.): Neurology and Psychiatry: A Meeting of Minds,
pp. 14–30 (Karger, Basel 1989)

The Relationship between Psychiatry and Neurology

A British Perspective with Particular Reference to Neuropsychiatry

Michael R. Trimble

National Hospitals for Nervous Diseases and Institute of Neurology, London, England

Psychiatry is a much older subject than neurology, and its foundations lie in the earliest of medical writings. Although reference is made to hysteria in the Egyptian papyri [Veith, 1965], the Greeks provide us with the most important early statements on psychiatry, and perhaps on what might now be termed biological psychiatry. Hippocrates, born in 460 BC, protested against the a priori speculations of his predecessors, advocating the importance of a naturalistic approach and the value of clinical experience in medicine. When writing on 'The Sacred Disease', the name which was given to epilepsy, he pointed out that it was no more sacred than any other disease and had a natural cause [Adams, 1939]. In one passage he describes the appearance of the brain in man and continues '...and men ought to know that from nothing else but thence (from the brain) come joys, delights, laughter and sports, and sorrows, griefs, despondency and lamentations..., and by the same organ we become mad and delirious, and fears and terrors assail us...' There can be no clearer statement on the biological origin of psychiatric illness than that.

It is generally accepted that between the time of the Greeks and the Renaissance in Europe, with singular exceptions, such as the contributions of the Arab world, medicine abandoned any semblance of a scientific approach and retreated under the combined influences of theology and demonology into the Dark Ages. In the 17th century a clear revival of the singular idea that the brain was the seat of many mental diseases occurred. To illustrate this one may consider the works of Thomas Willis (1621–1675), the founder of modern neurology. Willis, who had early interests in chemistry, believed that some handed-down descriptions of the brain were inaccurate and in 1655 published *Cerebri Anatome* [Dewhurst, 1982a]. In

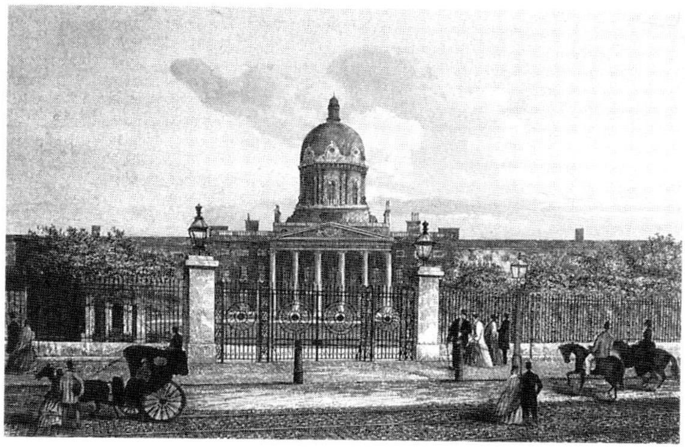

Fig. 1. The Bethlem Hospital as it was in the 19th century after it moved from the Moorfield's site. The world's most famous psychiatric hospital, later joined with the Maudsley Hospital.

contrast to the beliefs of some medieval scholars that mental functions were localized in the ventricles of the brain, Willis insisted that the substance of the brain itself had specific functions. He also argued that the brain, rather than the uterus, was the origin of the condition hysteria. Since both hysteria and epilepsy were related to disturbances of 'spirits', Willis continued a theme, initiated by the Greeks, which closely linked epilepsy to some psychiatric disturbances. This theme persists through to the present day. Willis, in addition to his neurological contributions, not only discussed conditions such as delirium, phrenzy, melancholia and mania, but also equated many mental disorders with brain diseases.

The 18th century saw great advances with regard to both classification of illness and the attribution of disease to various localizations within the body. With the possibility that psychiatric illnesses were related to brain disease, it was inevitable that physicians began to seek changes in the brains of patients at post-mortem examinations. Haslam (1764–1844), apothecary to the Bethlem Hospital (fig. 1), which at that time was situated at Moorfield's (the current site of Liverpool Street Station, London), reported an extensive series of post-mortems in mental illness. He is credited with one of the first pathological descriptions of general paralysis of the insane [Haslam, 1809]. Another important British contributor was Robert Whytt (1714–1766). A fellow of the Royal Society and physician to George II, Whytt examined the concept of reflex action and introduced such terms as stimulus and response. His book *On Nervous, Hypochon-*

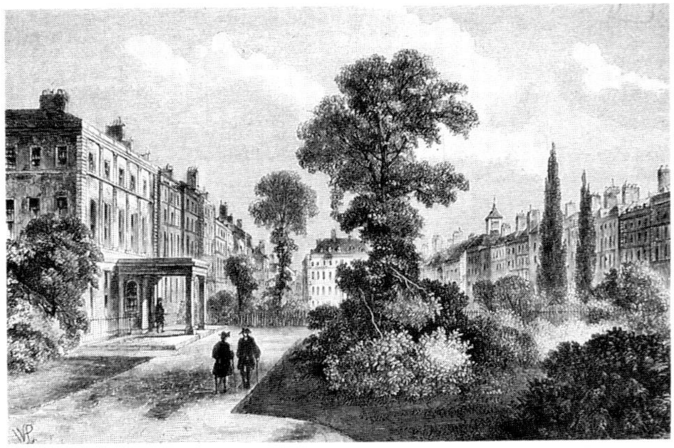

Fig. 2. Queen Square in 1810, before the hospital was founded there.

driacal or Hysterial Diseases was probably the first important treatise on psychiatric diseases since Willis [McHenry, 1969]. In it he gave a definition of the term nervous: 'Those disorders may peculiarly deserve the name nervous, which, on account of an unusual delicacy, or unnatural state of the nerves, are produced by causes, which in people of a sound constitution, would either have no such effects, or at least in a much less degree.' This term was later changed by the Scotsman William Cullen (1712–1790) to 'neurosis'. Both authors emphasized the clear relationship between disturbance of brain function and various conditions which would now be called psychiatric. Cullen in particular elevated the brain to a central position in the pathogenesis of many diseases.

In Cullen's terminology the neuroses were subdivided into comata, adynamiae, vesaniae and spasmi. Hypochondriasis was one of the adynamiae, while hysteria was one of the spasmi, and the vesaniae were 'the disorders of intellectual functions'. This included impaired judgement, amentia, mania, melancholia and disturbed imagination during sleep [Cullen, 1800]. Over time, during the next century in particular, many of Cullen's 'neuroses' evolved into distinct neurological entities, but the term continued to mean essentially a disturbance of nerve function without structural pathology. This concept, as noted below, continued to occupy an interesting position in the relationship between neurology and psychiatry.

The 19th century saw a rapid expansion of knowledge in medicine and continued growth of the anatomico-clinical method. This approach was

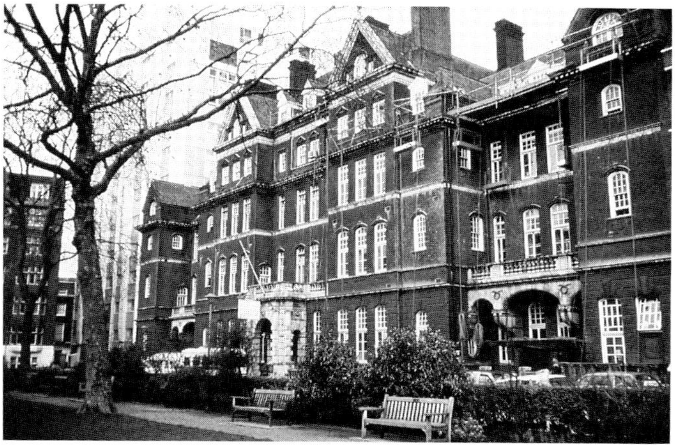

Fig. 3. The National Hospital, Queen Square, as it is at the present time.

especially noted in attempts to localize mental functions within the brain. Thus, apart from the various speculations regarding the origin of the seat of the soul, and the medieval principal of attribution to various ventricular systems of certain mental functions, the localization theories that we are familiar with today did not emerge until the rise of the phrenological movement. Although this did not originate in the British Isles, the main exponents being Gall (1758–1828) and Spurzheim (1776–1832), the general theme was taken up in France by neurologists such as Broca and in England by Ferrier. Ferrier (1843–1928) became a physician to the National Hospital, Queen Square (fig. 2, 3), but carried out his early work at the West Riding Lunatic Asylum where Dr. Crichton-Brown was the superintendant. Ferrier's extensive animal experiments provoked such hostility that the anti-vivisectionists of the day eventually took him to court in an unsuccessful law suit. *The Functions of the Brain* [1886] describes in detail Ferrier's experimental attempts to localize functions precisely in terms of neuroanatomy. It is dedicated to Dr. Hughlings Jackson, whose importance in the history of neurology and psychiatry is taken up further below.

The middle to late 19th century was a crucial era in the history of the neurosciences with regards to the relationship between neurology and psychiatry. The continuing pursuit of localization, and anatomic-pathological correlations based on these ideas, crystalized the discipline of neurology and led to distinctions with psychiatry. One reason for their separation was that localization failed to provide a satisfactory explanation for mental disorders. Another was that alienists, the physician superintendants of asylums who dealt with much severe psychiatric illness, remained aloof from the general stream of medicine. There were two outstanding figures of this era of relevance to the theme of this chapter, one a neurologist, the other a psychiatrist. The 150th birthdays of both of them were celebrated in 1985. The first was Hughlings Jackson, the second Henry Maudsley.

Hughlings Jackson

John Hughlings Jackson (1835–1911) (fig. 4) was born in Yorkshire. He apprenticed in a medical practice in Stonegate, York, before coming to London and studying briefly at St. Bartholomew's Hospital. In 1856 he received his licenciate of the Society of Apothacries and membership of the Royal College of Surgeons. He then worked for three years as House Physician at the York Dispensary. Although he had attended ward rounds at the York Country Asylum while in training, he was also introduced to mental illness by Daniel Tuke. The latter was the son of Samuel Tuke (1784–1857) who himself was the grandson of William Tuke, founder of the famous retreat in Yorkshire. Jackson also came under the influence of Thomas Laycock, whose ideas had been much influenced by the doctrine of reflex action, a concept of growing importance in neurology at that time.

Jackson came to London in 1859 and lived for a while with Jonathan Hutchinson, who was already established there. They jointly reported various medical events for the Medical Times and Gazette. Although it is often stated that at this time Jackson's preference was to study philosophy, Dewhurst [1982b] has recently concluded that by philosophy was meant a rather vague hinterland 'between philosophy, emergent psychology and psychiatry... (which would now include) psychology, abnormal psychology or neuropsychiatry' [p. 11].

It was Brown-Sequard (1817–1884) who stimulated Jackson's interest in neurology. In 1862 Jackson was appointed Assistant House Physician to the National Hospital for the Paralysed and Epileptic, Queen Square. Five years later he was promoted to full Physician, while also having appointments at the Metropolitan Hospital and the London Hospital.

Jackson's contributions to psychiatry and neurology have been discussed by several authors [Ey, 1978; Dewhurst, 1982b]. It is known that he married his cousin, who died in 1876 from thrombophlebitis of the brain.

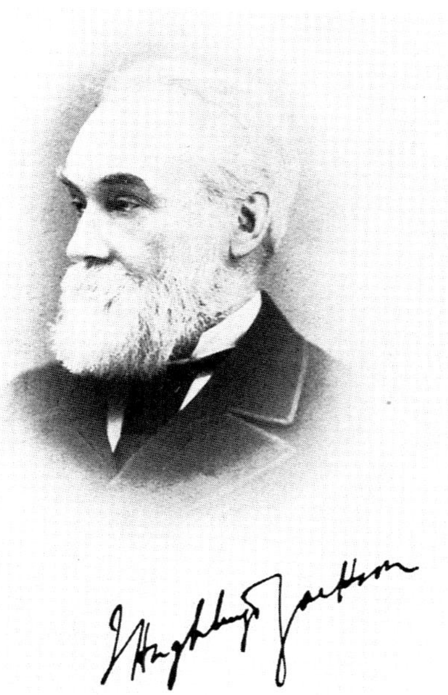

Fig. 4. John Hughlings Jackson. (From the archives of the National Hospital, Queen Square.)

Her illness had been complicated by a form of partial epilepsy which Jackson himself observed and described in great detail. Indeed, epilepsy became one of the cornerstones for the development of his theories of brain function, and the particular form of epilepsy from which his wife suffered came to be referred to as 'Jacksonian epilepsy' by the French neurologist Charcot. With post-mortem studies Jackson achieved accurate localization of lesions in the nervous system. He also described another form of partial epilepsy, 'a peculiar variety of epilepsy' [Jackson, 1888], associated with 'dreamy states' which affected the uncinate gyrus and adjacent areas of the temporal pole. From these descriptions arose the concept of 'the uncinate group of seizures', later to be revived under such concepts as temporal lobe epilepsy, psychomotor seizures and, in modern terminology, complex partial seizures.

Jackson's other writings on nervous disorders were considerable. They were more concerned with underlying principles of brain dysfunction in relationship to signs and symptoms than they were with classification and description of diseases. Jackson's interest in underlying principles was much influenced by Herbert Spencer (1820–1903), a very popular philosopher of the time. Indeed, it is said that Jackson corresponded with Spencer for some 40 years, although it is not known if they ever met. Spencer, who was influenced by authors such as von Baer, attempted to synthesize development in the sciences based upon evolutionary theory. Spencer saw organization in the cosmos ascending from homogeneity to heterogeneity, a principal that could be applied to a hierarchical organization within organisms and societies. Jackson wrote, 'I believe that Mr. Spencer's doctrines of evolution and dissolution are of very great value in the methodical analysis of cases of insanity, and further that, on the basis these doctrines apply, relations of different kinds of disease of the highest cerebral centres to one another can be traced, and also relations of disease of these centres to lower centres of the nervous system' [Swash, 1985]. Jackson went on to develop his scheme of nervous dysfunction which included four main principles. These were the evolution of nervous functions, the hierarchy of those functions, the negative and positive symptoms of dissolution, and the distinction between local and uniform dissolution [Ey, 1978].

Jackson refers to mental disorders throughout his writings. His continuing interest in psychiatry is shown by his joining the Medico-Psychological Association in 1866 and his assertion that mental disorders should be studied in general hospitals, where Jackson felt slight departures from normality could more readily be seen and investigated. Further, he attended ward rounds at the Bethlem Hospital with Sir George Savage, had regular visits to the West Riding Asylum at Wakefield (which James Crichton-Browne had turned into a world famous research center), and had contact with Sir John Bucknill. Bucknill, Jackson, Ferrier and Crichton-Browne were the first editors of the journal *Brain.*

Jackson influenced neurological thought far less than his contemporary, Charcot, and until recently has not been widely quoted. His influences in psychiatry and neurology in the UK are also not as great as some of those who followed him. However, authors such as Head, Riddoch and more recently Brain bear witness to Jackson's influence. Head's work on sensation particularly reflected Jacksonian evolutionary theory. This was done in close conjunction with W.H.R. Rivers, the psychiatrist and anthropologist who did much to popularize psychoanalysis in England. In Europe, Pick dedicated his book on aphasia to Jackson. Von Monakov quotes Jackson frequently, and his theories of diaschisis have a clear relationship to Jacksonian views. Jackson also influenced Foerster, and both Spencer and Jackson had influence on Ribot, who taught both Janet and Freud. In the USA, two of the founding fathers of neurology, namely Weir-Mitchell and Hammond, acknowledged Jackson's contributions. James Jackson Putnam, who was deeply influenced by Freud, also visited London and studied under Jackson, whose ideas impressed him.

Jackson's contributions to psychiatry have not been extensive. It is clear that he influenced Freud although the extent of this is debatable [Dewhurst, 1982b]. In particular, the French psychiatrist Henri Ey tried to combine Jacksonian neurodynamics with Freudian psychoanalysis. In America, references to Jackson's hierarchies are found in Jelliffe and White's [1915] *Diseases of the Nervous System,* a towering monument to the cooperation at the time between neurologists and psychiatrists. The 'father of American psychiatry', Adolf Meyer (1866–1950) acknowledged that Jackson exerted a profound influence on his ideas.

For those seeking evidence of Jacksonian thought in contemporary writings, it should be noted that the terms 'positive' and 'negative' symptoms derive almost directly from Jackson's phraseology. It is hoped that the rejuvenation of these terms will lead to a reanalysis of at least some of Jackson's ideas within psychiatry [Trimble, 1986]. Perhaps no better concluding comment on Jackson can be made than that by Golla [1932], who reviewed the *Selected Writings of Hughlings Jackson,* published by James Taylor (Jackson's best friend during his later years and another senior physician to the National Hospitals, Queen Square). Golla states: 'Valuable as are the lessons the neurologist may still gather from Jackson's writings, it is the psychiatrist, who, at the present epoch, is most likely to benefit from their teaching. Psychiatry has yet to find for itself a scientific basis, and there is no greater stimulus to clear thinking than the utterances of Jackson. His fundamental conception of the real significance of symptoms as the evidence of release of control is never lost sight of, and provides the clue to much that has been hopelessly entangled by the irrational contribution of positive symptoms to nervous matter that has undergone destruction.'

Henry Maudsley

Like Jackson, Maudsley (1835–1918) (fig. 5) was also born in 1835 and was a Yorkshireman. He took up an appointment at University College Hospital in 1850, but for career reasons spent six months as Assistant

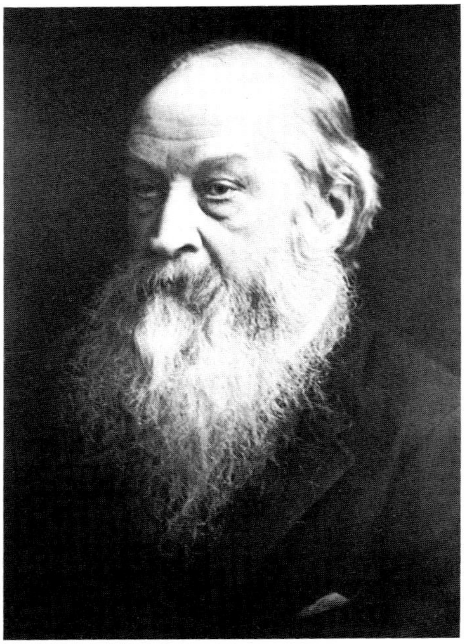

Fig. 5. Henry Maudsley. (From the archives of the Bethlem Hospitals, with permission.)

Medical Officer at an asylum in Wakefield. This led him to abandon ideas of taking up surgery and to commit himself to psychiatry. He was appointed as Medical Superintendant of Cheadle Royal where he stayed for three years before returning to London where he became physician to the West London Hospital and then Professor of Medical Jurisprudence at University College.

Maudsley's [1867] textbook, *The Pathology of the Mind,* was a landmark in British psychiatry. He was influenced by authors such as Pritchard, Griesinger, and Esquirol, and firmly held the opinion that mental diseases were due to diseases of the brain. Maudsley was firmly against metaphysical speculation and argued that constitutional diathesis was an important and often neglected factor in mental illness. Although Maudsley, like Jackson, was a philosophical enquirer, he emphasized a positivist view that was influenced by Darwin, Spencer, and John Stuart-Mill. For him the science of psychology had to be firmly based on

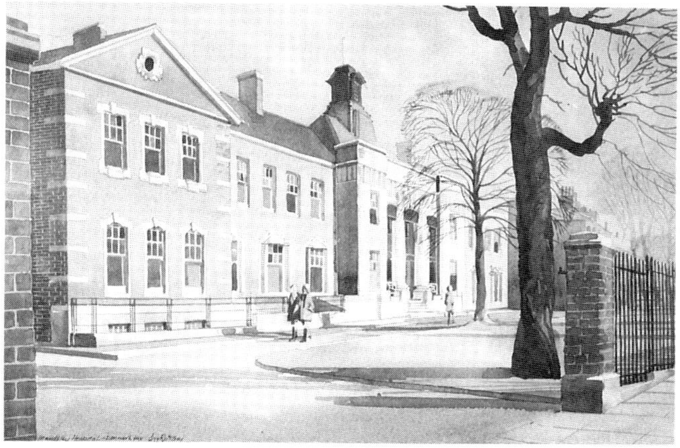

Fig. 6. A contemporary painting of the Maudsley Hospital. (From the author's collection.)

physiology, mental action being 'surely dependent on the nervous structure' [p. 44]. The fact that overt pathological changes were often not found in the brains of insane patients did not deter him from referring to important molecular and chemical changes that may take place 'in those inner recesses to which we have not gained access' [p. 428]. Such statements herald the important development of biological psychiatry in the 1960s. Maudsley believed that psychiatric illness did not merit the stigma so prevalent then as well as now and should be treated as any other bodily disease. His dislike of Cartesian dualism and his view that consciousness was an adjunct to brain function led him to rail against the notion that a man could be have a dual composition with the mind unrelated to the body. As early as 1870, Maudsley anticipated the introduction of convulsive therapy in this century when he speculated that a generalized convulsion might cure some cases of insanity. It is interesting that Maudsley, who shared with Jackson a common background, the influence of Spencer, and residence in London, does not quote Jackson's work.

Maudsley's writing should be considered an important stepping stone in the history of British psychiatry based, as it was, in neuroanatomy and neurophysiology rather than in psychology and sociology.

Through an intermediary, Dr. Frederick Mott, then pathologist to the London County Asylum, Maudsley offered £ 30,000 to the London County

Council to establish a hospital for patients with psychiatric illness, where the study of mental diseases and neuropathology might flourish. This living institution, the Maudsley Hospital, London (fig. 6), stands with the National Hospitals, Queen Square, as one of the twin pillars where succeeding generations of neurologists and psychiatrists have converged to attend lectures and ward rounds, in many cases coming from distant parts of the globe.

Psychiatrists and Neurologists, the First Half of the 20th Century

The early part of this century may properly be referred to as the golden age of British neurology. British contributions in psychiatry during this period, however, were limited. Instead, major developments took place in continental Europe and America. More specifically, the division between psychiatry and neurology at this time grew to become a huge chasm, more extensive in some countries than others. With regard to neurology, Gowers (1845–1911), whose *Manual of Diseases of the Nervous System* (1886) is still referred to as 'the bible of neurology', was clearly oustanding. He kept company with such notables as Ferrier, Horsley, and a succession of physicians at the National Hospital including Holmes, Kinnier Wilson, Walsh, and others whose names are prominent in the neurological honors list.

On the continent the development of somatic therapies proceeded at a rapid pace, including: the diagnosis and treatment of general paralysis of the insane (the latter brought Wagner-Jauregg in 1927 the only Nobel prize ever given to a psychiatrist); the development of convulsive therapies by von Meduna; and the introduction of insulin therapy by Sakel. This biologically based psychiatry may be contrasted with the contemporaneous flowering and proliferation of psychoanalytical theories in Europe and America.

It should be recalled that in Britain many of the early psychiatrists were asylum doctors, unlike in continental Europe where neuropsychiatry was represented in some university teaching hospitals. Many of the earlier British contributions had thus been directed towards establishing better treatment for institutionalized patients (see, for instance, the writings of Conolly, Tuke and Gardener-Hill). However, following Jackson's notion that the study of mental diseases is best carried out in general hospitals, there arose in some British hospitals the concept of 'psychological medicine', a forerunner of what is today referred to as consultation-liaison psychiatry. A close link between neurology and psychiatry was formed at the National Hospitals, Queen Square. One of the earlier exponents of this was Bernard Hart, physician in psychological medicine to the National Hospitals. His small book, *The Psychology of Insanity* [1941], went through many editions.

Outstanding contributions, particularly with reference to neurological disease, have emerged from authors such as Slater, Hunter, and Pratt. Slater, who with Sargant wrote *An Introduction to Physical Methods of Treatment in Psychiatry,* the first edition of which appeared in 1944, emphasized the importance of organic treatments in psychiatry. The introduction of the book makes a convincing case for a constitutional and biological approach to psychiatric illness. Such a theme is taken up later in Meyer-Gross et al.'s [1959] *Clinical Psychiatry,* for many years a core textbook for British psychiatric students. Slater's work on the schizophreniform psychoses of epilepsy reflects the link between psychiatry and neurology through epilepsy, and his work on genetics has helped reshape our ideas of a constitutional basis for psychopathology. Pratt, who was appointed Slater's registrar at Queen Square in 1952, developed his own special interest in the genetics of neuropsychiatric conditions. Pratt's [1967] book, *The Genetics of Neurological Disorders,* was the first monograph on this subject in the English language. Hunter, a contemporary of Pratt, devoted much of his writings to the history of psychiatry, but emphasized an understanding of psychopathology through neurology. Some of his ideas, such as the possible encephalitic origin of various neuropsychiatric conditions, preceded hypotheses currently in vogue. Lishman, who also practiced for a brief period at the National Hospitals, published his influential textbook *Organic Psychiatry* in 1978. This volume must be considered a substantial contemporary landmark illustrating the close links between neurology and psychiatry.

Thus, from the turn of the century up to the present day, there has been a continuing thread in the British Isles of certain physicians taking an active interest in the relationship of psychiatry to neurology. In the USA, however, other factors have emphasized differences between the two fields. At least for the first half of the century, psychoanalysis took over as the main method of psychiatric exploration in America. Thus, in spite of Adolf Meyer's early important psychobiological contributions, prior to and during the second world war, American psychiatry was dominated largely by European emigrees who brought with them the psychoanalytic legacy.

The situation in North America can be contrasted with that in Great Britain, where refugees such as Mayer-Gross, Guttmann, and Alfred Meyer influenced English psychiatric thinking so strongly that Slater himself commented: 'It was because of the popularisation of physical methods of treatment in psychiatry that Britain was saved from following America down the psychoanalytical path' [Slater, 1981]. There were, however, two further obvious reasons why American psychiatry opted for the path of greater separation from neurology. The first of these must relate to the 'optimistic' climate which has always pervaded the USA. In contrast to the European emphasis, particularly in the 19th century, on hereditary factors and biological determinism, America represented an egalitarian society. Background was felt to make no difference to one's achievements, and mental illness tended to be seen in terms of sociological developments. Second, there was the financial aspect: psychoanalytic treatment was expensive. The economic climate of North America proved a fertile source for its growth, as it did later for neurologists and their new tool, the electroencephalogram.

The first half of this century was, however, not without its North American proponents of neuropsychiatry. It should be remembered, for instance, that the neurologist Putnam was interested in psychoanalysis and had been in part responsible for inviting Freud to deliver his lectures at the Clark University in Worcester in 1909. Jelliffe too was deeply influenced by psychoanalysis, and both Cobb and Schilder, in their own ways, sought some integration. Nonetheless, the middle ground was more wearily trod, and the division between psychiatry and neurology more obvious.

An Interesting Theme

Of the numerous themes that interrelate neurology and psychiatry, it is particularly informative to look briefly at the shifting ground of the neuroses over the last century.

The Neuroses

The historical origins of the concept of neurosis have been discussed in detail by others, and it is clear that such conditions as hysteria have been recognized since the beginning of medical writings [Pinero, 1983]. Although the alleged anatomical basis for the condition moved from the uterus to the brain, the influence of emotional factors was recognized as early as the time of Sydenham and Willis. French physicians, in particular Briquet and later Charcot, made outstanding clinical contributions to the subject. Charcot was probably the last neurologist to embrace hysteria as a serious subject for research. Nonetheless, in the last century, particularly in Britain, the majority of patients with neuroses were seen and treated by neurologists and hysteria was discussed by authors such as Gowers. In contrast, many patients who suffered from what would now be considered neurological illnesses (i. e. infections, tumors or the consequences of brain trauma) were treated in the asylums. In America, Beard's introduction of the diagnosis 'neurasthenia', along with Weir-Mitchell's 'rest cure', must have proved a great spur to the incomes of privately practicing neurologists, whose specialty was then in the early stages of its development. In contrast, the 20th century has seen the neuroses become very much the province of the psychiatrist, while many of the conditions previously treated by psychiatrists have moved to the neurologist.

Thus, Cullen's original concept of the neuroses, having been gradually whittled away at by the description of numerous distinct neuropathological entities, was provided with the brightly polished handle 'psycho' and embraced by a new psychiatry. Accompanying this was the assumption that such conditions could be understood in terms of psychodynamic theories and that the brain was irrelevant to both theory and practice. It has to be of interest that the Third Diagnostic and Statistical Manual (DSM-III) has abandoned the diagnostic class neurosis because Freud and his successors had used it to indicate an etiological process. In so doing they have virtually ignored over two thousand years of medical history.

The Relationship of Neurology to Psychiatry

The bridge between neurology and psychiatry has been the subject of discussion by authors such as Stengel and Hill. Hill [1964], whose own extensive works on epilepsy, the electroencephalogram, and psychiatry are a substantial contribution to the interface, set the beginning of neuropsychiatry with Wernicke's success in discovering both a specific language disturbance and memory disturbance in association with localized brain lesions. He was critical of Henry Maudsley, whom he also referred to as a neuropsychiatrist who had developed a version of 'brain mythology'. Hill contrasted the social and psychological database of the psychoanalyst with the physical and physiological data of the neuropsychiatrist. Nonetheless, his discussion of the shared ground includes study of such disorders as consciousness, sleep, memory, speech, perception and motility, with particular emphasis on epilepsy. Hill suggested in 1964 that new bridges would be built, and some of these have recently been outlined by Marsden [1985]. These include: (1) common patients – namely those with epilepsy, movement disorders, hysteria and dementia; (2) common sciences – in particular the discovery of neurotransmitters and their role in behavior, which has a direct bearing upon both neurological and psychiatric illness; (3) common scientists – namely those people on whom both disciplines depend for further progress in their field, amongst whom are neuropathologists, molecular biologists, neurochemists, and neurophysiologists; (4) common technologies – for example EEG, CAT, MRI and PET scanning, particularly relevant in the investigation of such conditions as schizophrenia and dementia, and finally (5) shared treatments including the use of drugs which influence monoamine and other neurotransmitter systems within the brain.

Indeed, our concepts of the brain, its function, its structure, and its relationship to many clinical phenomena have changed so radically in the past 25 years that the development of areas so long in the borderland or, better stated, wilderness between neurology and psychiatry, is only to be expected. Such has been the division, that new disciplines have grown up which themselves try to cross the bridges and are variously termed neuropsychiatry, organic psychiatry, biological psychiatry, and behavioral neurology.

Both neuropsychiatry and behavioral neurology may be differentiated from organic psychiatry (which embraces a far wider range of conditions, including the 'exogenous psychoses') and from biological psychiatry (where the emphasis is on investigating disturbances of brain function, in particular neurotransmitter function, in association with psychiatric illness). Behavioral neurology has been dominant on the North American continent. It derives principally from the school of Geschwind and colleagues, who view disturbances of behavior from a strictly neurological standpoint. For Hill, behavioral neurology did not differ from neuropsychiatry. An alternative approach, however, may perhaps more properly be referred to as neuropsychiatry: namely, the understanding of behavior through an attempted integration of knowledge in neurology and psychiatry. Indeed, there appear to be four major differences between the much older neuropsychiatry and the newer discipline of behavioral neurology. Neuropsychiatry has a tradition as firmly rooted in brain function and pathology as does behavioral neurology, but has in addition: (1) a greater reference to changes of function as opposed to structure; (2) a tendency to embrace holism rather than localizationist approaches as a preferred method of understanding brain-behavior relationships; (3) an interest in a wider spectrum of disorders, and (4) an understanding of the dynamics of human behavior. Whether or not these differences are summarized in the quotation of Prof. Aaron Smith, quoted by Critchley [1986, p. 91], 'Broca is alive and well, and living in Boston; Jackson still lives too, but all over the world', is a matter of opinion.

References

Adams, T.: The genuine works of Hippocrates (Williams & Wilkins, Baltimore 1939).

Critchley, M.: The citadel of the senses (Raven Press, New York, 1986).

Cullen, W.: Nosology; or a systematic arrangement of diseases, by classes, orders, genera and species; with the distinguishing characters of each, and outlines of the systems of Sauvages Linnaeus, Vogel, Sagar and MacBride (Creech, Edinburgh 1800).

Dewhurst, K.: Thomas Willis and the foundations of British neurology; in Clifford Rose, Bynum, Historical aspects of the neurosciences, pp. 327–346 (Raven Press, New York 1982a).

Dewhurst, K.: Hughlings Jackson on psychiatry (Sandford, Oxford 1982b).

Ey, H.: Hughlings Jackson's fundamental principles applied to psychiatry; in Riese, Historical explorations in medicine and psychiatry, pp. 204–219 (Springer, New York, 1978).

Ferrier, D.: The functions of the brain (Smith Elder, London 1886).

Golla, F.L.: Review. J. ment. Sci. *78:* 204–206 (1932).

Hart, B.: The psychology of insanity (Cambridge University Press, Cambridge 1941).

Haslam, J.: Observations on madness and melancholy: including practical remarks on those diseases, together with cases; and an account of the morbid appearances on dissection (Callow, London 1809).

Hill, D.: The bridge between psychiatry and neurology. Lancet *i:* 509–514 (1964).

Jackson, H.: On a particular variety of epilepsy ('intellectual aura'). Brain *11:* 179–207 (1888).

Jelliffe, S.E.; White, W.A.: Diseases of the nervous system (Lewis, London 1915).

Lishman, W.A.: Organic psychiatry, 2nd ed. (Blackwell, Oxford 1987).

Marsden, C.D.: The common problems of neurology and psychiatry. Presented at 'Scientific Open Day – Bethlem Royal and Maudsley Hospitals', 13th Nov. 1985.

Maudsley, H.: The pathology of the mind (MacMillan, London 1867).

McHenry, L.: Garrison's history of neurology (Thomas, Springfield 1969).

Meyer-Gross, W.; Slater, E.; Roth, M.: Clinical psychiatry (Balliere Tindall & Cassell, London 1959).

Pichot, P.: A century of psychiatry (Da costa, Paris 1983).

Pinero, J.M.L.: Historical origins of the concept of neurosis, translated by Berrios, D. (Cambridge University Press, Cambridge 1983).

Pratt, R.T.C.: The genetics of neurological disorders (Oxford University Press, Oxford 1967).

Sargant, W.; Slater, E.: Introduction to physical methods of treatment and psychiatry (Livingstone, Edinburgh 1944).
Slater, E.: In conversation with Eliot Slater. Bull. R. Coll. Psychiat. *5:* 160 (1981).
Swash, M.: John Hughlings Jackson. 150th Anniversary of John Hughlings Jackson (Abstracts). (in press).
Trimble, M.R.: Positive and negative symptoms. Br. J. Psychiat. *148:* 587–589 (1986).
Veith, I.: Hysteria, the history of a disease (University of Chicago Press, London 1965).

Michael R. Trimble, FRCP, FRCPsych, National Hospitals for Nervous Diseases and Institute of Neurology, Queen Square, London WC1N 3BG (England)

Neuromorphology

Mueller (ed.): Neurology and Psychiatry: A Meeting of Minds,
pp. 32–42 (Karger, Basel 1989)

Anatomic Evolution of Neural Networks Subserving Language

Arnold B. Scheibel

Departments of Anatomy and Psychiatry and Brain Research Institute,
UCLA Medical Center, Los Angeles, Calif., USA

Introduction and Background

If we accept Jonathan Mueller's [this volume] rousing reaffirmation of the obligatory relationship between clinical psychiatry and the structuro-functional substrate of brain, then it is interesting to consider who, among the seminal figures active at the dawn of this century, might appropriately have contributed to this volume. Ramon y Cajal, the great Spanish 'functionalist with a microscope', would certainly have belonged because of his reiterated belief in the relationship of structure on the one hand with function and behavior on the other. His insights were, in part, the product of his data base, incomparably smaller than that available today. Yet, who can deny the grandeur of his idea that consciousness is lost when astrocytes sweep their tails, temporarily breaking synaptic contacts between pairs of neighboring neurons [Ramon y Cajal, 1911]. Indeed, the equally 'primitive' idea that increased physiological activity should increase the size of neural components and the density of their connections now constitutes one of the most enthusiastically accepted and actively investigated areas of current nervous system research.

Charles Sherrington, the acknowledged father of modern physiology, might well have been passed over, however. Increasingly moved by the complexity and the endless levels of neural involvement that his research and insights uncovered, he spoke almost despairingly of 'mind that went more ghostly than a ghost' [Sherrington, 1937]. Such a point of view differed substantially from that of his contemporary, Freud [1946]. While developing a superstructure of psychological dynamics which still provides the most coherent available framework in which to interpret human behavior and motivation, Freud also looked forward with confidence to the time when broader knowledge of the basic biological sciences would reinforce, or replace, his pychodynamic insights. Indeed, the increasing insularization of dynamic psychiatry and psychoanalysis which characterized the early and mid decades of this century must be attributed not to Freud, but to the several generations of his followers who codified and rigidified what they had been bequeathed. Freud would have belonged at this meeting, and would have rejoiced at its orientation.

Neural structure and its allied physiological and chemical disciplines do, in fact, remain the logical matrix within which the wealth of presently available psychodynamic data must eventually be understood. This is said with full realization of the enormous range of levels of organization which will eventually have to be mastered before this type of correlative understanding can be achieved. In this regard, I frequently remind my students that we are in the position of someone who removes the back of his television set and, by examining the structure and connections among the chips and circuits thus revealed, tries to deduce the content of the Evening News program.

The paragraphs which follow detail a pilot study [Scheibel et al., 1985], which attempts to tease out possible structural correlates of a high level human behavior, e.g. speech. The topic has been of medical and psychological interest since the mid-19th century when Dax [1865] and Broca [1865] focused attention on the apparent functional asymmetry of speech activity and the dominance of one hemisphere, usually the left, in its maintenance. Correlative evidence of structural asymmetry has been longer in coming, despite several isolated observations on unequal length of the two Sylvian fissures [Cunningham, 1892; Eberstaller, 1890] and scattered qualitative descriptions of bilaterally asymmetric, temporal and parietal operculi [Connolly, 1950; von Economo and Horn, 1930; Shellshear, 1937].

Nonetheless, as recently as 1962, the distinguished neuroanatomist, Von Bonin [1962], questioned the evidence for any significant degree of structural nonsymmetry. Five years later, the modern period of interest in structural correlates of functional asymmetry began with the report of Geschwind and Levitsky [1968], which presented quantitative data demonstrating increased area of the left planum temporale in 62% of the brains they studied. Since that time, a large body of confirmatory data has substantiated this report. However, aside from a few cytoarchitectonic studies which essentially review and refine our view of the cellular architecture of the temporal lobe (already familiar from the earlier studies of Brodmann [1909] and von Economo [1929]), and a growing library of PET-scan studies [Mazziotta et al., 1982], virtually nothing is yet known about the histological particularities of speech-involved cortex (if they exist). Nor is it known whether the robust bilateral functional asymmetries are reflected in the fine structure of the neuronal matrix. Indeed, if correlative variation can be shown at the level of individual neural circuit elements, initial attempts might then be made to model relevant substrate circuits.

With these possibilities in mind, we selected Broca's speech area (i. e. the opercular and triangular zones of the frontal lobe, area 44–45), for comparison with its homologous sites on the propositionally nondominant side. These were, in turn, contrasted with tissue samples from the corresponding orofacial motor speech areas just behind (i. e. the inferior portion of the 'primary motor strip' or area 4). For convenience, we refer to the former (motor speech) cortical area as the opercular region, the latter (orofacial) as the precentral. Our initial working hypotheses included the following: (a) The level of computational 'sophistication' of a cortical area should be reflected somehow in the pattern and organization of the neuronal dendrite ensembles. (b) Higher levels of computational complexity should result in longer and/or more complexly branched dendrite systems. (c) Neurons in Broca's area of the propositionally dominant cortex should have more complex dendrite systems than those of the opposite side. (d) Functional differences between these 'strategic' zones for speech and the 'tactical' motor areas just behind them should also be reflected in structural variations in the respective dendritic ensembles. In the present context, 'strategic' is used to indicate the lexical or word-selection role of the opercular area. 'Tactical' refers to the role of the orofacial zone in generating patterns of muscle activity in the laryngopharyngeal complex, mouth, tongue and lips needed to articulate the words.

The Study and the Data

This study was based on examination of tissue from eight male patients from a major Veterans Administration Hospital who came to autopsy within 5–28 h after death. Their ages ranged between 58 and 77 years (mean age 65.9, SD 6.4), and they were free of known neurological disease. Tissue samples from left and right opercular and precentral areas were prepared for analysis with the Golgi impregnation method. Adjacent tissue sections were stained with cresyl violet as controls. Once the tissue was sectioned (120 μm for Golgi material) and mounted under coverslips, all slides were coded to preclude investigator bias. From each of the four regions selected for examination, i. e. left opercular (LOP), right opercular (ROP), left precentral (LPC) and right precentral (RPC), six neurons were chosen for study from each subject according to a group of predetermined criteria which included: (a) position of the cell vis-à-vis the cortical surface, i. e. 400–1,300 μm beneath the pial-glial margin; (b) position of the cell body approximately midway between the upper and lower surfaces of the tissue section, and (c) the presence of at least three well-stained primary basilar dendrites and their branches.

These data were gathered and analyzed in two ways. In the first, a series of concentric rings (ring interval –28 μm) etched in the ocular were superimposed over a neuron and centered on the midpoint of the soma (fig. 1, central inset diagram). The number of dendritic intersections with each ring was then counted, thereby providing in aggregate a profile of the complexity of that dendritic ensemble. The graphs in figure 1 exemplify the use of such data and demonstrate significant differences at and beyond 160 μm from the center of the soma. This represents an approximate zone of transition between third and fourth order dendrite branches. The unexpected reversal in case 5 where values for the right opercular (Broca) area exceeded those of the left became more reasonable when we learned at the conclusion of the study that this patient was one of two nonright-handers in the series.

Our second method of data analysis was based on computer-aided measurement of the dendrite systems, providing a considerable amount of quantitative information about each dendrite ensemble, including total dendrite length (tdl), the average number of dendrite segments of each order (asn) and the average length of dentrite segments of each order (asl), etc. When all of the data had been collected and processed, information about handedness was sought along with any outstanding behavioral characteristics which the often-meager histories could provide.

Several findings emerged from this study which seemed of more than passing interest to the problem of verbal behavior (fig. 2).

(1) To our surprise, there was no significant difference between the tdl of basilar dendrite systems of the left and right sides (i. e. left opercular, 2,714.5 μm vs right opercular, 2,540.8 μm [not significant]; and left precentral, 2,208.3 μm vs right precentral, 2,499.9 μm [not significant]). According to our a priori hypothesis, we would have expected tdl values for

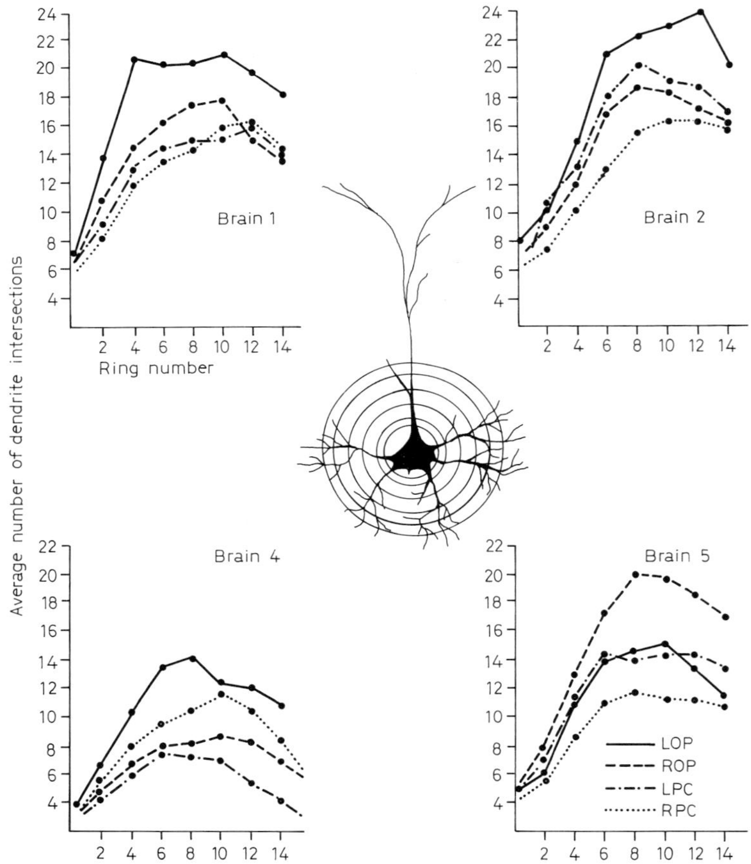

Fig. 1. Graphic representation of the average number of dendritic intersections per ring in the type of analysis described in the text. Dendritic trees from cells of the left opercular region (Broca's areas) consistently provide greater numbers of intersections (especially beyond ring No. 4) except in the case of brain 5. This patient with a reversed ring dendrite pattern (i. e. right opercular values greater than those of the left) was found to be a nonright-hander. The central inset diagram shows a single cortical neuron with superimposed concentric ring system providing the dendrite-ring intersection data on which these graphs are based.

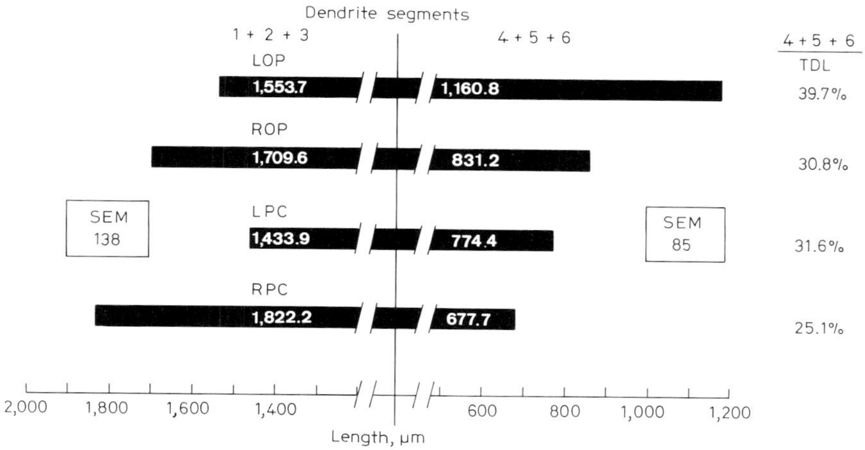

Fig. 2. Graphic comparison of total dendritic length (note breaks in the representational bars) and proportion of the dendrite tree composed of lower order (first, second and third) and higher order (fourth, fifth and sixth) dendrite segments in the four areas of study, i. e. left opercular, LOP; right opercular, ROP; left precentral, LPC; and right precentral, RPC regions. Standard error of the mean, SEM for left-right comparisons is 138; standard error of the mean for comparing opercular versus precentral regions is 85. The column of figures on the extreme right gives the percentage of total dendritic length (TDL) occupied by higher order dendrites in each area. From Scheibel et al. [1985], reproduced with permission.

opercular neurons on the propositionally dominant side to have been larger due to the presumably greater processing load engendered by speech-strategy activities.

(2) Segment-by-segment analysis revealed significant differences in the internal organization of dendrite ensembles on the two sides. In summary, a larger fraction of the dendrite arbor on the right side was made up of lower (first, second and third) order branches, whereas on the left, a larger fraction of the dendrite system was accounted for by branches of higher (fourth, fifth and sixth) order (fig. 3). These differences were also expressed in a distinctive manner. Lower order branches were longer on the right side; higher order branches were more numerous on the left side. It was particularly interesting to discover that these values were partially reversed in the two nonright-handed individuals, thereby suggesting that the histological differences might be related to behavior.

(3) The tdl of opercular neurons exceeded that of precentral cells by at least 10%, a difference which was found to reach significance ($p < 0.05$)

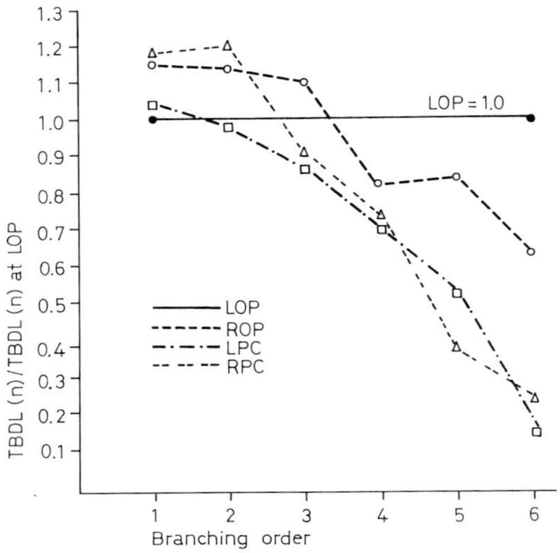

Fig. 3. Graphic representation of the increasing complexity of the dendrite system of the left opercular region (LOP) compared to all of the other regions studied. Total basilar dendritic length (TBDL) of LOP is maintained at 1.0 for each branch order and compared against that of similar branch orders of right opercular (ROP), left precentral (LPC) and right precentral (RPC) regions.

only in the left hemisphere. According to our hypothesis, we attribute this difference to the more extensive information processing activities of cells in the speech strategy (opercular) compared to the speech tactics (precentral) area.

Some Thoughts about the Data

In a series of challenging papers spanning the period of the mid-1940s to the early 1960s, and reprinted in bound form in 1965, McMulloch [1965] did much to refocus interest on the problems of experimental epistemology. Today, there is a rapidly growing subsection of the neuroscience literature which transcends the boundaries of neuroanatomy, neurophysiology, classic neurology, behavioral neurology, psychology and psychiatry. This is the challenging interface area where newer integrations are being attempted and where pilot attempts such as these to establish particularities of fine neural structure related to specific behavioral programs may eventually have a place.

These data may be evaluated in at least two frames of reference, one of which is essentially anatomico-physiological, the other, ontogenetic: both offer valid settings and either may contribute to the picture we are trying to sketch. Within the former, variations in dendrite structure may effect subtle, yet powerful constraints on processing operations of neurons. First order dendrites are usually the largest in diameter, have the lowest internal resistance values and the fewest dendrite spines [Marin-Padilla, 1967; Rall, 1967]. Correlative to the paucity of dendrite spines is a larger proportion of type-II synaptic terminals usually considered inhibitory in function [Uchizono, 1965].

Farther out along the dendrite tree, segments of higher order are characterized by progressively smaller shaft diameters, higher internal resistance values and greater spine density. In the most peripheral branch elements, the spine density begins to decrease again, and the morphology of the spines changes, often becoming longer-shafted and more filamentous [Marin-Padilla, 1967; Rall, 1967; Scheibel, unpublished]. The increasing density of dendrite spines is accompanied by enhanced numbers of type-I, probably facilitatory, synapses [Colonnier, 1967]. The number and pattern of dendritic bifurcations is also a significant factor in the overall physiology of the dendrite tree. Each branch point becomes, in effect, a decision point for patterns of local activity which are constantly waxing, summating and waning along the dendritic membrane. In the broadest sense, the greater the degree of branchedness, the higher the number of degrees of freedom in information processing.

The pattern of the dendritic tree also reflects the life history of the neuron, thereby encapsulating ontogeny with its complex admixture of genetic and epigenetic factors. There is an approximately time-linked progression in the successive development of the dendrite system, segment order by segment order. In the same way that climatic history can be 'read' in the rings of a felled tree trunk or in a sequence of geologic varves, so can the length of time and/or intensity of a certain neuroontogenetic epoch, to some extent, be inferred from the length of various dendritic segment order. Patterns of development and maturation in the human neocortex vary quite widely from area to area [Conel, 1939–1967], primary sensorimotor cortices developing appreciably earlier than cortical association areas. In general, however, dendritic elaboration begins during the early or mid-portion of the third trimester so that at birth, most cortical neurons bear first and second order branches while third and fourth order segments usually begin to develop almost immediately afterward. Between six months and one year of age, higher order branching becomes visible and by the second or third year of age, the cerebral cortex, to qualitative visual inspection at least, begins to approach the dendritic complexity of the mature brain [Conel, 1939–1967; Scheibel, unpublished]. In a limited sense, it is possible to view these dendrite patterns as a 'fossilized history' of early dendritic growth, modified only by our increasing appreciation of the capacity of dendrite systems to prune and reshape themselves to varying input patterns [Diamond and Connor, 1983].

With this caveat, we may interpret the presence of longer dendrite segments of lower order on the side nondominant for propositional speech as indicative of greater functional activity during the late prenatal and early postnatal (nonverbal) periods of life [Piaget, 1954]. In similar fashion, the marked increase in numbers of higher order branches on the left side compared to the right side, suggests enhanced dendritic growth at a somewhat later time when the beginnings of internalization and conceptualization mark the onset of language competence in the child. Assuming these interpretations have some validity, the data indicate that the right hemisphere (at least in the limited area of this study) initially leads the left in amount of available dendritic tissue during the initial preverbal period of life. During this time, the infant depends exclusively on sensory impressions of a highly concrete nature and appears limited to relatively large scale, undifferentiated motor acts [the sensory-motor period of Piaget, 1954]. The marked increase in numbers of higher order branches on the left side compared with the right suggests enhanced dendritic growth at a time when symbolic operations and other 'left hemisphere tasks' begin to emerge and motor actions become more discrete. It is of considerable interest to note that the apparent preponderance of dendritic tissue on the side nondominant for speech is gradually lost as speech function commences.

Despite the highly suggestive nature of these correlations, it is not possible to decide whether enhanced dendritic growth on the side dominant for speech reflects genetically determined preparation for the increased functional load of speech processing, or whether it represents, in fact, a response to the increased neural processing activity already accompanying the onset of speech function. In an attempt to answer this question, we have recently attempted quantitative analysis of dendritic development in the anterior speech and orofacial motor areas of 17 age-graded infant brains ranging from birth to 6 years of age [Simonds and Scheibel, submitted for publication]. Although these data have not yet been fully analyzed, initial evaluation of the material suggests that cortex nondominant for speech 'leads' the other in terms of tdl for only 3–6 months. Following this, the dendrite systems on the other side begin to increase more rapidly in length and complexity and soon exceed those of the nondominant hemisphere. These data provided another surprise for us insofar as the 'crossover' of dendrite growth patterns seem to occur substantially before the onset of what is generally considered infantile verbal language behavior (12–18 months). If so, this might suggest innate (genetic) preparation for language function.

However, preliminary reading of the data also suggests a second burst of dendrite building activity at 12–18 months, differing both in location of origin of dendrite growth on the nerve cell body, and in the hierarchic order of dendrite segment sequence. These developments might represent response to the demands of early language learning and utilization and, consequently, the epigenetic component of the development of speech cortex. Clearly no single measure can provide the insights necessary to grasp the relationships between neural substrate and behavior – and certainly not a high order behavior like speech. Nonetheless, it can be hoped that information vignettes of this sort may eventually provide clues, at least to the next step in the search for the biologic matrices of behavioral neurology and neuropsychiatry.

References

Broca, P.: Du siège de la faculté du langage articulé. Bull. Mem. Soc. Anthropol., Paris *6:* 377–393 (1865).

Brodmann, D.K.: Vergleichende Lokalisationslehre der Grosshirnrinde in ihren Prinzipien dargestellt auf Grund des Zellenbaues. (Barth, Leipzig 1909).

Colonnier, M.: The fine structural arrangement of the cortex. Archs Neurol., Chicago *16:* 651–657 (1967).

Conel, J.: The postnatal development of the human cortex (Harvard University Press, Cambridge 1939–1967).

Connolly, G.J.: External morphology of the primate brain (Thomas, Springfield 1950).

Cunningham, D.F.: Contributions to the surface anatomy of the cerebral hemispheres (Royal Irish Academy, Dublin 1892).

Dax, G.: Lesions de la moitié gauche de l'encéphale coïncidant avec trouble des signes de la pensée (lu á Montpellier en 1836). Gaz. Hebd. Med. Chir. *2:* 2nd ser., p. 259 (1865).

Diamond, M.C.; Connor, J.R.: A search for the potential of the aging cortex; in Enna et al.,

Brain neurotransmitters and receptors in aging and age-related disorders, vol. 17 (Raven Press, New York 1981).
Eberstaller, O.: Das Stirnhirn (Urban & Schwarzenberg, Vienna 1890).
Economo, C. von: The cytoarchitectonics of the human cerebral cortex (Oxford University Press, New York 1929).
Economo, C. von; Horn, L.: Über Windingsrelief, Masse und Rindenarchitektonik der Supratemporalfläche, ihre individuellen und ihre Seitenunterschiede. Zentbl. ges. Neurol. Psychiat. *130:* 687–757 (1930).
Freud, S.: Collected papers, vol. I–V (International Psycho-Analytical Press, London 1946).
Geschwind, N.; Levitsky, W.: Left-right asymmetries in temporal speech area. Science *161:* 186–187 (1968).
Marin-Padilla, M.: Number and distribution of the apical dendritic spines of the layer V pyramidal cells in man. J. comp. Neurol. *131:* 475–489 (1967).
Mazziotta, J.C.; Phelps, M.E.; Carson, R.E.; Kuhl, D.E.: Tomographic mapping of human cerebral metabolism. Auditory stimulation. Neurology *32:* 921–937 (1982).
McCulloch, W.D.: Embodiments of mind. (MIT Press, Cambridge 1965).
Piaget, J.: The construction of reality in the child (Basic Books, New York 1954).
Rall, W.: Distinguishing theoretical synaptic potentials compiled for different soma-dendritic distributions of synaptic input. J. Neurophysiol. *30:* 1138–1168 (1967).
Ramon y Cajal, S.: Histologie du système nerveux de l'homme et des vertébrés (Maloine, Paris 1911).
Scheibel, A.B.; Paul, L.; Fried, I.; Forsythe, A.; Tomiyasu, U.; Slotnick, J.: Dendritic organization of the anterior speech area. Expl Neurol *87:* 109–117 (1985).
Shellshear, J.L.: The brain of the aboriginal Australian: a study in cerebral morphology. Phil. Trans. R. Soc. ser. B. *227:* 293–409 (1937).
Sherrington, C.S.: Man on his nature. The Gifford Lectures, Edinburgh (Mcmillan, New York 1937).
Uchizono, K.: Characteristics of excitatory and inhibitory synapses in the central nervous system of the cat. Nature, London *207:* 642–643 (1965).
Von Bonin, G.: Anatomical asymmetries of the cerebral hemispheres; in Mountcastle, Interhemispheric relations and cerebral dominance, pp. 1–6 (Johns Hopkins University Press, Baltimore 1962).

A. B. Scheibel, MD, Department of Anatomy, UCLA Medical Center,
Los Angeles, CA 90024 (USA)

Mueller (ed.): Neurology and Psychiatry: A Meeting of Minds,
pp. 43–63 (Karger, Basel 1989)

Reciprocal Links of the Corpus striatum with the Cerebral Cortex and Limbic System: A Common Substrate for Movement and Thought?

Walle J. H. Nauta

Department of Psychology and Brain Science, Massachusetts Institute of Technology, Cambridge, Mass., USA

Broadly speaking, the cerebral hemisphere of mammals can be said to be composed of three major anatomical and functional realms: the neocortex, the limbic system, and the extrapyramidal system (also referred to as basal ganglia or corpus striatum). Traditionally, and not without good physiological and clinicopathological reason, the neocortex is considered to embody the highest level of sensory analysis and perceptual integration, as well as certain of the more differentiated mechanisms subserving somatic motor function. Last but not least, it is regarded as the staging ground for ideational processes. The limbic system, by contrast, is generally viewed as the main cerebral representative of the internal milieu, expressing its functions, in part at least, in the form of affects and motivation. And finally, the basal ganglia are generally considered to be essential components of the brain's somatic motor system.

Useful as the notion of a tripartite composition has been (and still is) as a broad-scale first approach to the functional organization of the cerebral hemisphere, recent findings suggest that it may require some qualification. Among the more compelling reasons for revision is an anatomical one: observations accumulated over the past decade or so indicate that the three subdivisions are more closely interconnected than they once seemed to be. More in particular, several places have been identified in which their respective circuitries converge and thus could lead into communal or parallel effector channels. One, and apparently the most extensive of such confluences, occurs in the striatum. In recent years its remarkable pattern has begun to raise the question whether the extrapyramidal system, beside its well-documented role in skeletomotor function, could play a part in perceptual and ideational processes as well [Teuber, 1976].

In the following account the anatomical foundation of this notion will be dealt with in some detail. No comprehensive survey of extrapyramidal circuitry is intended here. For more encompassing reviews of that circuitry reference can be made to a recent Ciba Foundation symposium [Evered and O'Connor, 1984]. The striatum, however, being so much of a nodal intersection of cortical, limbic and extrapyramidal circuits, will be given somewhat more extensive coverage.

General Terminological Remarks

The term, extrapyramidal system, introduced by S. A. K. Wilson in 1912, has never been satisfactorily defined anatomically. Although literally the term can be interpreted so as to denote all of the brain's suprasegmental motor mechanisms not transmitting their discharge by way of the pyramidal tract, convention over the years has made it nearly synonymous with the basal ganglia and their efferent connections. The much older term, basal ganglia, originally subsumed all of the gray masses at the base of the cerebral hemisphere, including even the thalamus, but gradually became restricted to the corpus striatum (striatum and globus pallidus), and only later came to include also the subthalamic nucleus and substantia nigra, both linked to the corpus striatum by reciprocal fiber connections.

The Striatum

A survey of extrapyramidal circuitry most conveniently begins with the striatum, for it is this structure rather than the globus pallidus (or pallidum) that receives the principal extrinsic afferents converging upon the basal ganglia.

In all primates and many nonprimate mammals the striatum is subdivided by a plate-like internal capsule into two main districts, the dorsomedially situated caudate nucleus and the ventrolateral putamen. In other mammalian forms, including the rat, the internal capsule passes through the striatum in the form of a brush rather than a plate; in such species the striatum lacks an overt bisection and is therefore often referred to as caudatoputamen. In either case, however, the anterior part of the striatum includes two further subdivisions that require separate mention.

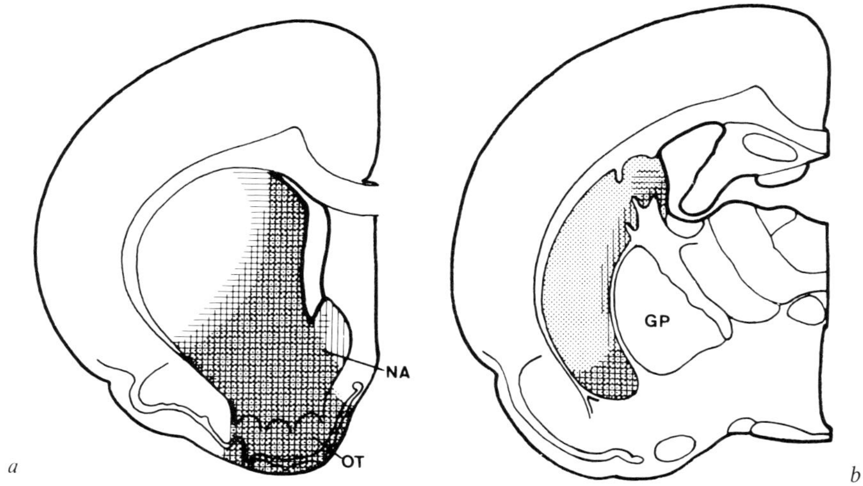

Fig. 1. Semidiagrammatic representation of three limbic system-associated projections to the striatum in rat brain: the dopamine projection from the ventral tegmental area (vertical lines), the projection from the frontal and cingulate cortices (horizontal lines), and the projection from the amygdala (stipple pattern). Not included in the figure (to avoid crowding) is the projection from the hippocampal formation to the nucleus accumbens. Left blank in the more rostral section *(a)* is the anterior, dorsolateral striatal region receiving only sparse limbic afferents but heavily projected upon by the sensorimotor cortex (cf. fig. 2). NA = Nucleus accumbens; OT = olfactory tubercle; GP = globus pallidus. Reproduced from Kelley et al. [1982] with permission of Pergamon Press, Oxford.

One of these, the ventromedial region nearest the base of the septum, and known as the nucleus accumbens septi (fig. 1a), was the first striatal region found to receive afferents from the limbic system, namely, fibers from the precommissural fornix [Fox, 1943; Sprague and Meyer, 1950; Swanson and Cowan, 1977]. On its ventral side the accumbens region extends into the olfactory tubercle, providing the latter with its core population of striatal cells [Heimer, 1978].

All districts of the striatum exhibit basically the same cytoarchitecture. Throughout its extent, more than 98% of its neurons are small to medium-sized, while the remaining 1–2% are large, cholinergic, multipolar cells that were long regarded as the source of the striatum's extrinsic efferents but are now believed to be intrinsic, or 'local-circuit' neurons.

On account of its lack of any broad-scale regional differentiation obvious on cursory inspection of preparations stained by routine survey techniques, the striatum has traditionally been described as a homogeneous structure. More recent studies, however, have disclosed a more covert, smaller-scale stereometric pattern of compartition that subdivides the striatum into an intricate labyrinth of small compartments ('striosomes') embedded in a more homogeneous cell matrix, and distinguished from the latter by peculiarities of histochemistry and cell-packing density [Graybiel and Ragsdale, 1983; Graybiel, 1984]. The relationship of this mosaic to the intrastriatal distribution of extrinsic afferents, to circuits intrinsic to the striatum itself, and to the sites of origin of striatal efferents is currently under intensive investigation. The findings reported thus far strongly suggest that the mosaic reflects a spatial ordering of striatal afferents and efferents of various neurotransmitter and/or neuropeptide content [Graybiel, 1984]. It appears likely, moreover, that intrinsic striatal neurons may provide an orderly system of cross-links between the striosomal and the matrix compartment, and thus between various classes of afferent and efferent conduction lines.

Afferent Connections of the Striatum

The striatum, the main entrance portal for neural inputs to the basal ganglia, receives its most voluminous afferent connections from the entire expanse of the cerebral cortex (including the hippocampal formation and the olfactory cortex), from the intralaminar thalamic nuclei, and from the substantia nigra (including the dopamine neurons of the ventral tegmental area). Additional substantial inputs originate from the amygdala, as well as from the serotonin neurons of the dorsal raphe nucleus of the midbrain. It is important to note that several of these afferent channels come from major limbic structures (hippocampal formation, amygdala, and cingulate cortex), whereas others arise from structures implicated in the subcortical circuitry of the limbic system: ventral tegmental area and dorsal raphe nucleus. The afferents from the cerebral cortex are distributed in the striatum in an intricate stereometric pattern that by and large preserves the topology of the cytoarchitectural subdivision of the cortical mantle but is considerably less sharply defined than the latter. Moreover, as will become evident below, the intrastriatal distribution of the projection from the neocortex as a whole must widely overlap that of projections from the limbic system, especially in the caudal half of the striatum.[1] A somewhat more detailed accounting of the afferentation of the striatum by the limbic system is necessary at this point. It is unfortunate that such an accounting can at present be given only for the rat brain. Even in that species, moreover, no complete description of the pattern of the corticostriatal projection can be given.

The Limbic Innervation of the Striatum

Recent studies in the rat by the aid of the autoradiographic fiber-tracing method [Kelley et al., 1982] have led to the conclusion that the anterior half of the striatum (the large part rostral to the level at which the anterior commissure crosses the midplane) can be subdivided into (a) a ventral and medial region including, but far exceeding, the nucleus accumbens and olfactory tubercle, and (b) a dorsolateral region. The reason for the distinction is that the former, anteroventromedial striatal subdivision is characterized by being densely innervated by several substantial and partially overlapping afferent fiber systems, each originating either from a major component of the limbic system such as the hippocampal formation, amygdala, or cingulate cortex, or from a structure involved in the circuitry of the limbic system, such as the ventral tegmental area and the prefrontal cortex. The remaining, anterodorsolateral striatal sector, by contrast, receives only sparse inputs of limbic origin and is, instead, massively innervated by the sensorimotor cortex. The subdivision of the anterior striatum here described is illustrated by figure 1a in which the limbic-afferented striatal region (for the sake of convenience to be called 'limbic striatum') is indicated by a variety of line and stipple patterns. The dorsolateral, 'nonlimbic' striatal sector heavily innervated by the sensorimotor cortex has been left open in the same drawing. At more caudal levels, as shown by figure 1b, the striatal region in which multiple limbic afferents overlap retains its medial position, but at these levels no 'nonlimbic' sector can be delineated, for the reason that the massive amygdalostriatal projection (indicated by stippling) here expands over the entire

[1] As here used, the term, overlap, solely refers to a convergence of afferent lines upon a large volume of striatal tissue; it carries no implications regarding communal or differential termination within either the matrix or striosomal compartment of the striatum.

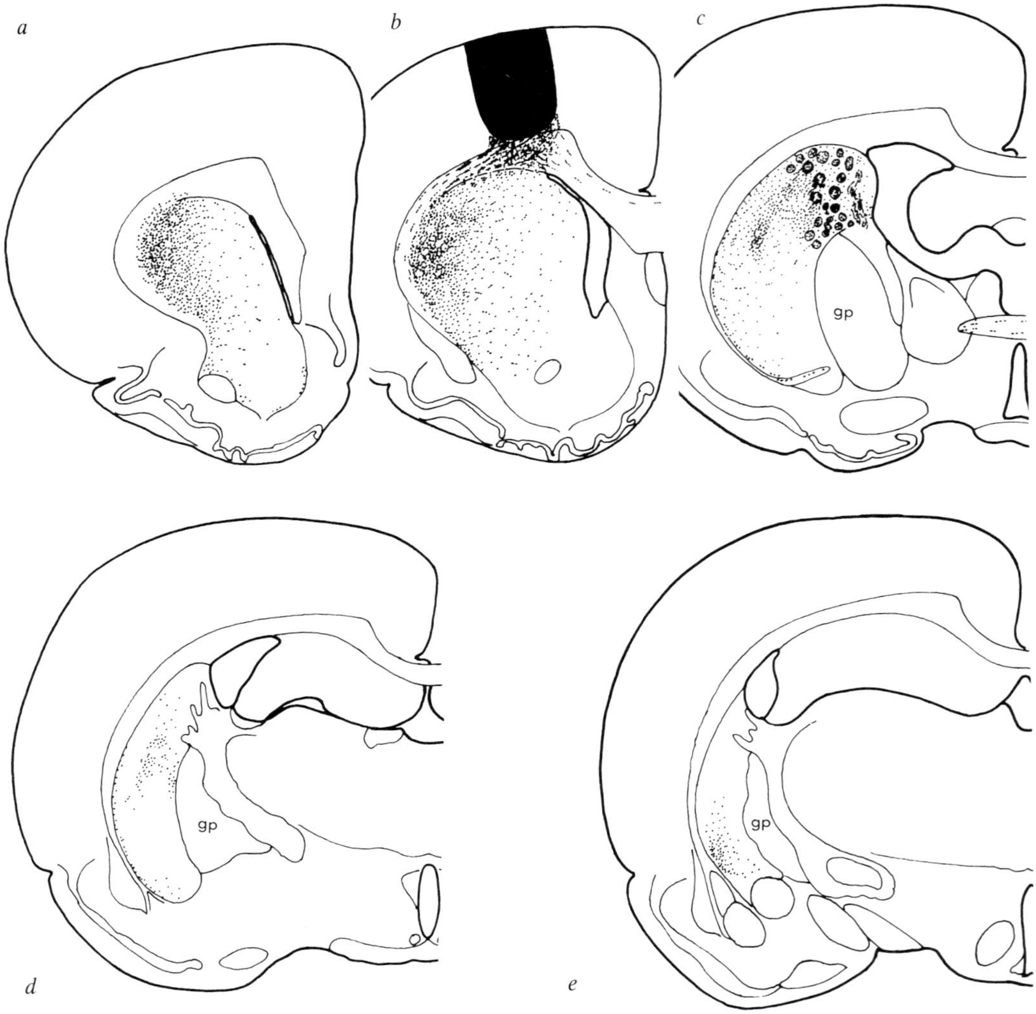

Fig. 2. Radioactive fiber labeling in the rat striatum following an injection of tritiated leucine-and-proline in the sensorimotor cortex. The injection site is shown in jet black in *b*. At the rostral levels shown in *a* and *b* note that the bulk of the projection involves the dorsolateral, relatively 'nonlimbic' striatal sector (left blank in figure 1a). Farther caudally *(d, e)* the motocortical projection overlaps the projection from the amygdala (cf. fig. 1b). gp = Globus pallidus. Reproduced from Kelley et al. [1982] with permission of Pergamon Press, Oxford.

cross-section of the striatum, and thereby overlaps the caudal extent of the corticostriatal projection arising from the motor cortex. (As shown by figure 2, the projection from the motor cortex continues from its major distribution area, a–b caudally and ventrally far enough to involve the entire antero-posterior dimension of the striatum.)

The evidence that the striatum – or at least its rostral half – comprises a limbic-innervated and a 'nonlimbic' district raised the question whether this dualism might not be reflected somehow in the distribution of the massive striatofugal projection to the globus pallidus. In more general terms, the question would be: Could the two striatal districts be the respective origins of two separate and distinct striatal exit lines to the pallidum?

Further study produced an affirmative answer. Comparison of a large number of cases, in each of which a small injection of tritiated leucine had been placed in one or the other striatal locus and the resulting anterograde fiber labeling had been recorded autoradiographically, clearly showed that the limbic-afferented anteroventromedial striatal region indicated in figure 1a projects exclusively to an only recently identified ventral component of the globus pallidus, the so-called *ventral pallidum* (vp). The 'nonlimbic' striatal sector, by contrast, projects to a larger pallidal subdivision, here to be called *dorsal pallidum* (dp) that forms most of the globus pallidus as conventionally outlined in atlases of the rat brain. This subdivision of the globus pallidus into two distinct parts needs some further comment.

The Ventral Pallidum

The vp was first described by Heimer and Wilson [1975] in the rat as an extension of the globus pallidus, stretching ventrally and rostrally beneath the anterior commissure. Its identification as a pallidal subdivision of the infracommissural forebrain region was originally based on cytological characteristics, as well as on the finding that it receives a massive striatal projection originating in particular from the nucleus accumbens [Wilson, 1972; Williams et al., 1977; Nauta et al., 1978]. Its pallidal nature was further documented by evidence that it also shares with the main mass of the globus pallidus a substantial projection from the subthalamic nucleus [Ricardo, 1980] as well as the histochemical characteristics of a high iron content [Switzer and Hill, 1979; Hill and Switzer, 1984] and a strong enkephalin-like [Haber and Nauta, 1981, 1983; Switzer et al., 1982] and glutamic acid decarboxylase-like immunoreactivity [Fallon and Ribak, 1980].

Despite these similarities, the vp must be viewed as distinct from the main mass of the globus pallidus. A principal reason for this distinction is histochemical: Whereas both the vp and the main mass of the globus pallidus are infiltrated by a dense plexus of enkephalin-positive fibers, the vp is pervaded by an additional and almost equally dense plexus of substance-P-positive fibers that extends over only a short distance into the main pallidal mass. For a proper understanding of the criteria followed in defining the vp for the purposes of the present account, a brief elaboration of this last point is necessary.

It is important to note that intrapallidal enkephalin and substance P are not intrinsic to the globus pallidus proper, but are associated with the striatopallidal projection. As first observed by Fox et al. [1974] in Golgi material, striatopallidal fibers enmesh the dendrites of pallidal neurons individually in sleeve-like plexuses. The characteristic histological picture reflecting this junctional arrangement in material immunoreacted for enkephalin ['woolly fibers', Haber and Nauta, 1983] provides a light-microscopic criterion for determining the extent of the globus pallidus. In such material the dense plexus of enkephalin-positive 'woolly fibers' filling the main mass of the globus pallidus is seen to continue without interruption ventrally into the infracommissural region where it extends rostrally over a wide area bordering the ventral side of the striatum and bed nucleus of the stria terminalis [Switzer et al., 1982; Haber and Nauta, 1983]. Interestingly, such material also shows that this infracommissural plexus extends around the lateral border of the nucleus of the diagonal band into the deep, fibrocellular layer of the olfactory tubercle [Switzer et al., 1982; Haber and Nauta, 1983]: this is in agreement with an earlier suggestion, made by Heimer [1978] on cytoarchitectural grounds, that the tubercle is a striatopallidal complex, as well as with the description by Ribak and Fallon [1983] of large cells associated with the islands of Calleja and electron microscopically indistinguishable from pallidal neurons.

Since the density of the enkephalin-positive intrapallidal fiber plexus varies little throughout its extent, it cannot serve to delineate the vp from the main, supra- and retrocommissural mass of the globus pallidus. Such a demarcation is, however, possible in sections processed for substance-P-like immunoreactivity. Such material reveals a dense plexus of substance-P-positive 'woolly fibers' that, with minor exceptions, is coextensive with the infracommissural enkephalin-positive plexus. But, unlike the latter, it extends over only a short distance into the main pallidal mass, then abruptly declines in density and only sparsely extends through the large remainder of the globus pallidus. The curved line along which this decline in density of the substance-P-positive 'woolly-fiber' plexus occurs suggests itself as the border between the vp and the remaining part of the globus pallidus, here for purposes of contrast to be referred to as dp [Haber and Nauta, 1981; cf. also the present fig. 3 in which the extent of the substance-P-positive plexus is indicated by a stippled pattern].

In summary, the vp is here defined as the largely infracommissural region massively pervaded by enkephalin-positive and substance-P-positive (and probably additional) striatofugal fibers terminating in the peridendritic-plexus fashion characteristic of the striatopallidal projection.

One further peculiarity of the vp must be mentioned here. The region corresponds to that part of the globus pallidus which contains the densest population of large, cholinergic neurons (fig. 3). Such cells are more sparsely scattered throughout the remaining parts of the globus pallidus; collectively, they form the intrapallidal component – or subgroup Ch 4 [Mesulam et al., 1983] – of the magnocellular nucleus of the basal forebrain.[2]

Differential Projections from Dorsal and Ventral Pallidum

The evidence that the subdivision of the striatum into a limbic-afferented and a 'nonlimbic' district is mirrored in a ventral versus dorsal dualism in the intrapallidal distribution of the striatopallidal projection raises the question whether the separateness of the two striatal exit lines might not extend even beyond the globus pallidus. To investigate this question, a small deposit of tritiated leucine was placed in either the dorsal or the vp in a large number of rats; the distributions of fibers radioactively

[2] In the human and other primates the magnocellular nucleus of the basal forebrain forms a large, compact group of large cholinergic cells, the basal nucleus of Meynert, located in the substantia innominata just ventral to the globus pallidus. Even in these more highly differentiated species, however, trails of cholinergic cells extend from the basal nucleus dorsally into the medullary laminae of the overlying globus pallidus. In rodents and carnivores the cholinergic cells of the magnocellular nucleus are more widely and diffusely distributed, and lack the circumscript local aggregation that enabled Meynert to recognize a basal nucleus in the human brain.

a 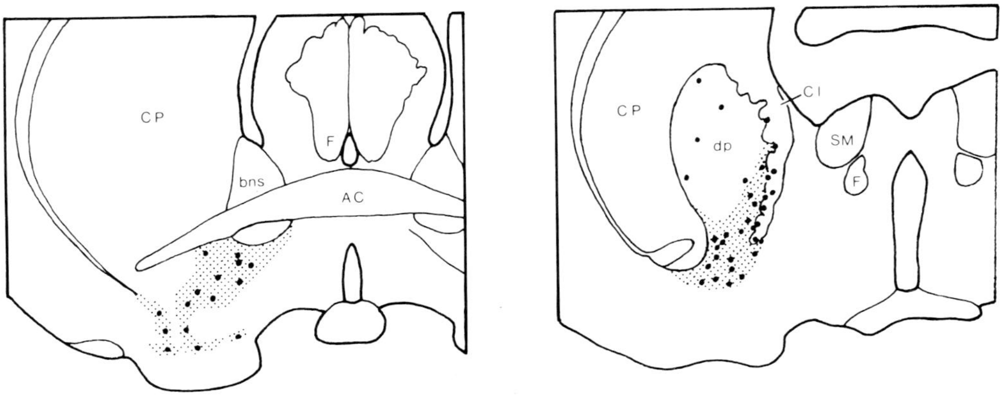 b

Fig. 3. Drawings of two frontal sections at the level of, respectively, the anterior commissure *(a)* and rostral part of the retrocommissural globus pallidus *(b)*. The extent of the dense substance-P-positive fiber plexus, coextensive with the vp of Heimer and Wilson [1975], is indicated by stippling (cf. Haber and Nauta, 1983]. Coarser black dots each represent a strongly acetylcholinesterase (AChE)-positive intrapallidal neuron; together, these neurons compose the intrapallidal subdivision, celled subgroup Ch4 by Mesulam et al. [1983], of the magnocellular nucleus of the basal forebrain. The numerous further cells of the magnocellular nucleus, distributed in the nucleus of the diagonal band and other sublenticular structures [cf. Butcher, 1983; Mesulam et al., 1983] have been omitted in these drawings. Note that such cells are much sparser in the dorsal (dp) than in the vp. AC = Anterior commissure; bns = bed nucleus of stria terminalis; CI = capsula interna; CP = caudatoputamen; dp = dorsal pallidum; F = fornix; SM = stria medullaris. Reproduced from Haber et al. [1985] with permission from Alan R. Liss, New York.

Fig. 4. Semischematic illustration of the two partly segregated striatofugal conduction lines described in the text. *a* 'Limbic' (shaded) and 'nonlimbic' striatal subdivisions and their respective main telencephalic afferents. *b* The striatofugal line leading from the motor cortex-innervated 'nonlimbic' striatal subdivision to the dorsal pallidum (heavy arrow) which in turn projects to the subthalamic nucleus and substantia nigra. *c* The line leading from the limbic-afferented striatal subdivision to the vp (heavy arrow) and from there not only to the subthalamic nucleus and substantia nigra but also to the frontocingulate and medial sensorimotor cortex, lateral habenular and mediodorsal thalamic nucleus, amygdala, hypothalamus, ventral tegmental area and more caudal regions of the midbrain tegmentum. abl = Amygdala; AC = anterior commissure; CC = cerebral peduncle; cgs = central gray substance; CI = capsula interna; dp = dorsal pallidum; ep = entopeduncular nucleus (internal segment of globus pallidus); FCC = frontocingulate cortex; H = hippocampus; hl = lateral habenular nucleus; ht = hypothalamus; md = mediodorsal nucleus; na = nucleus accumbens; rt = reticular nucleus of thalamus; SMC = sensorimotor cortex; sn = substantia nigra; st = subthalamic nucleus; vp = ventral pallidum; vta = ventral tegmental area. Reproduced from Haber et al. [1985] with permission from Alan R. Liss, New York.

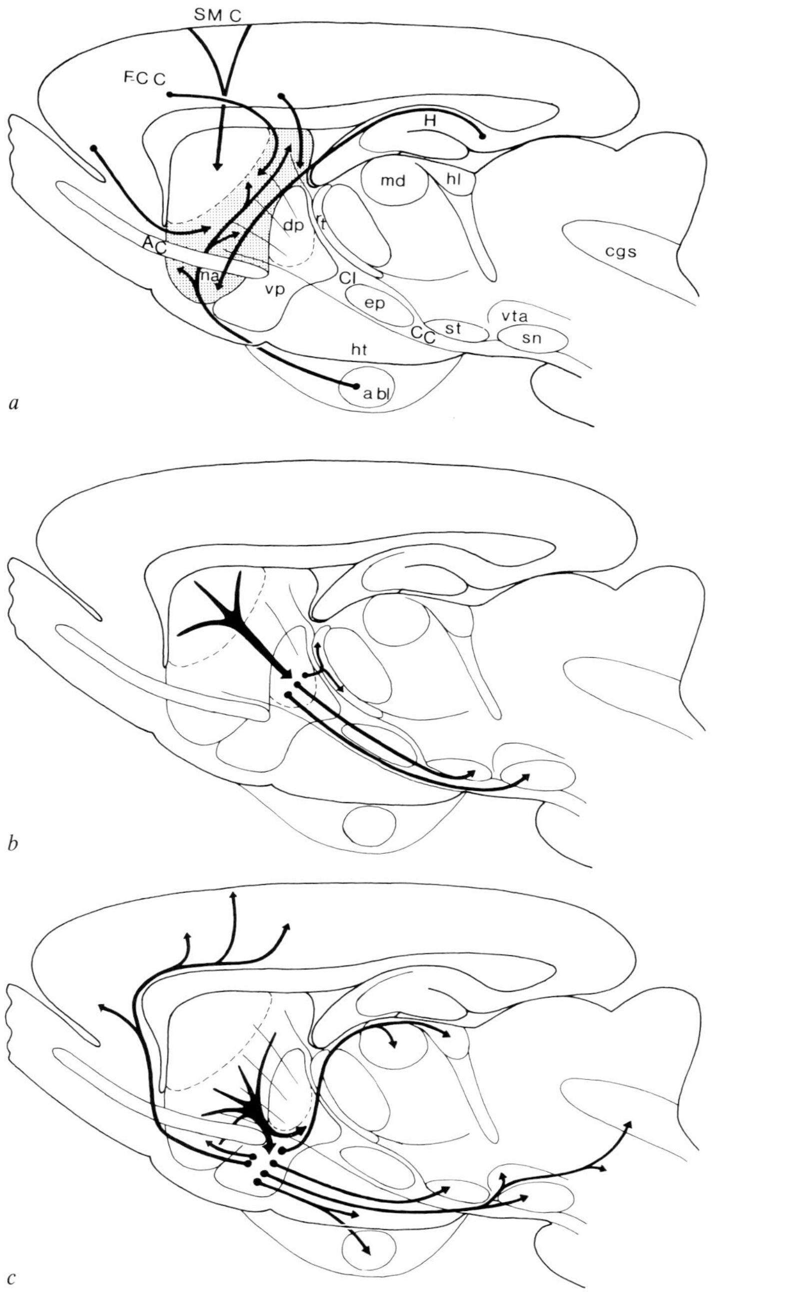
SM C
F.C C
H
md
hl
dp
AC
na
Cl
vp
ep
CC
st
vta
sn
ht
a bl
cgs
a
b
c

labeled by each of these isotope placements were then recorded autoradiographically, carefully charted, and compared. Since a documented account of the findings has been published previously elsewhere [Haber et al., 1985], only the main conclusions will be reported here.

The results of the study showed pronounced differences between the exit lines from the dorsal and vp, respectively. The findings are illustrated by figure 4 and can be summarized as follows:

(1) The efferent connections of the dorsal pallidum (fig. 4b) compose the classical projection from the external pallidum segment and involve primarily the subthalamic nucleus and substantia nigra. This pallidal exit line appears to lie in the extension of the striatopallidal projection arising from the 'nonlimbic' dorsolateral striatal sector (heavy arrow in fig. 4b), the striatal region that in turn receives its main telencephalic input from the sensorimotor cortex (fig. 4a).

(2) The vp projects, like the dp, to the subthalamic nucleus and substantia nigra, but it has further projections to several structures implicated in the circuitry of the limbic system, particularly the amygdala, the lateral habenular nucleus, and the mediodorsal nucleus of the thalamus (fig. 4c). It projects more sparsely to the hypothalamus, to the ventral tegmental area, and to more caudal regions of the midbrain tegmentum, including the region of the pedunculopontine nucleus. Of some special interest are those projections of the vp that ascend to the prefrontal cortex and an adjoining region of the sensorimotor cortex: There is evidence suggesting that this projection, as well as the one to the amygdala, originates largely, at least, from the cholinergic cells of the so-called magnocellular basal nucleus that lie embedded in the vp [Grove et al., 1983]. All these exit lines from the vp, however, appear to lie in the transsynaptic extension of that component of the striatopallidal projection (heavy arrow in fig. 4c) which originates from the limbic-afferented striatum, that is to say, the large striatal region densely innervated by a variety of afferents from within the circuitry of the limbic system (the shaded region in fig. 4a).

Discussion

One of the principal realizations to emerge from the anatomical findings of the past few years is that the striatum, a common target for voluminous projections from the cerebral cortex and the limbic system, has multiple exit channels available that could serve as 'return loops' to the cerebral cortex. Up until about ten years ago only one such loop was generally recognized: the extrapyramidal motor circuit leading from the striatum over, successively, the pallidum and the thalamic VA-VL complex back to areas within the motor domain of the neocortex. Naturally, the discovery of this loop (a step-wise disclosure that was not completed until 1945; cf. Nauta and Mehler, 1966] added further support to the prevalent view of the basal ganglia as a central somatic motor mechanism.

Evidence of further trans-striatal loops to the cortex, not specifically targeted on the motor cortex, is of more recent date. The first such loop to be recognized turned out to lead from the striatum over the pars reticulata of the substantia nigra – rather than over the globus pallidus proper[3] – to the ventromedial nucleus of the thalamus and from there to most of the extent of the neocortex [Cole et al., 1964; Carpenter et al., 1976; Herkenham, 1976]. A second potential return loop to the cortex was found to lead from the striatum over the globus pallidus to the reticular nucleus of the thalamus [Nauta, 1979a; Haber et al., 1985], a thalamic cell group that is unique in the sense that it lacks a projection to the cortex and instead projects to many – if not indeed all – other thalamic nuclei [Scheibel and Scheibel, 1966]; it thus could be suspected of being able to affect the functional state of virtually the entire expanse of the cerebral cortex by modulating the latter's inputs from the thalamus. (The pallido-reticular connection is schematically indicated in fig. 4b.)

It must be emphasized that neither of these two striato-pallido-thalamo-cortical return loops is at present known to be directed at any functionally specified cortical area in particular. On the contrary, both seem likely to involve most if not all of the neocortex. Since it appears to be unknown whether they originate throughout the striatum or from any particular striatal subdivision, nothing can be said at present concerning the functional nature of the corticostriatal input the two loops could 'feed back' to the cortex. This is not as categorically true for the two cortico-striato-pallido-thalamo-cortical circuits to be discussed next.

A distinction between the latter two circuits became possible only after Heimer and Wilson [1975] had recognized the vp, and Kelley et al. [1982] had noted that the anterior half of the striatum comprises a predominantly

[3] On both anatomical and physiological grounds the pars reticulata of the substantia nigra can be interpreted as a caudalmost component of the globus pallidus [cf. Nauta, 1979b; DeLong and Georgopoulos, 1981].

motor cortex-innervated (or 'nonlimbic') and a convergently limbic-innervated subdivision. The evidence presented in a foregoing section of this paper indicates that the limbic versus nonlimbic dichotomy in the innervation of the striatum reflects itself in the existence of two largely segregated striatofugal conduction lines. The present evidence of this dualism is schematically illustrated by figure 4, and can be summarized as follows.

A dorsolateral sector of the anterior striatum receiving only sparse afferents of limbic origin but instead heavily innervated by the sensorimotor cortex [Kelley et al., 1982] projects to an antero-dorsolateral region of the main, supra- and retrocommissural (i.e. conventionally recognized) mass of the globus pallidus; this pallidal region ('dorsal pallidum') in turn gives rise to the classical pallidofugal pathway descending to the subthalamic nucleus and substantia nigra (fig. 4b). By contrast, the heavily limbic-innervated antero-ventromedial striatal region (shaded in fig. 4a) projects to the largely infracommissural, but partly also supra- and retrocommissural vp (fig. 3), from which in turn efferents pass not only to the subthalamic nucleus and substantia nigra but also to various limbic-system-associated structures, in particular the amygdala, frontocingulate (and adjoining sensorimotor) cortex, mediodorsal thalamic nucleus, lateral habenular nucleus, hypothalamus, ventral tegmental area, and more caudal and dorsal regions of the midbrain tegmentum (fig. 4c).

As thus defined, the two striato-pallidofugal lines share the subthalamic nucleus and substantia nigra as common distribution targets. If it is assumed that both these target structures are first and foremost components of the somatic motor system, the present findings suggest both as sites where central skeletomuscular mechanisms are accessible to striatopallidal output of limbic antecedents, conveyed by the line leading from the limbic afferented striatum over the vp. It is likely that further sites of such access lie farther caudally in the midbrain. A small part of the great exit pathway from the globus pallidus (the ansa lenticularis), instead of recurving dorsally into the thalamic VA-VL complex, continues on a straight course into the midbrain tegmentum where it terminates mainly in the region of the so-called pedunculopontine nucleus. On the basis of physiological findings Grillner and Shik [1973] have referred to this tegmental area as the 'mesencephalic locomotor region'. Interestingly, fibers from the region of the vp have been found distributed here as well; Swanson et al. [1984] have interpreted this finding as evidence of a limbic innervation of Grillner and Shik's somatic motor mechanism.

A third route by which the limbic system could be thought to have access to central somatic motor mechanisms could lead from the limbic-innervated striatum over the strongly AChE-positive cells embedded in the vp. The present anterograde evidence suggesting that at least some of these cells project to the sensorimotor cortex only confirms earlier findings in retrograde-labeling experiments [McKinney et al., 1983; Saper, 1984].

Even more difficult to interpret from a functional point of view are the limbico-striato-pallidofugal lines leading to various limbic and limbic-system-associated structures, summarized in figure 4c. From one vantage point, these connections could be viewed collectively as a differentiated 'return loop' enabling the limbic system to monitor the effect of its outputs to the striatum (and thus possibly acting as an aid in adjusting the organism's motivational set to the output efficacy of the central somatic-motor system). But other possibilities must be considered. The question arises, for example, if one significance of the much-interrupted limbico-striato-pallido-limbic circuit here proposed may not lie in the fact that the striatum is the site of an unusually wide variety of intricately interspersed neurotransmitters and neuromodulators [Graybiel and Ragsdale, 1983], particular combinations of which might be required no less stringently for optimal functioning of limbic and cognitive-cortical mechanisms than the same or other combinations are required for optimal somatic-motor function. The possibility of such a more general functional role of the corpus striatum suggests itself from a remarkable parallel between the 'limbic' and 'nonlimbic' trans-striatal conduction lines: both prominently include channels over which part of their impulse flow can be led back to the domain of its origin in the cerebral hemisphere. To be more explicit: the familiar 'extrapyramidal motor circuit', motor cortex → striatum → pallidum → thalamic VA-VL complex → premotor cortex → motor cortex (fig. 5a) appears to have limbic counterparts in the sequences: limbic system → striatum → vp → amygdala, and: limbic system → striatum → vp → thalamic mediodorsal nucleus → frontal and anterior limbic cortex (fig. 5b). If it is considered likely on the basis of long-known anatomical connections that the motor function of the corpus striatum expresses itself in part at least through a major transthalamic circuit affecting the mechanisms of the motor cortex, the more recent anatomical data here reviewed make it appear no less likely that the corpus striatum, through analogous though less massive circuits involving the amygdala and prefrontal cortex, can affect a class of functions that is cognitive rather than primarily skeletomuscular.

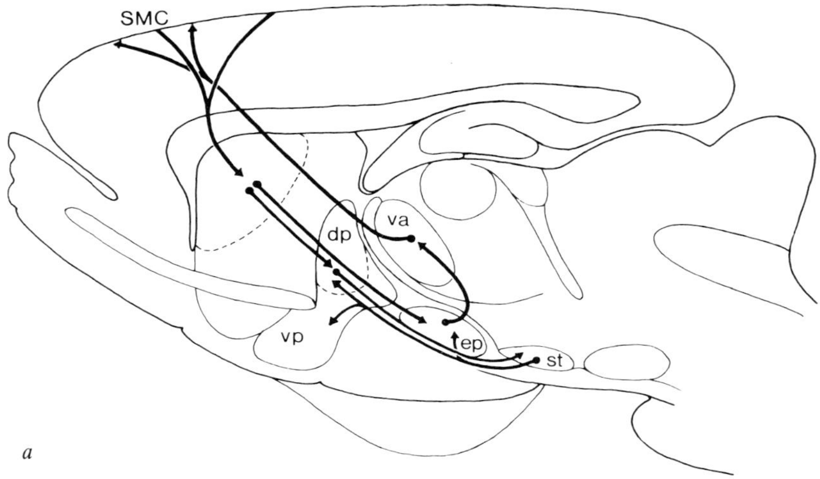

a

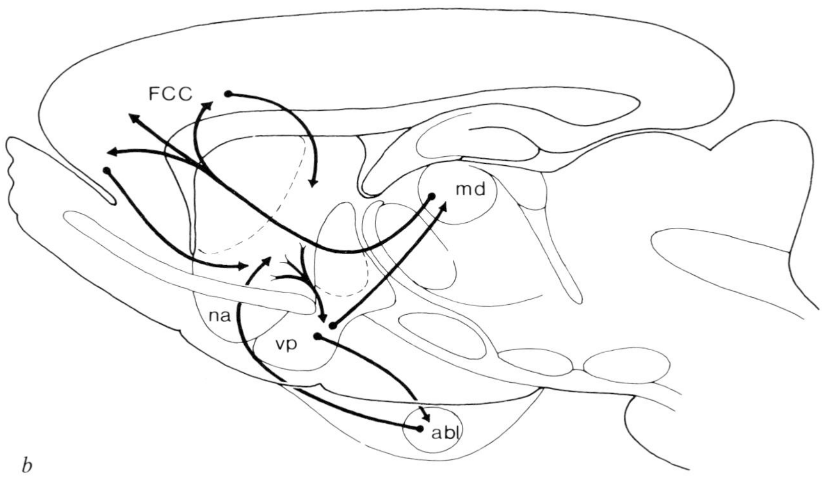

b

Fig. 5. Semidiagrammatic illustration of the two cortico-striato-pallido-thalamo-cortical circuits associated with, respectively, the motor cortex *(a)* and the frontocingulate cortex *(b)*. Note that the extrapyramidal motor circuit shown in *a* sequentially involves the 'nonlimbic' striatum, dp as well as internal pallidal segment (ep), and thalamic VA-VL complex (va). By contrast, the analogous circuit associated with the frontocingulate cortex, shown in *b,* involves the 'limbic' striatum, vp and thalamic mediodorsal nucleus (md); note also the shorter loop

General Comment

The recent evidence that the corpus striatum has various transthalamic exit lines available over which it could be thought to modulate the function not only of the motor cortex, but of most or all of the remaining cortical areas as well, does not come entirely unexpected. That the basal ganglia are implicated not only in motor but also in cognitive functions had been suspected for some time from findings in neurobehavioral experiments [Teuber, 1976], as well as from the frequent concurrence of extrapyramidal-motor and mental disorder. Most unambiguously perhaps, from detailed behavioral studies evidence had been reported of impaired frontal-lobe function in Parkinson's disease [Bowen, 1976] and, more recently, certain lesions of the striatum have been found to cause aphasia with marked impairment of language comprehension [Damasio, 1985].

Exactly which aspects of cognitive function could be influenced by the basal ganglia is at present unknown. One would be inclined to search for a functional attribute that is shared in common by cognition and movement, and affected in common by basal ganglia disorder. It is of interest in this connection to recall John Hughlings Jackson's vigorous argumentation against the notion, prevalent before the discovery of the motor cortex by Fritsch and Hitzig in 1870, that the 'convolutions' (i. e. the cerebral cortex) were the 'organ of mind', and thus exclusively for 'ideas', while 'movements' were represented solely in lower parts of the brain. Jackson's views are illustrated by the following quotations from his selected writings [Taylor, 1958]:

'But of what "substance" can the organ of mind be composed, unless of processes representing movements and impressions; and how can the convolutions differ from the inferior centres, except as parts representing more intricate coordinations of impressions and movements in time and space than they do?' [Hughlings Jackson, 1870].

'There is . . . proof, although indirect, of the opinion that faint and central excitation of sensori-*motor* processes suffices in thought' [italics as in original; Hughlings Jackson, 1872].

---

associated with the amygdala (abl). To avoid excessive complexity of the diagrams, only one of several possible cross-links between the *a* and *b* circuits has been indicated: as shown in *a,* the subthalamic nucleus – innervated by both dp and vp – projects back to both dp and vp, as well as to the internal pallidal segment (ep). For further labels see legend to figure 4. Reproduced from Haber et al. [1985] with permission from Liss, New York.

It is, of course, difficult to say how literally Jackson's view should be taken. Is ideation really the internal expression of the same sensori-motor mechanisms which, when activated more forcibly, would manifest themselves as movements? On the other hand, it is easy to see at least parallels between thought and movement. To begin with, both seem to require a motivational vis a tergo to be initiated and to be kept in progress. It takes an effort to change from a state of relaxed daydreaming – a sort of resting tonus perhaps – to one of goal-directed thinking, and it is something like an act of endurance to keep such a thought process going. Movement and thought share with each other a need for 'feedback' allowing for corrective adjustments. Thought often spills over into the motor sphere, in the form of unintentional changes in body posture and facial expression, pacing the floor, or thinking aloud. More similarities could be mentioned, including the evidence that the physiological substrates of both movement and thought embody a dopamine-dependent mechanism. The 'primary thought disorder' of schizophreniform psychoses may respond well to dopamine-receptor blocking agents, and the protracted use of such drugs can result in dyskinesia.

From all this it could be suspected, as Hughlings Jackson did, that the central motor mechanism and the neural apparatus of ideation have elements in common and may even be in partial overlap. At present, however, any suggestion as to where the two mechanisms might intersect must remain very largely hypothetical. A main reason for this is that it is still impossible to state where in the brain the impetus to a deliberate movement arises, and by what sequence of steps it is ultimately transduced into the requisite pattern of motoneuronal activation and inhibition. The neural substrate for thought processes, needless to say, is even more obscure. It seems reasonable to assume that ideation is primarily a function of the neocortex, but even if it were exclusively a cortical phenomenon it would be continuously affected by subcortical inputs varying from the selectively targeted specific-sensory thalamocortical radiations on the one extreme to the pervasively distributed serotonergic and cholinergic innervations of the cortex by, respectively, the mesencephalic raphe nuclei and the basal nucleus of Meynert on the other extreme. The striato-pallido-thalamo-cortical circuits are among this diversity of afferents to the cortex. Two of the four such circuits described in the foregoing account – the ones leading over, respectively, the ventromedial and the reticular nucleus of the thalamus – are at least potentially diffuse in the sense that they appear to be distributed to much if not all of the neocortex. The two remaining circuits, however, are more selectively targeted. One of these (fig. 5a) is the classical 'extrapyramidal motor circuit' leading over the thalamic VA-VL complex to the motor domain of the cortex, the other (fig. 5b) the more recently identified parallel loop leading over the mediodorsal thalamic nucleus to the frontal and anterior limbic cortex. Even though hypothetical, it seems reasonable to postulate that the loop involving the frontal cortex could play a role in cognitive functions that is comparable to the role of the 'extrapyramidal motor circuit' in bodily movement. In line with this hypothesis, it is tempting to suggest that movement and ideation share with each other a need for propulsion and timing, and that the basal ganglia might be for both functions a source of such dynamic properties.

References

Bowen, F.P.: Behavioral alterations in patients with basal ganglia lesions; in Yahr, The basal ganglia (Raven Press, New York 1976).

Butcher, L.L.: Acetylcholinesterase histochemistry; in Björklund, Hökfelt, Handbook of chemical neuroanatomy, vol. 1 (Elsevier, Amsterdam 1983).

Carpenter, M.B.; Nakano, K.; Kim, R.: Nigrothalamic projections in the monkey demonstrated by autoradiographic technics. J. comp. Neurol. *165:* 401–416 (1976).

Cole, M.; Nauta, W.J.H.; Mehler, W.R.: The ascending efferent projections of the substantia nigra. Trans. Am. Neurol. Ass. *1964:* 74–78.

Damasio, A.R.: Language and the basal ganglia; in Evarts, Wise, Bousfield, The motor system in neurobiology (Elsevier Biomedical Press, Amsterdam 1985).

DeLong, M.A.; Georgopoulos, A.P.: Motor functions of the basal ganglia; in Brooks, Motor control, part 2, pp. 1017–1061 (Am. Physiological Society, Bethesda 1981).

Evered, D.; O'Connor, M. (eds): Functions of the basal ganglia. Ciba Fdn Symp., No. 107 (Pitman, London 1984).

Fallon, J.H.; Ribak, C.E.: Multiple neurotransmitter studies in the islands of Calleja complex of the basal forebrain. III. Connections, correlations and reservations. Soc. Neurosci. Abstr. *6:* 114 (1980).

Fox, C.A.: The stria terminalis, longitudinal association bundle and precommissural fornix fibers in the cat. J. comp. Neurol. *79:* 277–295 (1943).

Fox, C.A.; Andrade, A.N.; Lu Qui, I.J.; Rafols, J.A.: The primate globus pallidus: a Golgi and electron microscopic study. J. Hirnforsch. *15:* 75–93 (1974).

Graybiel, A.M.: Neurochemically specified subsystems in the basal ganglia; in Evered, O'Connor, Functions of the basal ganglia. Ciba Fdn Symp., No. 107, pp. 114–144 (Pitman, London 1984).

Graybiel, A.M.; Ragsdale, C.W.: Biochemical anatomy of the striatum; in Emson, Chemical neuroanatomy (Raven Press, New York 1983).

Grillner, S.; Shik, M.T.: On descending control of lumbosacral spinal cord from the 'mesencephalic locumotor region'. Acta physiol. scand. *87:* 320–333 (1973).

Grove, E.A.; Haber, S.N.; Domesick, V.B.; Nauta, W.J.H.: Differential projections from AChE-positive and AChE-negative ventral-pallidum cells in the rat. Soc. Neurosci. Abstr. *9:* 16 (1983).

Haber, S.N.; Groenewegen, H.J.; Grove, E.A.; Nauta, W.J.H.: Efferent connections of the ventral pallidum: evidence of a dual striato-pallidofugal pathway. J. comp. Neurol. *235:* 322–335 (1985).

Haber, S.N.; Nauta, W.J.H.: Substance P, but not enkephalin, immunoreactivity distinguishes ventral from dorsal pallidum. Soc. Neurosci. Abstr. *7:* 916 (1981).

Haber, S.N.; Nauta, W.J.H.: Ramifications of the globus pallidus in the rat as indicated by patterns of immunohistochemistry. Neuroscience *9:* 245–260 (1983).

Heimer, L.: The olfactory cortex and the ventral striatum; in Livingston, Hornykiewicz, Limbic mechanisms, the continuing evolution of the limbic system concept (Plenum Press, New York 1978).

Heimer, L.; Wilson, R.D.: The subcortical projections of the allocortex: Similarities in the neural associations of the hippocampus, the piriform cortex, and the neocortex; in Santini, Golgi Centennial Symp., pp. 177–193 (Raven Press, New York 1975).

Herkenham, M.: The nigro-thalamo-cortical connection mediated by the nucleus ventralis medialis thalami: evidence for a wide cortical distribution in the rat (Abstract). Anat. Rec. *184:* 426 (1976).

Hill, J.M.; Switzer, R.C.: The regional distribution and cellular localization of iron in the rat brain. Neuroscience *11:* 595–603 (1984).

Hughlings Jackson, J.: see Taylor (1958).

Kelley, A.E.; Domesick, V.B.; Nauta, W.J.H.: The amygdalostriatal projection in the rat – an anatomical study by anterograde and retrograde tracing methods. Neuroscience *7:* 615–630 (1982).

McKinney, M.; Coyle, J.T.; Hedreen, J.C.: Topographic analysis of the innervation of the rat neocortex and hippocampus by the basal forebrain cholinergic system. J. comp. Neurol. *217:* 103–121 (1983).

Mesulam, M.-M.; Mufson, E.J.; Wainer, B.H.; Levey, A.I.: Central cholinergic pathways in the rat: An overview based on an alternative nomenclature (Ch 1-Ch 6). Neuroscience *10:* 1185–1201 (1983).

Nauta, H.J.W.: Projections of the pallidal complex: an autoradiographic study in the cat. Neuroscience *4:* 1853–1873 (1979a).

Nauta, H.J.W.: A proposed conceptual reorganization of the basal ganglia and telencephalon. Neuroscience *4:* 1875–1881 (1979b).

Nauta, W.J.H.; Mehler, W.R.: Projections of the lentiform nucleus in the monkey. Brain Res. *1:* 3–42 (1966).

Nauta, W.J.H.; Smith, G.P.; Faull, R.L.M.; Domesick, V.B.: Efferent connections and nigral afferents of the nucleus accumbens septi in the rat. Neuroscience *3:* 385–401 (1978).

Ribak, C.E.; Fallon, J.H.: The islands of Calleja complex of rat basal forebrain. I. Light and electron microscopic observations. J. comp. Neurol. *205:* 207–218 (1983).

Ricardo, J.: Efferent connections of the subthalamic region in the rat. I. The subthalamic nucleus of Luys. Brain Res. *202:* 257–271 (1980).

Saper, C.B.: Organization of cerebral cortical afferent systems in the rat. II. Magnocellular basal nucleus. J. comp. Neurol. *222:* 313–342 (1984).

Scheibel, M.E.; Scheibel, A.B.: The organization of the nucleus reticularis thalami: a Golgi study. Brain Res. *1:* 43–62 (1966).

Sprague, J.M.; Meyer, M.: An experimental study of the fornix in the rabbit. J. Anat. *84:* 354–368 (1950).
Swanson, L.W.; Cowan, W.M.: An autoradiographic study of the organization of the efferent connections of the hippocampal formation in the rat. J. comp. Neurol. *172:* 49–84 (1977).
Swanson, L.W.; Mogenson, G.J.; Gerfen, C.R.; Robinson, P.: Evidence for a projection from the lateral preoptic area and substantia innominata to the 'mesencephalic locomotor region' in the rat. Brain Res. *295:* 161–178 (1984).
Switzer, R.C.; Hill, J.: Globus pallidus component in the olfactory tubercle: evidence based on iron distribution. Soc. Neurosci. Abstr. *5:* 79 (1979).
Switzer, R.C.; Hill, J.; Heimer, L.: The globus pallidus and its rostroventral extension into the olfactory tubercle of the rat: a cyto- and chemoarchitectural study. Neuroscience *7:* 1891–1904 (1982).
Taylor, J.: Selected writings of John Hughlings Jackson, vol. I (Basic Books, New York 1958).
Teuber, H.-L.: Complex functions of the basal ganglia; in Yahr, The basal ganglia (Raven Press, New York 1976).
Williams, D.J.; Crossman, A.R.; Slater, P.: The efferent projections of the nucleus accumbens in the rat. Brain Res. *130:* 217–227 (1977).
Wilson, R.D.: Efferent connections of the nucleus accumbens in the rat; Master thesis, MIT, Cambridge, Mass. (1972).

W.J.H. Nauta, MD, PhD, 196 Kent Road, Newton, MA 02168 (USA)

Mueller (ed.): Neurology and Psychiatry: A Meeting of Minds, pp. 64–87 (Karger, Basel 1989)

The Search for an Anatomic Basis of Schizophrenia: Review and Update

Janice R. Stevens

National Institute of Mental Health, Saint Elizabeth's Hospital, Washington, D.C., USA

Psychiatrists at the turn of this century, all trained as they were in neurology and neuropathology, were convinced that dementia praecox (only later to be named schizophrenia) was a disease of the brain. This point of view nearly vanished during the middle of the century under the powerful influence of psychodynamic and social psychiatry.

Three discoveries in the two decades between 1954 and 1974 set the stage for the return of psychiatrists' interest in functional anatomy of the brain. First was the development of two new classes of antipsychotic drugs, the neuroleptics and the antidepressants. Both groups of drugs not only relieve psychotic symptoms in a majority of patients treated, but because of their effects on specific brain systems led to new hypotheses concerning the etiology of both affective and schizophrenic psychoses. In the case of schizophrenia, the ubiquitous dopamine (DA) blocking effect of all effective neuroleptic agents led to the hypothesis that the symptoms and signs of schizophrenia were due to overactivity of a DA system of the brain. The beneficial effects on depression of monoamine protagonists (agonists, precursors and degradation blockers) similarly initiated several monoamine hypotheses of mood disorder.

A second major contribution to the psychiatric revolution of the 1950s and 1960s was the discovery of previously unknown monoamine pathways in the brain and application of new detection techniques for quantitative estimation of these amines and their metabolites in brain and various body fluids.

Finally, techniques for quantitative measurement and autoradiographic visualization of neurotransmitter-specific binding sites turned attention to receptor chemistry, physiology and potential pathology. The very large number of studies measuring the monoamines, their metabolites, precursors and binding sites in brain of patients with schizophrenia has, however, provided rather few replicable abnormalities. The more recent measurement of an ever-increasing number of peptides in brain, comparing schizophrenics with normal controls, has provided equally equivocal results.

In the last decade, there has been renewed interest in investigation of brain morphology and pathology in schizophrenia. Stimulated by development of noninvasive imaging techniques, a number of investigators have shown mild to moderate ventricular dilatation in 15–20% of schizophrenic patients, thus confirming the all but forgotten reports of similar changes shown by pneumoencephalography five decades ago. This rediscovery has greatly accelerated the interest of psychiatrists in the morphology and pathology of the brain.

This chapter will briefly review the present status of work with both old and new investigative techniques. An attempt will be made to integrate laboratory studies with the clinical picture, course and possible pathogenesis of schizophrenia.

The Clinical Syndrome: Psychiatric and Neurologic Analysis

Similarities of Schizophrenic Symptoms to the Auras of Temporal Lobe Epilepsy

Examination of the details of schizophrenic illness, as in other neurologic disorders, reveals several consistent themes which suggest clues to the underlying anatomy and pathophysiology. A number of striking similarities have been noted between the early symptoms of schizophrenia and the auras of temporal lobe epilepsy [Stevens, 1973]. Disordered perceptions, intermittent preemption of consciousness by suspicion, fear, and feelings of unreality are common in both illnesses. Apparently irrelevant memories of recent and remote events intrude insistently on consciousness and in schizophrenia, unlike epilepsy, are separated with difficulty from thoughts or ideas to which they are tangentially or allegorically associated. Stereotyped automatisms, a peculiar faraway stare and psychomotor blocking in schizophrenia are highly reminiscent of brief psychomotor or petit mal absence seizures, but in contrast to epilepsy are not associated with loss of consciousness or visible changes in the scalp EEG. Particularly striking in both the auras of some temporal lobe seizures and the subjective reports of schizophrenia are feelings of intense fear, the altered quality of sensory experience, and the sense of strangeness, uncanniness, hidden significance, or danger.

Similar sensations can be evoked from electrical stimulation of sharply localized areas of amygdala or hippocampus through intracerebral electrodes chronically implanted in patients with temporal lobe epilepsy [Stevens et al., 1969; Gloor et al., 1982; Halgren, 1982].

Thought Processes, Attention, Blocking, Stereotypic Thinking. Thinking defects are an early hallmark of the schizophrenic illness. The onset of such symptoms may be abrupt but is more often subtle and progressive. Headaches, insomnia, change of disposition, loss of ability to concentrate, preoccupation, restlessness or withdrawal are followed by disturbance in goal-directed thinking, by repeated loss of thought train, intrusion of unwanted percepts or stereotyped repetitious ideas and compulsions. The result is that thinking becomes bizarre, confused, incorrect, 'ataxic'. Sometimes all associative threads fail and the thought chain is totally interrupted. After such blocking, ideas may emerge which have no recognizable connection with the preceding ones.

Case 1. A 34-year-old former Fulbright scholar, ill for a dozen years with schizophrenia, complained of the radio in his rooming house continually broadcasting reports accusing him of homosexuality. He wrote long, incoherent letters to his physician in which sexual references were interlaced with odds and ends of French history, politics and other remnants of his former scholarly career.

Examination revealed a disheveled man with marked external strabismus, paresis of the medial rectus of the right eye, monotonous, poorly modulated speech, and episodic, prolonged psychomotor blocking. Delays in speech or reply could be aborted if the patient was touched on the shoulder. Following this he immediately resumed muttering poorly articulated fragments of tangentially connected information. During episodes of psychomotor blocking there were spontaneous horizontal nystagmoid movements of the eyes in mid-position.

Stereotypic Thoughts. Fragmentation of goal-directed thinking and intrusion of bizarre ideas are characteristic of the early stages of the illness. In chronic progressive schizophrenia, perseverated thoughts and utterances appear to dominate the stream of consciousness, preventing intellectual effort, but can usually be interrupted for the performance of daily tasks or exchange of conventional conversational pleasantries. Patients so afflicted are to be found in large numbers on the back wards of state hospitals and it is among these individuals that evidence of neurologic as well as psychologic deterioration is usually readily demonstrated.

Case 2. A 37-year-old former truck driver was well until age 28 when he became depressed, agitated, preoccupied, and had many somatic complaints. Treatment with high doses of phenothiazines and with ECT induced little improvement. Progressive deterioration of speech, thought and behavior ensued. His days and evenings were now spent in almost continuous conversation with hallucinated voices; 'they can't get workers enough to get in the hay, instead of going down to us and spending a thousand bucks sometimes I bought a Singer sewing machine; had to buy a chopped thing, get a bag big enough, you know why they sputter 'cause they're mounted on the body around to the left, but come to bed at my house, meat, bread, butter, eggs, peanuts, can't even find the damn thing 'cause it ain't big enough to get in, jump on it and the competition lost the whole goddam game, lost the red automotive wheel, ya know? Why? Cause if you don't do what I ask you I can't get started. Watch the plate glass, it'll jump out the window.' Neurological examination revealed a striking vacant stare associated with tonic contraction of the periorbital musculature, absent glabella reflex, incessant rocking, pacing and talking. Attention could be briefly obtained for following simple motor commands.

Affective and Emotional Disturbance. The incongruity between affect and behavior frequently emphasized in schizophrenia reflects the difficulty in distinguishing apparently senseless motor acts or expression from behavior based on responses to underlying change in perception, feeling, and loss of recognition of social signals from others. This distinction becomes increasingly difficult to determine late in the illness when the patient may be nearly totally uncommunicative, but continues to perform incomprehensible, impulsive acts despite blunting of affect and apparent loss of human empathy. In contrast to psychomotor epilepsy, consciousness may be altered but is usually not lost during assaultive or self-destructive episodes and total amnesia is rare.

Case 3. A 21-year-old boy with chronic paranoid schizophrenia entered the hospital after smashing up all the furniture in his home. Mute and remote, his expression was that of a hunted animal. His eyes darted fearfully from side to side as he stood tensely in the examining room. When the attendant caring for him turned his back momentarily the patient struck him brutally on the side of the head, afterwards explaning that he had interpreted the behavior as a homosexual gesture. Remanded to a hospital for the criminally insane, he lapsed into mute, expressionless withdrawal.

An intense subjective sense of fear or dread is a striking feature of many patients with schizophrenia and, as in psychomotor epilepsy, appears to reflect either an inexplicable inner visceral 'paresthesia' of terror, or response to the extraordinary sense of perceptual change, personal estrangement, disordered thought control, or alterations in signification which cause the most banal stimulus to assume signal portent.

Memory. In the realm of memory, great variability is noted. Many patients can recall events prior to the illness exactly as though they had occurred the day before, and the memories rouse many of the affects with which they were originally associated. A 32-year-old patient, chronically hospitalized for nearly 16 years, remained preoccupied much of the time with the same erotic fantasies described in the record of her first admission. Perplexed and irritable, she was mute and constantly pacing throughout the day, but at night she giggled and whispered as she sat on the edge of her bed: 'Johnny, don't do that, Johnny stop.'

Motor Disturbances. Kraepelin [1907], who was the first to distinguish dementia praecox from other major mental ills, was also the first to describe the motor disturbances associated with the disorder. The dyskinesia that he described so vividly and that he considered characteristic of dementia praecox must be considered indistinguishable from tardive dyskinesia. Catatonia, the most dramatic motor manifestation of the illness, appears to have been more common in Kraepelin's time than now. However, catatonic schizophrenia, usually characterized by excitement and violence, is still the most frequent subtype diagnosed on admission to mental wards in much of the Third World. Often abrupt in onset, catatonic stupor or excitement is commonly associated with good prognosis. Catatonia can result from a number of different pathologic events and reflects the site or chemistry of the compromised area of brain more than it relates to any single diagnostic entity. Thus, Mettler and Crandell [1959] reported that signs of catatonic stupor are faithfully replicated by bilateral lesions of globus pallidus and Nielsen [1948] reported catatonic stupor following bilateral destruction of the cingulate gyri. Herpes encephalitis [Raskin and Frank, 1974], third ventricle tumors, subarachnoid hemorrhage and a variety of pharmacologic agents can also induce catatonic states [De Jong, 1945]. Catatonic excitement, although it can resemble an epileptic seizure, is usually not associated with frank convulsions and responds best to neuroleptic medication and convulsive therapy. Catatonic stupor of schizophrenia also clears temporarily following sodium amytal [Bleckwenn, 1930].

Others have described a variety of less dramatic motor disturbances in schizophrenic patients. These include dyskinesias of face and limbs (considered a particularly grave prognostic sign) [Yarden and Discipio, 1971], stereotyped motor acts (patting, tapping, circling, rocking, pacing) and a variety of oculomotor signs [Stevens, 1978]. Dyskinesias were reported in schizophrenia well before the phenothiazine era. Owens et al. [1982]

maintain that dyskinetic movements are as common in schizophrenics never treated with neuroleptics as they are in patients who have received treatment. Although most psychiatrists would dispute this claim, dyskinesias indistinguishable from today's 'tardive dyskinesia' certainly occurred in patients prior to introduction of phenothiazines, as illustrated in the following history:

Case 4. A 17-year-old high school student, previously sociable and at the top of his class, gradually withdrew from normal contacts, became restless, irritable, and complained that people looked at him in a peculiar fashion. He developed periodic rage attacks, suffered accusatory and obscene auditory hallucinations, gave up his studies and threatened his family. On admission to Saint Elizabeths Hospital in 1944 he was fearful, untidy, preoccupied, slow of speech with marked staring and psychomotor blocking. His illness followed a progressive deteriorating course. Gradually he became mute, isolated, idle, manneristic, masturbated openly and intermittently was impulsively assaultive. In 1952, he was described as blank-faced, mute, squinting, grimacing and with 'marked tics of face and head'. Chlorpromazine 100 mg daily was started in 1956. He died suddenly the following year from food aspiration. The brain was unremarkable grossly. Histologic examination revealed intense gliosis of the basal forebrain including the preoptic area, lateral hypothalamus, tuber cinereum, substantia innominata, head of caudate nucleus and dorsomedial thalamus. There was capillary proliferation in the floor of the third ventricle.

Speech. Although schizophrenia is not usually considered to entail a disturbance of motor function, dysarthric, flat, scanning speech and altered modulation of speech are commonly observed in individuals with chronic schizophrenia. Mutism is a frequent presenting sign in acute schizophrenia and is usually readily ameliorated by intravenous sodium amytal or rapid neuroleptization. End-stage schizophrenia is often characterized by almost total loss of speech or by verbigeration, gibberish or word salad.

This brief review suggests that the signs and symptoms of schizophrenia can be associated with similar symptoms associated with known cerebral pathology, a view amplified by examination of Davison and Bagley's [1969] monumental study of schizophrenia-like psychosis associated with organic brain disorders. These authors calculated correlation coefficients between individual symptoms and sites of brain lesions in 150 cases of schizophrenia-like illness associated with organic disease collected from the published literature. Although correlation coefficients were very low (generally less than 0.20), they found statistically significant correlations between catatonia and pathology of the left hemisphere and basal ganglia, between primary delusions and lesions of the left hemisphere and

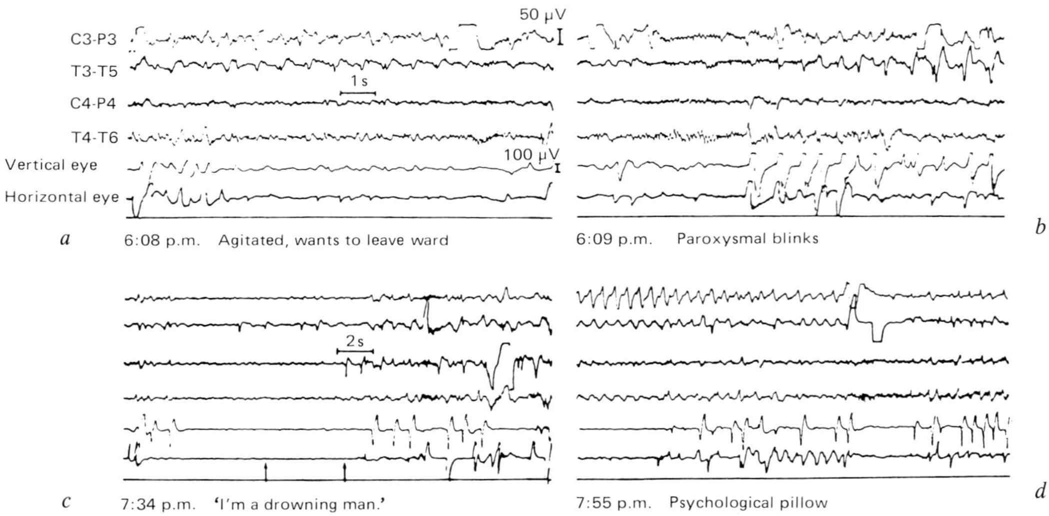

Fig. 1. Telemetered scalp EEG from 24-year-old male with severe chronic paranoid schizophrenia during a period of intense delusional activity. *a* Steady, rhythmic, slow (0.8/s) spike-wave discharge recorded by telemetry from left centroparietal and temporal regions during period of agitation. *b* Paroxysmal blinking coincides with a burst of left centroparietal and temporal slow spike and wave activity. *c* Small left temporal spikes during bizarre speech fragments. *d* Rhythmic, 2.5 cps, notched high-voltage slow waves appeared and then disappeared over left centroparietal and temporal regions while patient remained in characteristic 'psychological pillow' posture, lying supine, with head raised from surface of couch for nearly 5 min. From Stevens et al. [1979].

temporal lobe, and between auditory hallucinations, thought disorder, and first rank Schneiderian symptoms and lesions of the brain stem and diencephalon. Flattening and incongruity of affect, catatonic symptoms and thought disorder were associated with early age of onset, while paranoid delusions were associated with later onset of disease. Etiologically, only four potential pathologic antecedents of the illness were found in significant excess among patients with schizophreniform illness compared with a nonschizophrenic population: Huntington's chorea, pituitary adenoma, glioma (12 of 19 were in temporal lobe) and narcolepsy. Multiple sclerosis, cerebrovascular disease and Parkinson's disease were underrepresented among those with schizophreniform illness. Epilepsy was neither significantly increased nor decreased in this sample compared with a nonschizophrenic population. Their evidence and ours suggest a subcortical pathology.

Electroencephalogram

Twenty-five to 30% of patients diagnosed schizophrenic show some abnormalities in the conventional EEG [Hill, 1957; Abenson, 1970]. These may take the form of focal paroxysmal slow or spike activity (usually over one or both temporal regions of the scalp) or diffuse mild slowing as in catatonia. Computer analysis of the EEG of unmedicated schizophrenic patients reveals decreased alpha and increase in both slow and fast frequencies [Itil, 1974]. Scalp records and computer-analyzed EEGs made during hallucinatory or catatonic periods generally reveal no evidence of cortical seizure activity [Stevens et al., 1979; Stevens and Livermore, 1982]. During prolonged telemetered recordings made in ambulatory psychotic patients, one schizophrenic patient demonstrated a paroxysmal discharge over the temporal lobes during a period of severe delusory behavior (fig. 1). However, Heath [1954] and others [Sem-Jacobsen, 1957; Hanley et al., 1979] have reported random spike activity from chronic intracerebral electrodes implanted in subcortical nuclei of the basal forebrain or thalamus during active psychosis of schizophrenic patients. Evoked potential studies [Shagass et al., 1984], feature extraction and significance probability mapping of power spectra show some promise in discerning pathologic changes [Morihisa et al., 1983; Morstyn et al., 1983; Duffy, 1985]. The frontal slowing reported in schizophrenia from several sources with these techniques is probably, however, a result of the excessive eye movement shown by many schizophrenic patients.

Findings from Radiology and Other Brain Imaging Techniques

Pneumoencephalographic demonstration of large ventricles in schizophrenic patients was first reported by Jacobi and Winkler [Jacobi and Winkler, 1977]. More recently Johnstone et al. [1976], Weinberger et al. [1979] and many others have made similar observations by computerized axial tomography. Crow [1981] divided schizophrenia into two subgroups on the basis of clinical symptoms. Those with 'positive symptoms' (e.g. hallucinations, delusions and labile affect) generally had normal size ventricles, while those with 'negative symptoms' (e.g. poverty of speech, dementia and flat affect) tended to have larger ventricles. In my experience, most patients have a mixture of 'positive' and 'negative' symptoms in the course of their illness. Furthermore, the constellation of so-called

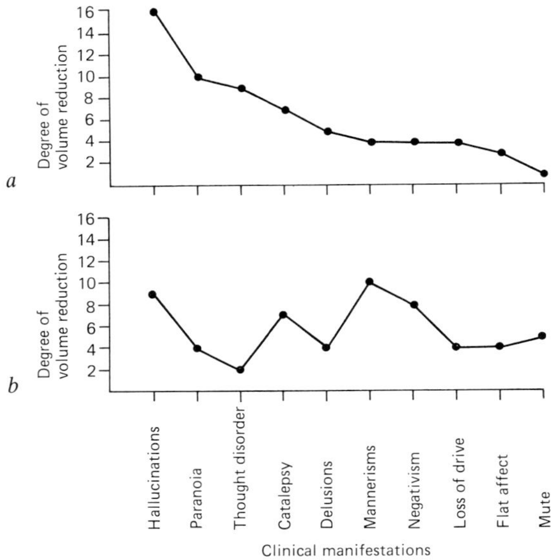

Fig. 2. Relationship between symptoms and signs of schizophrenia and degree of volume reduction in amygdala, hippocampus, parahippocampal gyrus *(a)* or caudate, putamen, globus pallidus *(b)* as measured in postmortem brains by Bogerts et al. [1985]. Degree of volume reduction derived by summing numerical value of standard deviation from normal control brain means [Stevens, 1986]. Note that the decreased volume of temporal lobe structures appears more related to hallucinations, paranoia and thought disorder 'positive' symptoms of Crow [1981], while the decrease in volume of the basal ganglia appears to be associated more with 'negative' symptoms.

positive or negative symptoms generally corresponds to the course and stage of the illness and, as in other neurologic disorders, doubtless reflects both localization and stage of progression of the pathology of the disease (fig. 2). Thus, Crow's 'positive symptom' patients are significantly younger than those with negative symptoms. Reveley et al. [1984] reported a negative correlation between ventricular size and a positive family history of schizophrenia. A larger percentage of older patients with chronic deteriorated schizophrenia have increased ventricle size [Woods and Wolf, 1983]. Although not apparent in studies of chronic or older patients, a positive correlation between ventricular size and duration of illness has been shown in a few studies [Tanaka et al., 1981; Woods and Wolf, 1983].

Recent studies with the functional imaging techniques of cerebral blood flow (CBF) and positron emission tomography (PET) have produced some conflicting results. The early evidence for hypoperfusion and hypometabolism in frontal regions at rest in schizophrenia [Ingvar and Franzen, 1974] appears to be related to reversible frontal lobe 'turnoff' seen in some schizophrenic patients during specific tasks or at rest [Weinberger et al., 1986]. Sheppard [1983] reported no decrease in frontal metabolism in schizophrenics at rest with (PET) using ^{13}O while Kishimoto et al. [1987], using ^{18}F fluorodeoxy-glucose, found decreased parieto-temporal metabolism in a group of paranoid schizophrenics and frontal hypometabolism in a group with nonparanoid undifferentiated schizophrenia. Differences in subject condition during testing, medication status, time for resolution of the isotopes used, and type of the illness doubtless account for some of these inconsistencies and delay interpretation of the findings in relation to a pathophysiology of the illness.

Dopamine Hypothesis of Schizophrenia

It is now more than 30 years since the introduction of chlorpromazine for the treatment of schizophrenia and the recognition that this drug could cause most of the symptoms and signs of Parkinson's disease. Twenty years ago, Carlsson and Lindquist [1963] and Randrup and Munkvad [1965] pointed out that pharmacologic agents effective against schizophrenia all share the property of increasing DA turnover, while DA agonists and precursors can exaggerate schizophrenic symptoms. In a particularly influential report, Creese et al. [1976] showed that the DA (D_2) binding affinity of antipsychotic agents is directly related to their clinical potency against the symptoms of schizophrenia. These studies form the basis of the DA hypothesis of schizophrenia and have led to a very large number of investigations of DA and its metabolites in various bodily fluids and in brains of schizophrenic patients and controls.

Although there have been sporadic reports of elevation or decrease in one or more neurotransmitters in various brain regions, the only replicated findings have been the evidence for increased binding of several DA antagonists in both neo and limbic striatum of patients with schizophrenia [Seeman et al., 1976; Owen et al., 1978]. Since these studies are confounded by past or current treatment with neuroleptics in a majority of the subjects concerned, and since such treatment is a well-known cause of increased neuroleptic binding in the brains of animals, the significance of this finding remains moot [MacKay et al., 1980].

Interest in DA and thus in the nigrostriatal network in schizophrenia has important precedents. Thus, following the encephalitis lethargica pandemic of the early decades of this century, many patients who recovered showed not only parkinsonism, but also typical schizophrenic manifestations such as echopraxia, akinesia, sleep disturbances, chorea flexibilitas, echolalia, catalepsy, staring, pouting ('Schnauzkrampf') and 'psychological pillow' [Jelliffe, 1927].

Demonstration of specific DA containing neurons in substantia nigra (SN) and ventral tegmental area (VTA) of midbrain, the axons of which project principally to neostriatum (caudate putamen) and limbic striatum (nucleus accumbens, olfactory tubercle, bed nucleus of stria terminalis and central amygdala nucleus) focused attention on these striatal structures where more than 85% of the DA in the brain is found. Discovery of specific bindings sites for each of the monoamines and, in particular, demonstration of increased DA binding in neo and limbic striatum of patients with schizophrenia appeared to support the conjecture that schizophrenia was due to overactivity in brain DA systems.

Of the three DA systems in the brain, the nigrostriatal, mesolimbic-mesocortical and tuberoinfundibular, the mesolimbic-mesocortical system is of special interest in psychiatry. The terminals of this system project to the cerebral cortex and to ventral striatal nuclei that receive afferents from amygdala, hippocampus and allocortex. In parallel to neostriatum, which projects via globus pallidus and SN to ventral lateral thalamus and then to motor cortex, limbic striatal nuclei project via ventral pallidum to substantia innominata, hypothalamus, and via dorsomedial thalamus to frontal lobe. The high ratio of input to output through the DA-biased system suggest that neo and limbic striata filter, compress, modulate or 'gate' information from sensory to motor systems in neostriatum and from amygdala-hippocampal affect and memory processing regions projecting to limbic striatum en route to thalamus, hypothalamus and frontal lobe [Stevens, 1973].

Because so many of the symptoms and signs of schizophrenia resemble the experiences and behaviors of individuals with abnormal excitation of limbic structures (e. g. as in patients with temporal lobe epilepsy), attention has been focused on limbic striatum and its DA system. However, despite hundreds of quantitative analyses of monoamines, their precursors, metabolites, enzymes of synthesis and degradation, few consistent results have emerged with respect to increase or decrease of DA or its metabolites in the schizophrenic brain or CSF. Only the increased binding of DA antagonists in neo and limbic striatum has been replicated by several groups and, as noted above, may (or may not) reflect previous treatment with DA-blocking neuroleptics. There the matter rests, seemingly incapable of resolution by postmortem studies and now under scrutiny by new methods for assessment of DA binding sites in previously untreated patients using in vivo quantitative imaging of brain neuroreceptors [Sedvall et al., 1986].

Experimental Investigations

In an early attempt to prepare a model of DA hyperactivity in limbic striatum, we blocked the GABAergic inhibitory feedback pathway from striatum to VTA by infusing micro amounts of the GABA-blocking agent bicuculline on cells of the VTA in freely moving cats chronically implanted with electrodes and cannulas [Stevens et al., 1974]. Introduction of 2–4 μl of a solution containing 10–30 mg of bicuculline in the VTA caused the animals to display an extraordinary state consisting of intense arousal, stare, withdrawal, waxy flexibility, statuesque posture, searching, sniffing, and hiding stereotypies. Several animals exhibited stalking, crouching, or abrupt visual searching behaviors as though something unusual was seen or heard. These behaviors were accompanied by spike activity limited to the superior terminus of the VTA-DA projection in nucleus accumbens, the same region from which spike activity has been recorded in schizophrenic man. Similar disturbances were not obtained from injection of bicuculline in nearby substantia nigra. Instead, GABA blockade of this region induced ipsilateral circling, cutaneous hyperesthesia or ipsilateral self-biting and grooming suggestive of somatosensory disturbances associated with spike activity in caudate nucleus and medial and lateral geniculate nuclei. The responses to bicuculline were blocked or attenuated by systemic haloperidol and potentiated by systemic pretreatment with *L*-dopa or apomorphine, supporting the hypothesis that the behavior and EEG changes induced by bicuculline in SN and VTA may be elicited through DA release. However, excitation of non-DA pathways is not excluded.

Although this is the best animal model of schizophrenia I know, in the 15 years since these experiments were carried out the search for evidence of enhanced release of DA in striatum of schizophrenic patients has been unrewarding. GABAergic agents have not been found useful in treatment. Moreover, the evidence for increased DA binding cited above, while readily produced in experimental animals by neuroleptic treatment, is not

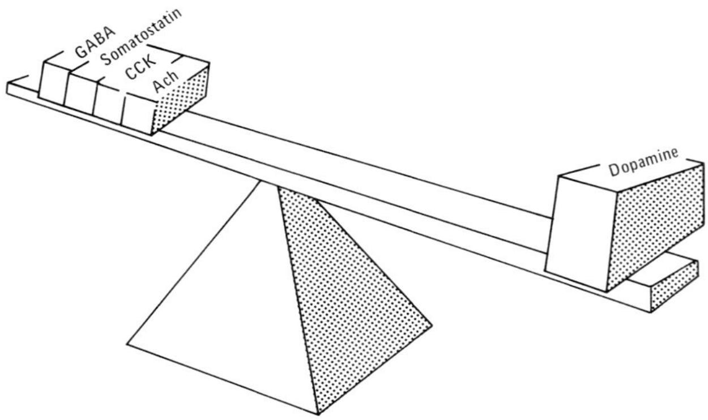

Fig. 3. The physiologic balance that regulates DA activity in the brain can be disturbed by either overactivity of a DA system or underactivity in opposing neurotransmitter systems, such as γ-aminobutyric acid (GABA), somatostatin, cholecystokinin (CCK) and acetylcholine (Ach).

associated with manifestations of psychosis. In the absence of firm evidence of DA hyperactivity, it seems reasonable to propose as an alternative that one or more systems opposing DA activity in critical areas of the brain may be deficient in schizophrenia. This is an obvious analogy to the situation in Parkinson's disease where treatment with acetylcholine-blocking agents was the mainstay of effective treatment prior to the introduction of *L*-dopa, even though the deficiency lies in the DA system and not in overactivity of an acetylcholine system (fig. 3). We have explored this possibility further in neuropathologic studies that are described below.

Anatomic and Neuropathologic Findings: Clinical Correlations

From 1980–1982, I had the opportunity to examine sections of schizophrenic and control brains taken from cortex, basal ganglia, basal forebrain, thalamus, brainstem and cerebellum. These specimens, stained with hematoxylin and eosin, Nissl, Weigert's, Bodian's silver and Holzer's technique for glial fibrils, were obtained from 55 schizophrenic patients age 19–55 years and 46 nonschizophrenic patients aged 10–55 years.

Four general categories of pathologic change were recognized in the schizophrenic brains compared with controls: (1) patchy fibrillary gliosis maximum in periventricular, periaqueductal, and basal forebrain regions

(18 cases); (2) neuronal loss principally affecting large neurons of the globus pallidus (3 cases); (3) massive focal infiltration with corpora amylacea in the forebrains of young individuals (4 cases); (4) Purkinje cell loss in cerebellum (5 cases) [Stevens, 1982].

The distribution of pathology differed from case to case and no unique pathology emerged for any schizophrenia subtype. Although a number of the changes described are common in aging, no relationship between periventricular and forebrain gliosis and age at death could be discerned. In contrast, prominent mineralization of the pallidum, found in a number of schizophrenic brains, was much more common in the older age group.

Noting that routine cell or myelin stains reveal little pathology in schizophrenia, Nieto and Escobar [1972], using the lithium carbonate stain for glial fibrils, described similar pathologic gliosis in the diencephalon of schizophrenic patients. Also using a glial stain, Fisman [1975] reported 'glial knots' resembling those of a viral encephalitis in the brain stem in a group of older schizophrenic patients. However, in a recent photometric study of density of glial staining using an immunocytochemical method, Roberts et al. [1986] were unable to detect any increase in glia in schizophrenic brains. Loss of neurons from globus pallidus or nucleus basalis of substantia innominata was reported by Vogt and Vogt [1952] and was said to be associated especially with catatonic schizophrenia.

More recently, Bogerts et al. [1985] have measured the volumes of a number of limbic regions and subcortical nuclei in serial sections from schizophrenic and control brains in the Vogt collection. They reported a significant decrease in volume of parahippocampal gyrus, amygdala, hippocampus, internal pallidum and periventricular areas of the hypothalamus in schizophrenic brains. In an attempt to extract clinical pathological correlations from the material of Bogerts et al. [1985], I correlated the salient symptoms of each of their cases with the reported morphometric findings. The results of this exercise suggest a correlation between amygdala-hippocampal atrophy and paranoid hallucinatory symptoms (fig. 2) [Stevens, 1986]. Falkai and Bogerts [1986] have recently reported decreased cell counts in the pyramidal layer of Ammons horn in schizophrenic patients. Although hippocampal glia were somewhat decreased in males (n = 2) and increased in females (n = 11) in their material, atrophic hippocampi, in contrast to the case in epilepsy, did not display significant gliosis. Kovelman and Scheibel [1986] reported abnormal orientation of hippocampal pyramidal cells and Jakob and Beckman [1986] described dystrophic changes in entorhinal and ventral insular cortex in a number of brains from schizophrenic patients. Both groups consider these histologic malformations to represent disturbances in normal development during the 4th to 5th month of fetal life. As with gliosis and ventricular dilatation, there is no uniform distribution of cell loss or orientation in all patients with a diagnosis of schizophrenia. Benes et al. [1986] using innovative and imaginative techniques for cell enumeration and density, has recently reported a change in these parameters in prefrontal and cingulate cortices of the several schizophrenic patients she has studied so far.

What Has Happened to These Structures? When Did It Happen? Why the Limbic System?

If we accept the evidence (1) from brain imaging studies demonstrating enlargement of the ventricles of a subgroup of schizophrenics, (2) of gliosis in several brain areas, and (3) of decreased volume and loss of cells in cortex or one or more subcortical nuclei, then we must inquire what has caused this and when it happened? At least three theories can be usefully entertained at this time.

Genetic. For many years the existence of a genetic predisposition to schizophrenia has been well-accepted. This belief was based at first on the simple frequency of family histories of schizophrenia in patients seen in hospitals and clinics. More recently, elegant studies of patients separated from parents at birth have strongly supported the importance of genetic factors [Heston, 1966; Kety et al., 1976]. However, monozygotic twins are concordant for schizophrenia in only around 50% of cases. This implies that in addition to the genetic factors, or in the absence of genetic factors, other, presumably environmental, influences must play a part in a significant number of patients with this disorder.

Infectious or Immunologic Etiology. We have been particularly interested in the possibilitiy of infection as an important cause of schizophrenia for several reasons. First, the gliosis noted in periventricular regions and basal forebrain (structures that impinge directly on the spinal fluid filled spaces of the brain), resemble changes seen following other encephalitides. Second, several reports of increased antibodies in CSF of schizophrenic patients against viruses of the herpes family seemed to point to specific, perhaps active ongoing infection [Albrecht et al., 1980; Torrey et al., 1982]. Finally, a number of ancillary findings, including the waxing and waning course of the illness, reports of abnormal lymphocytes in blood similar to those seen in infectious mononucleosis [Hirata Hibi et al., 1982], and abnormal response of lymphocytes to mitogens [Liedeman et al., 1978] appeared to support an infectious or autoimmune etiology. Unfortunately, none of these studies have withstood attempts at replication [DeLisi and Crow, 1986]. A lower prevalence and better prognosis of schizophrenia has been reported from several less-developed countries [World Health Organization]. This finding, if confirmed, may suggest either a lower incidence of, or greater resistance to, a responsible organism. Seasonal variation of birth of future schizophrenics and seasonal peaks of admission to hospital are consistent with the possibility of an infectious basis for the illness.

Several attempts have been made to test this hypothesis. Inoculation of frozen brain specimens from schizophrenic patients into brains of non-human primates and guinea pigs has not thus far provided evidence for a transmissible agent [Kaufmann et al., 1983]. Tyrrell et al. [1979] reported a cytopathic effect of spinal fluid from some patients with schizophrenia, Huntingtons chorea and multiple sclerosis on embryonic fibroblasts. These workers were unable to demonstrate the presence of a replicating agent. Intracerebral inoculation at multiple sites of cytopathic CSF in marmosets was followed by reduced motor activity in animals receiving CSF from neurologic and schizophrenic patients compared with those injected with control CSF [Baker et al., 1983]. Search for antigens of herpes (HSV), cytomegalovirus (CMV) and a number of other common viruses in fixed and frozen brains of patients who died with their schizophrenic illness has yielded few positive results [Stevens et al., 1984] (table I). In situ hybridization for CMV and HSV have thus far proved negative [Aulakh et al., 1981]. Presently, in collaboration with Dr. Joan Schwartz and William Turner of the NIMH research unit at Saint Elizabeths Hospital, we are culturing schizophrenic brain and CSF on human neuroblastoma cells. As is usual in studies of schizophrenia, we have just enough positive results to keep us working at the project, but not enough to be sure of anything.

Developmental Changes. One of the most striking aspects of the schizophrenic syndrome is the common onset of the disorder in young adults. This fact has led all investigators to consider the relationship between schizophrenia and the onset and maintenance of reproductive

Table I. Results of immunoperoxidase studies with high titer antibodies against seven common viruses

	Age	Sex	Duration	PMI	CMV	HSV_1	HSV_2	VZV	Mumps	Rubella	Rubeola
Schizophrenia											
33B	25	M		21.5	=	–	–	±	+	–	±
32B	23	M	6	16.5	–	–	–	–	–	–	
32K	28	M		3.5	–	–	–	–		–	–
26F	21	F	4–5	14	±	±	+	±	–	–	
A16	28		?	6.7	–	–	–	–	–	–	–
26IJ	31	M	12	20	–	–	–	–	–	–	–
A264	45	F	20	24	–	–	–	–	–	–	–
1M	23	M	2.5	18	–	–	–	–		–	–
282	30	F	1		–	–	–	–		–	
21D	31	M		2.5	–	±	±	–	–	–	–
Controls											
30J	24	M		19.5	–	–	–	–	–	–	–
A108	22	M		18	–	–	–			–	–
A127	23	M		16	–		–			–	–
27A	30	M		23	–	–	–	–	–	–	–
24J	32	M		3	–		–				
3E	17	M		6.5	–		±	–	–	–	–
A247	26	M		6.5	–	–	–	–		–	–
A252	22	M		18	–		–	–	–	–	–
28F	25	M		22	–	–	–	–	–	–	–
A52	19	M		21				–	–		
A177	19	F		5.5	–	–	–	–	–		
1176	31	M		16.5	–	–	–	–	±	–	–
A179	18	M		12	–						

Duration = Duration of schizophrenia (years); PMI = postmortem interval (hours); CMV = Cytomegalovirus IgG 1:1,500; HSV = herpes simplex virus 1 (1:400) and 2 (1:600); VZV = varicella zoster virus 1:320; mumps IgG 1:3,000; rubella 1:500; rubeola 1:200; + = positive immunoreactivity in scattered neurons of amygdala and hypothalamus on repeated trials; ± = equivocal immunoreactivity, not replicable on repeated trials

Studies made on frozen sections of hippocampus, hypothalamus, amygdala, globus pallidus of 10 young schizophrenic patients, all of whom died by suicide, and 13 controls, most of whom were victims of homicide. All specimens courtesy of the Medical Examiner's office, Washington, D.C., and Dr. Joel Kleinman and Ingrid Phillips, St. Elizabeth's Hospital, Washington, D.C.

activity. In addition to the endocrinologic changes and psychological stresses that accompany young adulthood, there are a number of physiologic changes in the brain itself that accompany the onset and maintenance of reproductive life. The most prominent of these occur in the limbic system and hypothalamus. In the female, at least in the rat, there are marked changes in firing rates of neurons in amygdala, bed nucleus of stria terminalis and hypothalamus in relation to the estrus cycle. In the human female, distinct changes of convulsive threshold to photic stimulation occur over the monthly cycle. Humans, as well as other mammals, display paroxysmal microseizure-like discharges from electrodes implanted in amygdala or basal forebrain during orgasm [Heath, 1972].

The sexualization of the brain that takes place during and following puberty is associated with binding of the specific sex hormones and of cortisone to neurons in hippocampus, amygdala and other cerebral areas. If these structures are malformed in some schizophrenic patients as described above, their response to this hormone tide could also be highly abnormal.

There are other mechanisms for neuronal loss in hippocampi and related structures. The marked increase in firing rate of neurons of these regions during estrus and ovulation in rat resemble sharply localized microseizures. It has long been known to epileptologists and experimental neurophysiologists that hippocampus and amygdala have the lowest threshold for seizure discharge in the brain. This must serve some important functional purpose for Nature to have taken the risk of epilepsy in the natural selection of individual traits for survival. These focal microseizures and spikes in limbic nuclei and the low threshold for limbic seizure discharge represent a powerful information transmission system that must be protected by steep voltage gradients to prevent propagation to other areas of the brain of physiologic paroxysmal actively associated with sexual behavior, ovulation and perhaps gonadotropin release [Stevens, 1977].

As recently shown by Meldrum [1986] and others, sustained rapid neuronal discharge associated with focal seizures can cause self-destruction of rapidly discharging neurons and their targets due to excessive release of excitatory amino acids. It is thus reasonable to conjecture that loss of neurons in hippocampus and amygdala of some schizophrenics could follow prolonged excessive paroxysmal discharge in specific subcortical circuits, especially those limbic and hypothalamic circuits mediating reproductive activities. Reports by Heath [1954] and others of spikes with synchronous excessive discharge in these very regions in schizophrenic patients are consistent with other evidence of structural damage or functional disturb-

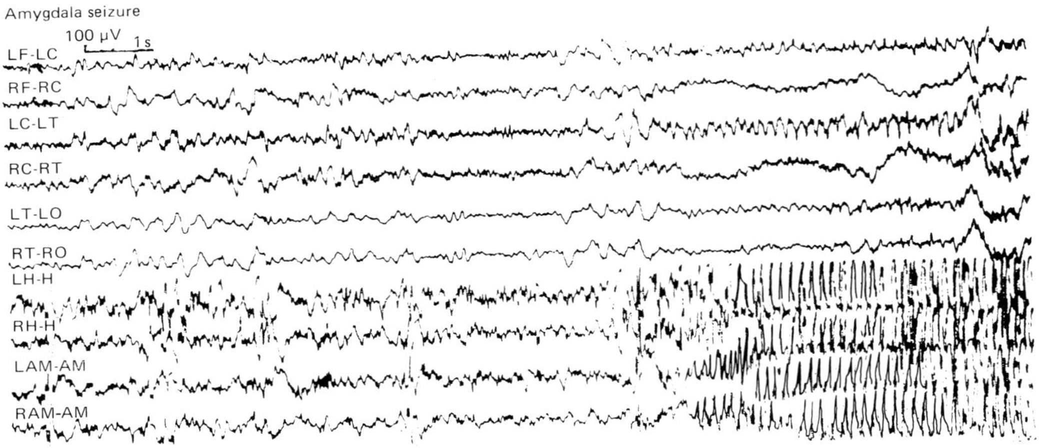

Fig. 4. 'Spontaneous' seizure in cat with epileptic focus produced by placing 100 μl aluminium hydroxide in amygdala several weeks earlier. EEG from chronic implanted electrodes records a high-voltage amygdala spike discharge that does not spread to dural electrodes only 1 cm distant; animal showed only hypervigilance and staring. Several minutes later, the 'inhibitory surround' failed; discharge spread to dural leads as focal limbic seizure spread to cortex and a generalized tonic clonic seizure ensued. L = Left; R = right; F = frontal; C = central; T = temporal; H = hippocampus; AM = amygdala; O = occipital.

ance in specific brain areas in schizophrenia. Because of the steep voltage gradients that protect the spread of subcortical microseizures, they are unlikely to be detected by any surface analytic technique (fig. 4). Studies showing increased local DA release following experimental amygdala-generated seizures in rats suggest that DA participates in maintaining this inhibitory wall [Csernansky et al., 1985].

Unfortunately, no subcortical electrophysiologic studies are now being done in man to replicate or refute the early pioneering work of Heath and others. Our hands have been tied by the antipsychosurgery lobby for more than two decades so that little progress has been made on this front. From many investigations of temporal lobe epilepsy, however, it is clearly evident that very small foci of spike discharges in amygdala or hippocampus, when associated with similar changes in specific sensory cortex and cingulate gyrus, can be associated with (1) auditory, visual and somatosensory hallucinations, (2) delusions, and (3) spontaneous mood and behavior changes in the absence of any other manifestations of epilepsy [Wieser, 1983]. The specific sensory nature of the delusion or hallucinatory experience appears to be determined by which primary or secondary sensory areas are activated by the seizure discharge at the same time that activation occurs in the amygdala, hippocampus, cingulum and perhaps certain subcortical areas.

In addition to the possibility of hippocampal or amygdalar cell loss occurring in response to hyperexcitability and excessive firing of specific units in these structures during the period of onset and maintenance of reproductive function, it is possible that sustained stress with associated hypercortisolemia could have a role in inducing focal cell death. Thus, Sapolsky et al. [1985] have shown that prolonged systemic glucocorticoid infusion in the rat reduces the number of hippocampal pyramidal cells, especially in the CA3 field, an area implicated in cell loss by Bogerts et al. [1985] and Falkai and Bogerts [1986].

The evidence noted above describes multiple sites of modest pathologic change (focal cell loss, focal gliosis, focal atrophy) in many schizophrenic brains, with particular involvement of sensory convergence areas such as parahippocampal gyrus, dorsal and ventral pallidum, amygdala, and hippocampus. It is not, therefore, surprising that the clinical syndrome is marked by misperceptions of signal significance, derailment of thinking and by hallucinations which may resemble those of temporal lobe epilepsy. Whatever the cause or causes of the schizophrenic syndrome, it appears at present that, as in other neurologic disorders, the symptoms and signs do relate, at least in part, to morphologic and functional pathology in specific brain areas. This encourages us to believe that clinical-pathological correlations between symptoms and pathology may eventually be possible.

References

Abenson, M.H.: EEGs in chronic schizophrenia. Br. J. Psychiat. *11:* 421–425 (1970).

Albrecht, P.; Torrey, E.F.; Boone, E.; Hicks, J.T.; Daniel, N.: Raised cytomegalovirus antibody level in cerebrospinal fluid in schizophrenic patients. Lancet *ii:* 769–772 (1980).

Aulakh, G.S.; Kleinman, J.E.; Aulakh, H.S.; Albrecht, P.; Torrey, E.F.; Wyatt, R.J.: Search for cytomegalovirus in schizophrenic brain tissue. Proc. Soc. exp. Biol. Med. *167:* 172–174 (1981).

Baker, H.F.; Ridley, R.M.; Crow, T.J.; Bloxham, C.A.; Parry, R.P.; Tyrrell, D.A.J.: An investigation of the effects of intracerebral injection in the marmoset of cytopathic cerebrospinal fluid from patients with schizophrenia or neurological disease. Psychol. Med. *13:* 499–511 (1983).

Benes, F.M.; Davidson, J.; Bird, E.D.: Quantitative cytoarchitectural studies of the cerebral cortex of schizophrenics. Archs gen. Psychiat. *43:* 31–35 (1986).

Bleckwenn, W.J.: Production of sleep and rest in psychotic cases. Archs Neurol. Psychiat. *24:* 365 (1930).

Bogerts, B.; Meertz, E.; Schonfeldt-Bausch, R.: Basal ganglia and limbic system pathology in schizophrenia: a morphometric study of brain volume and shrinkage. Archs gen. Psychiat. *42:* 784–796 (1985).

Carlsson, A.; Lindquist, M.: Effect of chloropromazine or haloperidol on the formation of 3-methoxytyramine and normetanephrine in mouse brain. Acta pharmac. tox. *20:* 140–144 (1963).

Creese, I.; Burt, D.R.; Snyder, S.H.: Dopamine receptor binding predicts clinical and pharmacological potencies of anti-schizophrenic drugs. Science *192:* 481–483 (1976).

Crow, T.J.: Positive and negative schizophrenia and the role of dopamine. Br. J. Psychiat *139:* 251–254 (1981).

Csernansky, J.G.; Csernansky, C.A.; Bonnet, K.A.; Hollister, L.E.: Dopaminergic supersensitivity follows ferric chloride-induced limbic seizures. Biol. Psychiat. *20:* 723–733 (1985).

Davison, K.; Bagley, C.R.: Schizophrenia-like psychoses associated with organic disorders. Br. J. Psychiat. suppl., pp. 140–183 (1969).

De Jong, H.H.: Experimental catatonia (Williams & Wilkins, Baltimore 1945).

DeLisi, L.E.; Crow, T.J.: Is schizophrenia a viral or immunologic disorder? Psychiat. Clin. N. Am. *9:* 115–132 (1986).

Duffy, F.H.: The BEAM method for neurophysiological diagnosis; in Nottebohm, Hope for a New Neurology. Ann. N.Y. Acad. Sci. *457:* 19–34 (1985).

Falkai, P.; Bogerts, B.: Cell loss in the hippocampus of schizophrenics. Eur. Arch. Psychiat. Neurol. Sci. *236:* 154–161 (1986).

Fisman, M.: The brain stem in psychosis. Br. J. Psychiat. *126:* 414–422 (1975).

Gloor, P.; Olivier, A.; Quesney, L.F.; Andermann, F.; Horowitz, S.: The role of the limbic system in experiential phenomena of temporal lobe epilepsy. Ann. Neurol. *12:* 129–144 (1982).

Halgren, E.: Mental phenomena induced by stimulation in the limbic system. Hum. Neurobiol. *1:* 251–260 (1982).

Hanley, J.; Rickles, W.R.; Crandall, P.H.; Walter, R.D.: Spectral characteristics of EEG activity accompanying deep spiking in a patient with schizophrenia. Electroenceph. clin. Neurophysiol. *28:* 90 (1979).

Heath, R.G.: Studies in schizophrenia (Harvard University Press, Cambridge 1954).

Heath, R.G.: Pleasure and brain activity in man: deep and surface electroencephalograms during orgasm. J. nerv. ment. Dis. *154:* 3–18 (1972).

Heston, L.L.: Psychiatric disorders in foster home reared children of schizophrenic mothers. Br. J. Psychiat. *112:* 819–825 (1966).

Hill, D.: The encephalogram in schizophrenia; in Richter, Schizophrenia: somatic aspects (Butterworth, London 1957).

Hirata Hibi, M.; Higashi, S.; Tachibana, T.; Natanabe, N.: Stimulated lymphocytes in schizophrenia. Archs gen. Psychiat. *39:* 82–87 (1982).

Ingvar, D.H.; Franzen, G.: Abnormalities of cerebral blood flow distribution in patients with chronic schizophrenia. Acta psychiat. scand. *50:* 425–462 (1974).

Itil, T.M.: Quantitative pharmaco-electroencephalography; in Itil, Psychotrophic drugs and the human EEG. Mod. Probl. Pharmaco-psychiat., vol. 8, pp. 43–75 (Karger, Basel 1974).

Jacobi, W.; Winkler, H.: Encephalographische Studien an Schizophrenen. Arch. Psychiat. NervKrankh. *84:* 208–226 (1977).
Jakob, H.; Beckmann, H.: Prenatal development disturbances in the limbic allocortex in schizophrenics. J. neural Transm. *65:* 303–326 (1986).
Jelliffe, S.E.: The mental pictures in schizophrenia and in epidemic encephalitis. Am. J. Psychiat. *6:* 413–465 (1927).
Johnstone, E.C.; Crow, T.J.; Frith, C.D.; Husband, J.; Kreel, L.: Cerebral ventricular size and cognitive impairment in chronic schizophrenia. Lancet *ii:* 924–926 (1976).
Kaufmann, C.A.; Stevens, J.; Torrey, E.F.: World Health Symposium on Psychovirology. Archs gen. Psychiat. *41:* 1184–1185 (1983).
Kety, S.S.; Rosenthal, D.; Wender, P.H.; et al.: Mental illness in the biological and adoptive families of adopted individuals who have become schizophrenic. Behav. Genet. *6:* 219–225 (1976).
Kishimoto, H.; Kuwahara, H.; Takazu, O.; Ohno, S.; Hama, Y.; Sato, C.; Ishii, T.; Nomura, Y.; Fujita, H.; Miyauchi, T.; Yokoi, S.; Iio, M.: The three subtypes of chronic schizophrenia using ^{11}C-glucose positron emission tomography (PET). Psychiat. Res. *21:* 285–292 (1987).
Kovelman, J.A.; Scheibel, A.B.: A neurohistological correlate of schizophrenia. Biol. Psychiat. *19:* 1601–1621 (1986).
Kraepelin, E.L.: Der Psychiater; 7th German ed.; vol. 88 (transl. Diefendorf Ar) (Macmillan, London 1907).
Liedeman, R.R.; Prilipko, L.L.: The behavior of T lymphocytes in schizophrenia; in Bergsma, Goldstein, Neurochemical and immunologic components in schizophrenia. Birth defects, Orig. Article Ser., No. 14, pp. 365–377 (1978).
MacKay, A.V.P.; Bird, E.D.; Spokes, E.G.; Rossor, M.; Iversen, L.L.; Creese, I.; Synder, S.H.: Dopamine receptors and schizophrenia: drug effect or illness? Lancet *ii:* 915–916 (1980).
Meldrum, B.S.: Cell damage in epilepsy and the role of calcium in cytotoxicity. Adv. Neurol. *44:* 849–855 (1986).
Mettler, F.A.; Crandell, A.: Relation between parkinsonism and psychiatric disorder. J. nerv. ment. Dis. *129:* 551 (1959).
Morihisa, J.M.; Duffy, F.H.; Wyatt, R.J.: Brain electrical activity mapping (BEAM) in schizophrenic patients. Archs gen. Psychiat. *40:* 719–728 (1983).
Morstyn, R.; Duffy, F.H.; McCarley, R.W.: Altered topography of EEG spectral content in schizophrenia. Electroenceph. clin. Neurophysiol. *38:* 262–271 (1983).
Nielsen, J.M.: The basic pathology of schizophrenia. J. nerv. ment. Dis. *107:* 340–357 (1948).
Nieto, D.; Escobar, A.: Major psychoses; in Minckler, Pathology of the nervous system, vol. III, pp. 2654–2665 (McGraw-Hill, New York 1972).
Owen, F.; Crow, T.J.; Poulter, M.; Cross, A.J.; Longden, A.; Riley, G.J.: Increased dopamine-receptor sensitivity in schizophrenia. Lancet *ii:* 223–225 (1978).
Owens, D.G.; Johnstone, E.C.; Frith, C.D.: Spontaneous involuntary disorders of movement: their prevalence, severity, and distribution in chronic schizophrenics with and without treatment with neuroleptics. Archs gen. Psychiat. *39:* 452–461 (1982).
Randrup, A.; Munkvad, I.: Special antagonism of amphetamine-induced abnormal behavior: inhibition of stereotyped activity with increase of some normal activities. Psychopharmacologia *7:* 416–422 (1965).

Raskin, D.E.; Frank, S.W.: Herpes encephalites with catatonic stupor. Archs gen. Psychiat. *31:* 544–546 (1974).
Reveley, A.M.; Reveley, M.A.; Murray, R.M.: Cerebral ventricular enlargement in nongenetic schizophrenia: a controlled twin study. Br. J. Psychiat. *144:* 89–93 (1984).
Roberts, G.W.; Colter, N.; Lofthouse, R.; Bogerts, B.; Zech, M.; Crow, T.J.: Gliosis in schizophrenia: a survey. Biol. Psychiat. *21:* 1043–1050 (1986).
Sapolsky, R.M.; Krey, L.C.; McEwen, B.S.: Prolonged glucocorticoid exposure reduces hippocampal neuron number: implications for aging. J. Neurosci. *5:* 1222–1227 (1985).
Sedvall, G.; Farde, L.; Persson, A.; Wiesel, F.-A.: Imaging of neurotransmitter receptors in the living human brain. Archs gen. Psychiat. *43:* 995–1005 (1986).
Seeman, P.; Lee, T.; Chau-Wong, M.; Wong, K.: Antipsychotic drug doses and neuroleptic/dopamine receptors. Nature *261:* 17–19 (1976).
Sem-Jacobsen, C.W.: Intra-cerebral electrographic studies in schizophrenic patients. Report 2nd Int. Psychiatric Congr., Zürich 1957, pp. 247–248.
Shagass, C.; Roemer, R.A.; Straumanis, J.J.; Josiassen, R.C.: Psychiatric diagnostic discriminations with combinations of quantitative EEG variables. Br. J. Psychiat. *144:* 581–592 (1984).
Sheppard, G.; Manchanda, R.; Gruzelier, J.; Hirsch, S.R.: ^{15}O positron emission tomographic scanning in predominantly never-treated acute schizophrenic patients. Lancet *ii:* 1448–1452 (1983).
Stevens, J.R.: An anatomy of schizophrenia? Archs gen. Psychiat. *29:* 177–189 (1973).
Stevens, J.R.: The EEG spike: signal of information transmission? Ann. Neurol. *1:* 309–314 (1977).
Stevens, J.R.: Disturbances of ocular movements and blinking in schizophrenia. J. Neurol. Neurosurg. Psychiat. *41:* 1024–1030 (1978).
Stevens, J.R.: Neuropathology of schizophrenia. Archs. gen. Psychiat. *39:* 1131–1139 (1982).
Stevens, J.: Clinicopathologic correlations in schizophrenia (ltr. to editor). Archs gen. Psychiat. *43:* 715–716 (1986).
Stevens, J.R.; Bigelow, L.; Denney, D.; Lipkin, J.; Livermore, A.H., Jr.; Rauscher, F.; Wyatt, R.J.: Telemetered EEG–EOG during psychotic behaviors of schizophrenia. Archs gen. Psychiat. *36:* 251–262 (1979).
Stevens, J.R.; Langloss, J.M.; Albrecht, P.; Yolken, R.; Wang, Y.-N.: A search for cytomegalovirus and herpes viral antigen in brains of schizophrenic brains. Archs gen. Psychiat. *41:* 795–801 (1984).
Stevens, J.R.; Livermore, A., Jr.: Telemetered EEG in schizophrenia: spectral analysis during abnormal behavior episodes. J. Neurol. Neurosurg. Psychiat. *45:* 385–395 (1982).
Stevens, J.R.; Mark, V.H.; Ervin, F.; Pacheco, P.; Suematsu, K.: Deep temporal stimulation in man. Archs Neurol. *21:* 157–169 (1969).
Stevens, J.R.; Wilson, K.; Foote, W.: GABA blockade, dopamine and schizophrenia: experimental studies in the cat. Psychopharmacologia *39:* 105–119 (1974).
Tanaka, Y.; Hazama, H.; Kawahara, R.; Kobalyashi, K.: Computerized tomography of the brain in schizophrenic patients. Acta psychiat. scand. *63:* 191–197 (1981).
Torrey, E.F.: Schizophrenia and civilization (Aronson, New York 1980).
Torrey, E.F.; Yolken, R.H.; Winfrey, C.J.: Cytomegalovirus antibody in cerebrospinal fluid of schizophrenic patients detected by enzyme immunoassays. Science *216:* 892–894 (1982).

Tyrrell, D.A.J.; Parry, R.P.; Crow, T.J.; Johnstone, E.C.; Ferrier, I.N.: Possible virus in schizophrenia and some neurological disorders. Lancet *i:* 839–841 (1979).

Vogt, C.; Vogt, O.: Alterations anatomiques de la schizophrenie et d'autres psychoses dites fonctionelles; in Rosenberg, Sellier, 1st Int. Congr. Neuropathology, vol. I, 516–532 (1952).

Weinberger, D.R.; Berman, K.F.; Zec, R.F.: Physiological dysfunction of dorsolateral prefrontal cortex in schizophrenia. I. Regional cerebral blood flow (rCBF) evidence. Archs gen. Psychiat. *43:* 114–125 (1986).

Weinberger, D.R.; Torrey, E.F.; Neophytides, A.N.; Wyatt, R.J.: Lateral cerebral ventricular enlargement in chronic schizophrenia. Archs gen. Psychiat. *36:* 735–739 (1979).

Wieser, H.G.: Depth recorded limbic seizures and psychopathology. Neurosci. behav. Rev. *7:* 427–440 (1983).

Woods, B.T.; Wolf, J.: A reconsideration of the relation of ventricular enlargement to duration of illness in schizophrenia. Am. J. Psychiat. *140:* 1564–1570 (1983).

World Health Organization: Schizophrenia: an international follow-up study (Wiley & Sons, Chichester 1979).

Yarden, P.E.; Discipio, W.J.: Abnormal movements and prognosis in schizophrenia. Am. J. Psychiat. *128:* 317–323 (1971).

Janice R. Stevens, MD, National Institute of Mental Health, Saint Elizabeth's Hospital, William A. White Building, Washington, DC 20032 (USA)

Mueller (ed.): Neurology and Psychiatry: A Meeting of Minds,
pp. 88–104 (Karger, Basel 1989)

The Quest for an Ideal Image of the Brain

Charles D. Yingling

Langley Porter Psychiatric Institute and Department of Neurological Surgery,
University of California, San Francisco, Calif., USA

Early attempts to image the brain directly in intact humans did not provide pictures of the brain itself, but instead provided images of associated tissues. For example, skull X-rays image bone; pneumoencephalography, the ventricular system (CSF); angiography, the vascular system (blood). Only with the advent of X-ray computed tomography (CT) in the early 1970s did a direct image of brain parenchyma become possible. Now, in the late 1980s, the variety of imaging methods is growing rapidly. This wealth of alternative approaches forces both clinicians and researchers to decide which method(s) are most appropriate for addressing a given clinical question.

In addition to providing an image of the brain itself rather than of other tissues (table I), an ideal system for imaging the brain would have several important characteristics. Obviously, spatial resolution and contrast sensitivity should be as high as possible in order to provide detailed *anatomical* information. However, *functional* information is also desirable, as many pathological conditions may alter brain function without producing grossly evident anatomical lesions. When functional information is desired, it also becomes important that the *temporal* resolution be high, so that changes in metabolic parameters can be associated with different behavioral states. Finally, the ideal method would be noninvasive, safe for use in children and normal controls as well as patients, inexpensive, and easy to use.

The quality with which anatomical structures are delineated is primarily a function of spatial resolution and contrast sensitivity. High spatial resolution permits visualization of small structures and provides anatomic detail. Contrast sensitivity, on the other hand, permits discrimination among regions of tissue that possess subtly different biophysical properties

Table I. Characteristics of an ideal imaging system for brain

1	Images brain directly, rather than associated tissues
2	Functional as well as anatomical information
3	High spatial resolution and contrast sensitivity
4	High temporal resolution for functional imaging
5	Noninvasive, safe for use in control subjects or children
6	Inexpensive and easy to use

(such as the percentage of water content), even though the anatomy per se may not be grossly different.

These ideal characteristics are desirable in any imaging technique, and apply equally well to pathological and normative studies. However, in the context of functional imaging, high temporal resolution becomes an important factor to consider. Behavior, after all, takes place rather rapidly. Even a simple reaction time task involves sensation, perception, cognitive decision processes, response selection and motor output – all of which happen within a few hundred milliseconds. An ideal method would be able to image information flow through the brain and depict the sequential activation of different anatomical structures on the same time scale as the behavior of interest. Methods which require even a few minutes to obtain a single image fail to capture dynamic patterns of activity which may be crucial in the understanding of functional disturbances.

The criteria of noninvasiveness and safety are, of course, particularly important for studies in populations such as children with dyslexia or other learning disabilities, where there is no reason to suspect gross pathology. Moreover, with new techniques it is especially important to obtain normative data from control populations. The more invasive a technique is, the more difficult it is to obtain an appropriate normative data base. Finally, an ideal imaging method should be inexpensive and easy to use so that it can be clinically practical rather than remaining an expensive research tool.

When the presently available methods are evaluated against these criteria, it becomes apparent that no one method can yet be termed ideal. Rather, each has its own strengths and weaknesses; the choice of an imaging modality for a particular instance must depend on exactly what information is needed. The remainder of this chapter will review the major imaging modalities in terms of the above-listed criteria.

To begin with a brief historical review, figure 1 illustrates the techniques which were available until the development of X-ray CT in the early 1970s. The plain skull film (fig. 1a), although it represents a considerable

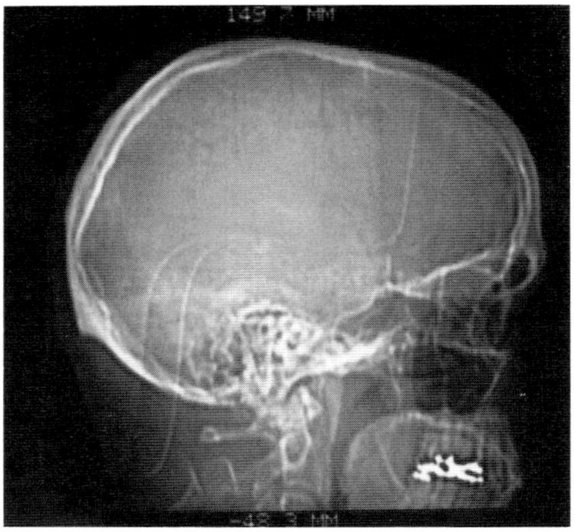

a

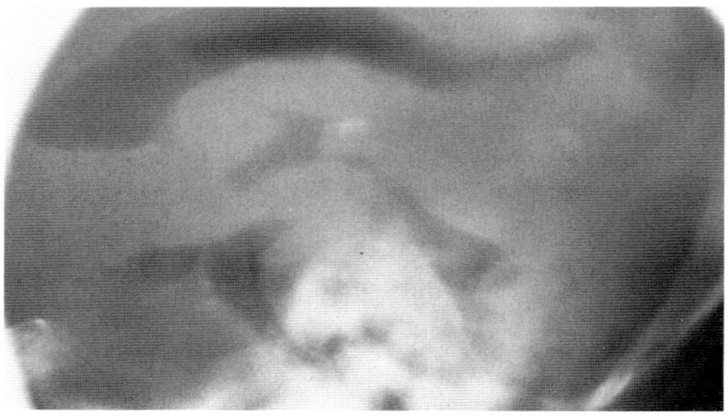
b

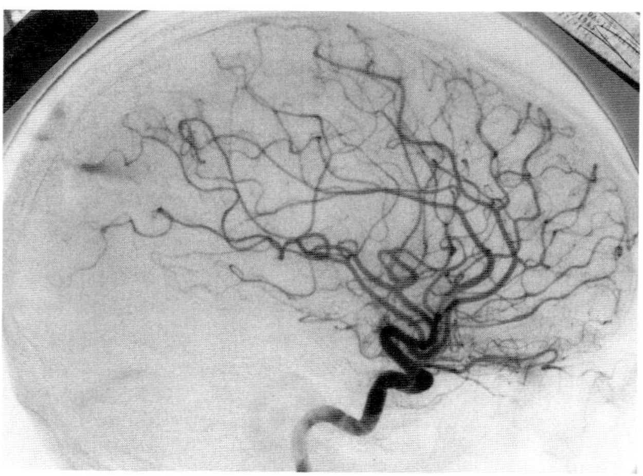
c

technical advance over the first X-rays, still essentially produces an image of the distribution of calcium in the skull, not the brain itself. Figure 1b shows a pneumoencephalogram, made by first injecting air into the ventricular system through a lumbar puncture and then allowing it to percolate up to the ventricles themselves. This is a highly invasive and painful procedure which, fortunately, has been rendered obsolete by the advent of the CT scan. Again, the pneumoencephalogram does not produce an image of the brain itself, but rather demonstrates where the CSF used to be in the ventricular system. Figure 1c is an angiogram obtained by injecting dye into the carotid artery and taking X-rays at fixed time intervals. This technique is still widely used in diagnosis of cerebral vascular disorders. It provides us with an image of the distribution of blood, but still not an image of the brain itself. Thus, as of the early 1970s, the best imaging techniques available provided only indirect pictures of the brain via its associated tissues. (For a highly readable account of the history of brain imaging techniques, see Oldendorf [1980].)

The major technical development which for the first time allowed a direct image of the living human brain arrived in the early 1970s. While associated with the development of X-ray CT, for which Cormack and Hounsfield were awarded the Nobel prize in 1979, CT is actually based on a more general analytical procedure known as projection reconstruction imaging. This technique also forms the basis for magnetic resonance imaging (MRI), positron emission tomography (PET), single photon emission computed tomography (SPECT), and undoubtedly other methods yet to be developed. It involves computer reconstruction of a 2-dimensional view of a slice of tissue, starting with a set of 1-dimensional projections taken at all possible angles. In the case of X-ray CT, the initial signals are density profiles derived from the relative attenuation of an X-ray beam directed through the brain from a series of points as the radiation source is rotated around the subject. The computer is then used to

---

Fig. 1. *a* Lateral skull X-ray of author's head. Note total absence of any evidence that a brain is contained therein. *b* Pneumoencephalogram obtained by substituting air for CSF in the ventricular system. The outline of the ventricular system can be clearly seen, but the presence of any abnormalities can only be inferred from ventricular displacement; the brain itself is not directly visualized. *c* Carotid angiogram showing distribution of blood flow in the middle cerebral artery. Again, the brain itself cannot be seen, and any abnormalities can only be inferred from displacement of the arteries, rather than being directly imaged. Figures 1b and c courtesy of Dr. David Norman, Department of Radiology, UCSF.

reconstruct the corresponding 2-dimensional density profile [Morgan, 1983]. The X-ray CT and most other tomographic techniques (MRI, PET, etc.) share the essential principles of this reconstruction, but differ in the origin of the initial signals.

X-ray CT is currently the most commonly used imaging modality, available at virtually every medical center. The images obtained are of medium spatial resolution but limited contrast resolution, although this can be improved by the use of contrast-enhancing agents. The spatial resolution is inherently limited, due to diffusion of the beam by the much greater density of bone relative to brain parenchyma. Artifact due to scattering by bony tissue is particularly a problem in imaging the regions of the posterior fossa and inferior surfaces of the frontal and temporal lobes. Due to the physical origin of the signals, images are limited to axial (horizontal) planes. Although coronal or sagittal reconstructions can be computed, their spatial resolution is quite low. Exposure to ionizing radiation is also involved.

Although CT is widely available, and despite the fact that substantial experience has been gathered over the last decade, the limitations described above are causing X-ray CT to be slowly supplanted by MRI. This technique produces images of equal or superior spatial resolution and provides greatly improved contrast sensitivity. Other advantages of MRI include: the absence of ionizing radiation (which makes the method more suitable for children, controls, and repeated studies), and the fact that coronal or sagittal planes can be obtained as easily as, and with equivalent resolution to, axial sections. Although the MRI technique is a relatively recent development, and therefore not yet as widely available as X-ray CT, its inherent advantages will undoubtedly lead to much greater utilization over the next few years.

While the principle of projection reconstruction imaging in MRI is essentially the same as that of X-ray CT, the origin of the signals is quite different. Magnetic resonance refers to the fact that any atomic nucleus with an odd number of protons has magnetic properties, i. e. that the nucleus of the atom acts as a small magnet. Normally these magnets are oriented randomly. If, however, they are placed into a strong externally applied magnetic field, they will line up parallel to the orientation of the external field. The field is then briefly perturbed with a radio-frequency pulse at the resonant frequency which is appropriate for the element to be imaged and is known as the Larmor frequency. This tilts the field and the nuclei very slightly. Following the external pulse the nuclei return ('relax')

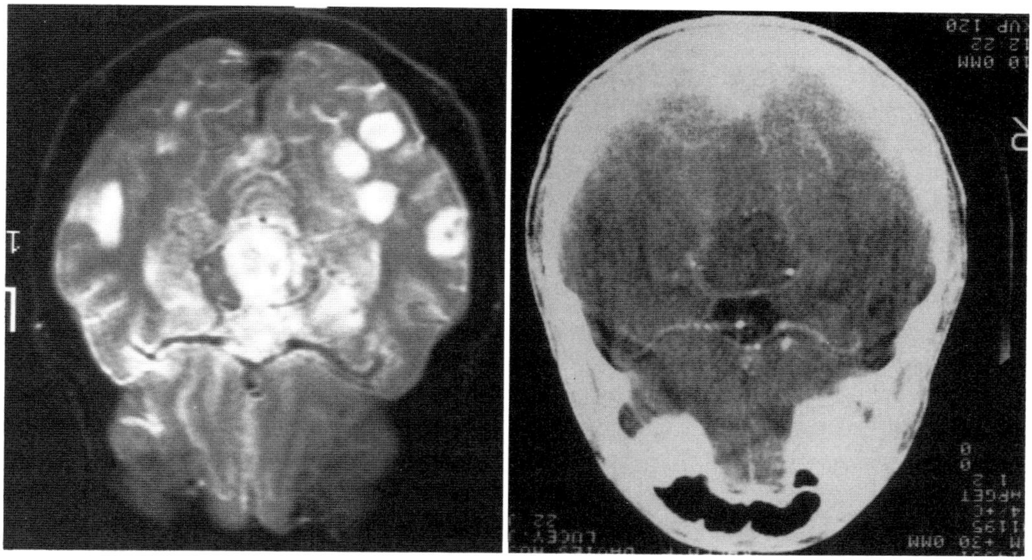

a b

Fig. 2. *a* X-ray CT of patient with toxoplasmosis; although brain parenchyma is now directly imaged, the scan is normal, revealing no visible pathology. *b* MRI of same patient as *a*; note multiple infectious foci in temporal and parietal lobes and brainstem; the pathology is much more clearly visualized than in the X-ray CT, due to the sensitivity of MRI to slight differences in water content between normal and diseased tissue. Courtesy of Dr. Michael Brant-Zawadski, Department of Radiology, UCSF.

back to the original orientation with the external field. As they do so, they emit a radio wave at the Larmor resonant frequency, hence the term 'magnetic resonance'. These radio waves are detected and used to create an image in much the same way as is done for X-ray CT image construction [Morgan and Hendee, 1984].

Current MRI systems usually image hydrogen, which is the most common element of the body. Essentially, MRI images the distribution of water in brain tissue. Since the concentration of water is altered differently in white matter, gray matter and CSF by many pathological processes, this may be exploited to obtain excellent delineation of internal structures.

Figure 2a shows an X-ray CT scan of the brain of a patient with toxoplasmosis. While certain structural aspects of the brain can be seen, even in this relatively poor quality scan, the picture is essentially normal, betraying no hint of pathology. In figure 2b, the same brain is seen imaged with MRI; multiple foci of infection can now be clearly seen in the temporal

a 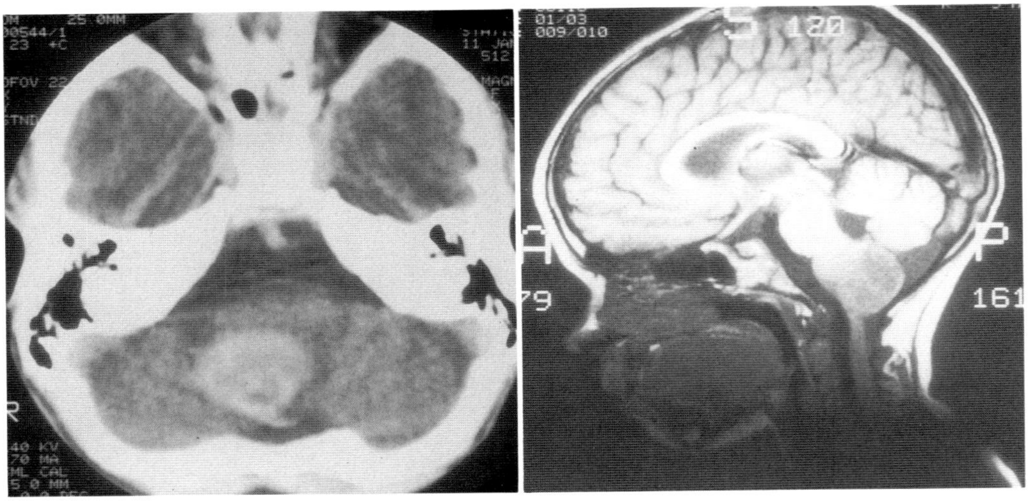 *b*

Fig. 3. a X-ray CT of patient with medulloblastoma in the posterior fossa. Note presence of artifact due to X-ray scattering from dense bone in this region. *b* Midsaggital MRI of same patient as *a*; in this plane, the tumor can be seen clearly on the posterior aspect of the medulla, below the cerebellum. Courtesy of Dr. Michael Brant-Zawadski, Department of Radiology, UCSF.

and parietal lobes and brainstem. The dramatic enhancement of the contrast between normal and diseased tissue is due to the ability of MRI to demonstrate differing concentrations of water in the normal and diseased tissue. The greater contrast sensitivity of MRI and its ability to detect a variety of disease processes, including most brain tumors, have made MRI the initial screening imaging technique of choice at UCSF for patients with suspected brain disorders.

Figure 3a shows another example of a tumor visualized with X-ray CT, this time in the posterior fossa. While the tumor can be seen quite easily with contrast enhancement, the significant amount of artifact (the streaky lines) in the image is due to scattering of the X-ray beam by the surrounding bone. In addition, the relationship of the tumor to the surrounding structures is not clear from this view, although more information could be obtained by examination of serial sections. Figure 3b shows the same case, now seen in midsagittal section with MRI. Since MRI does not image bone, the problem of artifact does not exist. Combined with the sagittal view, it is now possible to see clearly the tumor on the posterior aspect of the medulla. One of the great advantages of MRI over X-ray CT is that images can be obtained easily in any desired plane. In cases such as this, this feature considerably enhances the delineation of the tumor's exact anatomical location. This figure also demonstrates beautifully the exquisite anatomical detail available with MRI. One can see clearly the distinction between cortical gray matter and the underlying white matter, the folia of the cerebellum, the corpus callosum, and the various levels of the brainstem eventually leading into the spinal cord.

A potential future application of MRI is the possibility of obtaining functional, as well as anatomical, information. While current systems primarily image the distribution of hydrogen (mostly in water), any element with an odd atomic number, such as ^{31}P, can be used in principle. The advantage of ^{31}P is that its exact resonant frequency changes when the atom is in different chemical environments. Phosphorus is a very important element in energy metabolism. Adenosine triphosphate (ATP), adenosine 5′-diphosphate, cyclic 3′:5′-adenosine monophosphate, creatine phosphate and inorganic phosphate all produce different signals. This fact can be used to monitor the metabolic state of brain tissue. For example, it becomes possible to examine the ratio of ATP to other phosphates. Although research thus far has been limited to NMR spectroscopy of relatively large brain regions, it should be possible to use ^{31}P MRI to obtain images of regional brain metabolism. This promises to be an exciting area to watch for further developments.

Finally, a major advantage of MRI compared to X-ray CT is that it is noninvasive; there are no known ill effects of exposure to magnetic fields and therefore MRI can be used in imaging studies of children and control subjects without concern over radiation exposure. At this point, MRI is about 20% more but expensive than X-ray CT. However, since it is a growing technology that is becoming more widely available, the cost may well go down in the future. Improved spatial resolution and the ability to obtain multiple planes of section already make MRI clearly superior to X-ray CT for most anatomical imaging studies.

The first successful technique for functional imaging was the measurement of regional cerebral blood flow (rCBF). Since blood flow is related to local metabolic rate, rCBF measurements can be used to image cerebral metabolism during different behavioral states. As originally introduced by Lassen and Ingvar [1961], rCBF measurement involved intracarotid injection of (radioactive) ^{85}Kr, a procedure which certainly does not meet the ideal criterion for noninvasiveness! The method did, however produce striking images of differential patterns of rCBF during different behaviors.

The gamma rays were detected with an array of detectors placed over the scalp and the flow was calculated from the kinetics of the washout of radioactivity. Subsequent development of the technique utilized ^{133}Xe, and a more extensive array of detectors [Harper et al., 1964; Ingvar et al., 1965; Lassen et al., 1978]. Figure 4a illustrates the distribution of blood flow in the left hemisphere during reading aloud. It shows clear activation of the occipital visual association areas, Wernicke's aera, Broca's area, motor areas controlling the speech musculature, and the supplementary motor area. Spontaneous speech (fig. 4b) produces a similar pattern, but without the activation of the occipital area.

A number of alternate methods for imaging rCBF have been developed. These include inhalation of ^{133}Xe, inhalation of nonradioactive Xe, SPECT, and PET, a technique which is one of the most versatile imaging methods yet developed [Mazziotta, this volume; Phelps and Mazziotta, 1985]. Inhalation of ^{133}Xe was developed as a less invasive modification of the carotid injection procedure and uses the same array of surface detectors over the scalp that was employed with the injection method. With inhalation, however, the ^{133}Xe is distributed through the entire circulatory system. This leads to detection of nonspecific radioactivity from the scalp and other tissues, so that the spatial resolution suffers in contrast to intracarotid injection. The relatively recent development of SPECT [Lassen, 1985] overcomes some of this difficulty by combining radioactive Xe inhalation with projection reconstruction imaging to produce tomographic images of blood flow, allowing visualization of metabolic activity in subcortical as well as cortical structures. Figure 5a is a SPECT image of blood flow in a subject at rest with eyes closed, exhibiting a typical hyperfrontal pattern with some activity in the visual cortex. Figure 5b shows the same subject copying a text. Much more activity is seen now in the visual cortex. This is accompanied by activation of the left hemisphere regions responsible for linguistic processing and motor outflow through the right hand.

There are at least two other methods for imaging rCBF: PET (see below) and Xe enhanced X-ray CT. The latter method uses nonradioactive Xe as a contrast agent for X-ray CT. Thus, while no radioactivity is injected or inhaled in this technique, exposure to X-rays is entailed. This method can produce images of cortical and subcortical blood flow which change with behavioral state [Yingling et al., 1985], but it suffers from the drawback that the concentrations of Xe necessary are highly psychoactive and, similar to nitrous oxide, produce a dissociated state of consciousness. Unless the sensitivity of the technique can be increased enough to allow lowering the Xe concentration significantly, this effect will seriously constrain the applicability of this method, especially in any contemplated studies of children or cognitively impaired individuals.

When the various methods for imaging rCBF are evaluated in terms of the ideal criteria listed in table I, it is clear that these techniques address a different set of questions than X-ray CT or MRI. The spatial resolution is relatively poor, but this is offset by the fact that one obtains functional information which allows the visualization of regional brain activity during different behavioral states. The temporal resolution is relatively poor, as all the methods currently require several minutes to obtain a single image. This constraint limits the technique to functional measurement of either behaviors which can be sustained for extended periods (for example, speaking or other continuous motor activities), or continuous stimulation of a particular sensory modality. Finally, all the methods involve some degree of risk, and the instrumentation required is complex and costly.

A very exciting development in functional imaging is the advent of PET. This technique, which will be discussed in more detail by Dr. Mazziotta [this volume], is one of the most versatile methods available. PET imaging is based on the physical properties of positrons, which are positively charged particles with the same mass as the electron. When a positron collides with an electron, the particles are mutually annihilated and their mass is converted into two gamma rays which travel away from the site of the collision at an angle of exactly 180 degrees. Thus, gamma detections which occur simultaneously must have originated from a point on the line connecting the two simultaneously activated detectors. Collection of a large number of such events allows reconstruction of tomographic images reflecting the distribution of the positron-emitting compounds.

Unfortunately, there is an inherent limitation on the spatial resolution that can be obtained with PET. Positrons are emitted with such high velocity that they travel a considerable distance through the tissue before encountering an electron; while the distance varies slightly with different elements, the average distance is about 0.9 mm. Thus, the site of positron-electron annihilation and gamma ray formation (which is what is actually imaged) is at a variable distance from the actual site of the positron emission (which is the event of interest). Therefore, the image quality from PET is not quite up to the standards of X-ray CT or MRI; however, this limitation is more than offset by the incredible versatility of PET for functional imaging.

What makes this technique so versatile is that positron emitters such as ^{11}C or ^{18}F can be incorporated into a wide variety of biologically significant compounds and used to image many different metabolic processes. Examples include (^{18}F)2-deoxy-2-fluoro-*D*-glucose, to measure glucose transport and metabolism; ^{15}O to measure rCBF; ^{11}C-labelled amino acids to assess protein synthesis; and an extensive list of ^{11}C-conjugated neurotransmitters or pharmacological agents which can provide quantifiable images of the distribution of many neurotransmitters or receptors. (See Mazziotta [this volume] for details.) Because of this versatility, PET scanning will undoubtedly become a major research tool as the method becomes more widely available. Unfortunately, routine clinical use is likely to remain more limited in at least the near future. Production of the positron-emitting isotopes and their incorporation into biologically relevant compounds requires a cyclotron and highly trained chemists due to the short half-life of the isotopes. While 'baby cyclotrons', about the size of two office desks, have been developed, the method is very expensive. Although future developments will undoubtedly lessen these problems to some extent, it seems unlikely that PET scanning will become a routine clinical procedure in the near future.

In the light of the table I criteria, PET provides medium spatial resolution images, with unmatched versatility for functional studies. The temporal resolution is still low, on the order of several minutes per scan. Again, this limits the behaviors which can be studied in the same way as described above for measurements of rCBF. PET scanning is relatively invasive, requiring arterial catheterization and the injection of highly radioactive compounds. It is also very expensive and requires highly trained personnel. Despite these limitations, PET is probably the single most promising development in functional imaging. As the technology continues to be developed, it is hoped that PET will become more widely available for both research and clinical use.

A final imaging technique involves the production of topographical maps of electrical brain activity recorded with multi-channel electroencephalography (EEG). This method differs from those discussed so far in that it does not actually produce an image of the brain per se, but rather provides quasi-anatomical graphs of scalp-recorded EEG or event-related potential (ERP) activity. The numerical value of a chosen parameter of EEG or ERP activity, such as the power in the alpha band or the voltage at a chosen peak of a sensory evoked response, is assigned to the appropriate electrode location on a stylized top or side view of the head. Points lying between actual electrode locations are assigned values by interpolation from the values at neighboring electrodes. The numerical values are then assigned to

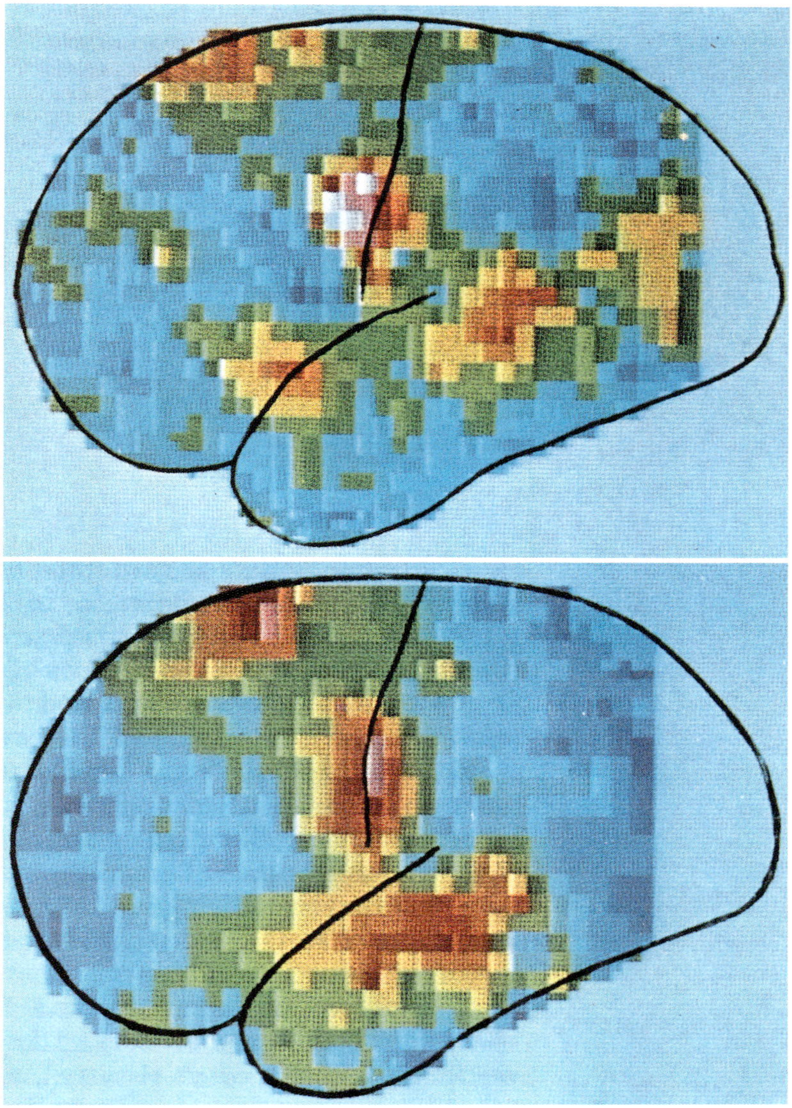

a

b

Fig. 4. a Regional cerebral blood flow (rCBF) in cortex of left hemisphere during oral reading. Increased flow relative to the resting state is mapped as warmer colors, showing increased metabolism in visual and language areas. *b* RCBF in same subject as *a*, during spontaneous speech. Note similar pattern of activation as in *a*, with notable exception of occipital visual area. From Lassen et al. [1978].

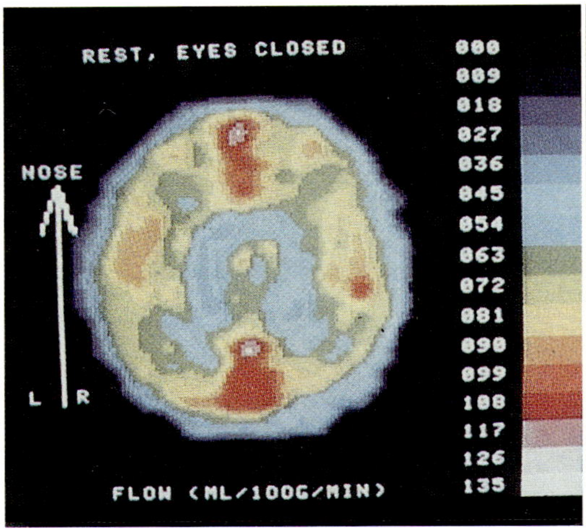

5a

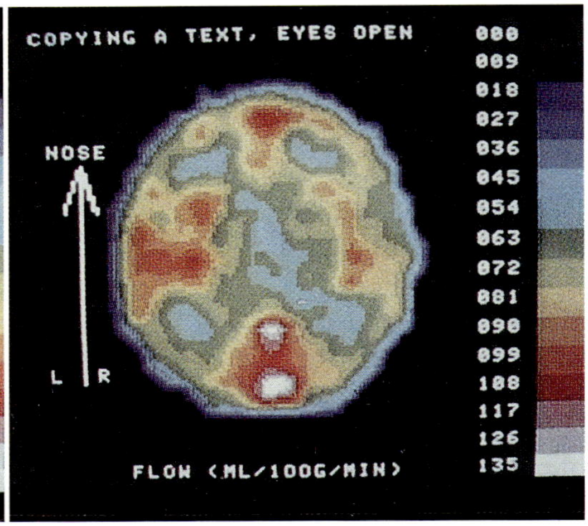

5b

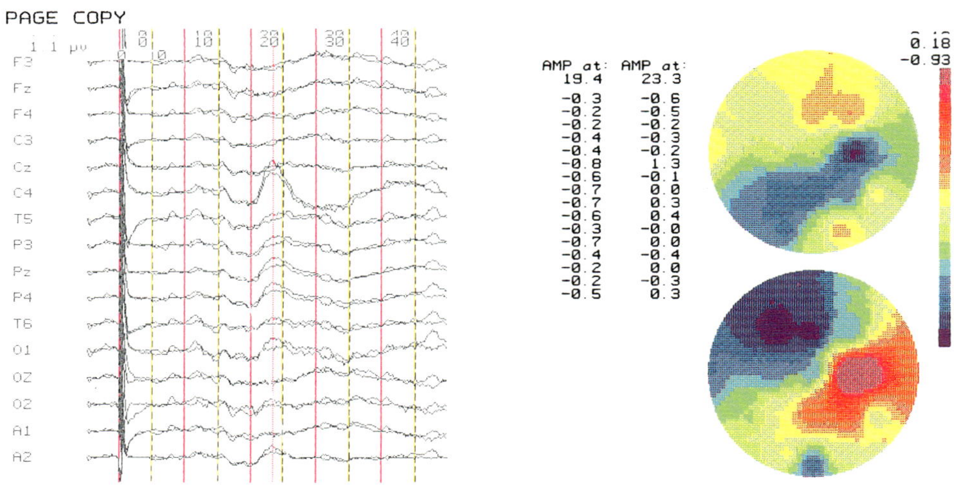

6

Fig. 5. a Single photon emission computed tomography (SPECT) showing cortical and subcortical rCBF of subject at rest, exhibiting typical 'hyperfrontal' pattern. *b* SPECT rCBF image of same subject as *a,* while copying text with the right hand. Activation of left hemisphere language and motor regions can be clearly seen. From Lassen [1985].

Fig. 6. Topography of somatosensory evoked potential to stimulation of the left median nerve. Two superimposed 16 channel averages are plotted at the left, with the actual voltages at 19.4 and 23.3 ms indicated in the center. On the right are bit-mapped color images of the distribution of voltages at the two latencies; the location of the central sulcus, where the activity changes polarity, can be clearly seen. Positivity is plotted up in the traces, and as warmer colors in the maps. Courtesy of Siegen Corporation, Sunnyvale, Calif.

either a gray scale or (more usually) a color scale, and the results are plotted to give a graphical representation of the scalp distribution of the chosen activity.

This method, initially popularized by Duffy and colleagues [1979] as brain electrical activity mapping (BEAM), has severely restricted spatial resolution due to the lateral spread of EEG currents across the scalp. The *temporal* resolution, however, is unsurpassed by any other imaging modality, since electrical events can be measured with sub-millisecond resolution (compared with several *minutes* for PET or rCBF). For example, figure 6 shows the distribution of evoked activity at 19.4 and 23.3 ms after the delivery of an electrical stimulus to the left median nerve at the wrist. At the first time point, the activity in the dorsal column-medial lemniscus pathway is just reaching the primary somatosensory cortex of the contralateral postcentral gyrus. Since the cortical pyramidal cells which generate the scalp-recorded potentials at this particular latency are oriented in the posterior bank of the central sulcus, parallel to the scalp, the electrical dipole resulting from their activation has a negative pole posteriorly, and a positive pole anteriorly, as can be seen from the upper map in the figure. Four ms later, the dipole has reversed polarity and appears with a posterior positivity and anterior negativity (lower map). With computer technology it is a simple matter to present a series of such figures representing successive time points and create a 'movie' of the patterns of activation as they spread across the scalp. When this 'movie' is played back slower than real time it allows the changing patterns to be visualized readily.

Similarly, it also is possible to visualize (1) the activation of the occipital cortices roughly 100 ms following a visual stimulus; (2) the cognitive P300 wave associated with stimulus discrimination in any modality, or (3) event-related desynchronization (ERD) of the EEG associated with different sensory or motor events [Pfurtscheller et al., 1984]. For example, figure 7a, which shows the distribution of alpha activity at rest with eyes closed in a normal subject, demonstrates the classical occipital maximum. Figure 7b shows not the distribution of alpha power itself, but rather a statistical comparison of the *change* in alpha power from the resting level during spontaneous movement of the right hand, with all other conditions the same as in figure 7a. Despite the higher *amplitude* of alpha at the occipital pole, the region of maximum movement-related *desynchronization* is over the contralateral motor hand area. Figure 8 illustrates the application of this method to a variety of behavioral conditions. Specifically, it shows ERD associated with photic stimulation, spontaneous counting, movement of the

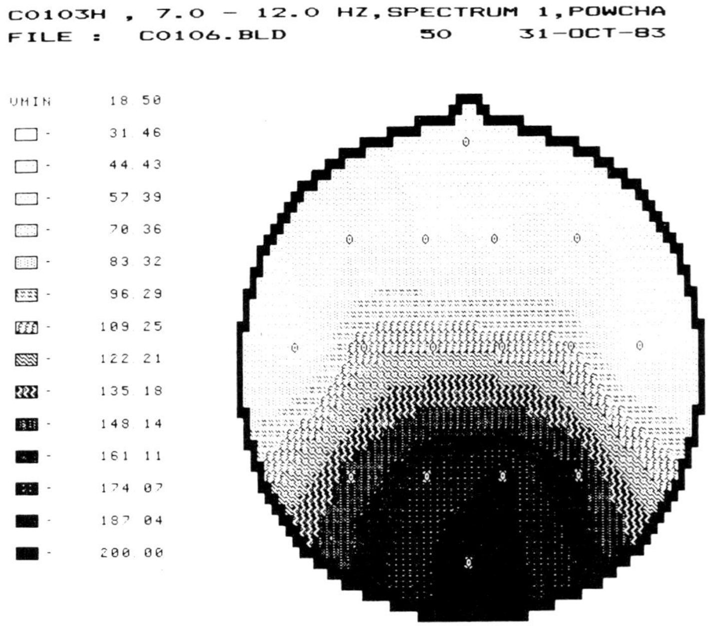
CO103H , 7.0 – 12.0 HZ,SPECTRUM 1,POWCHA
FILE : CO106.BLD 50 31-OCT-83
VMIN 18.50
31.46
44.43
57.39
70.36
83.32
96.29
109.25
122.21
135.18
148.14
161.11
174.07
187.04
200.00

a

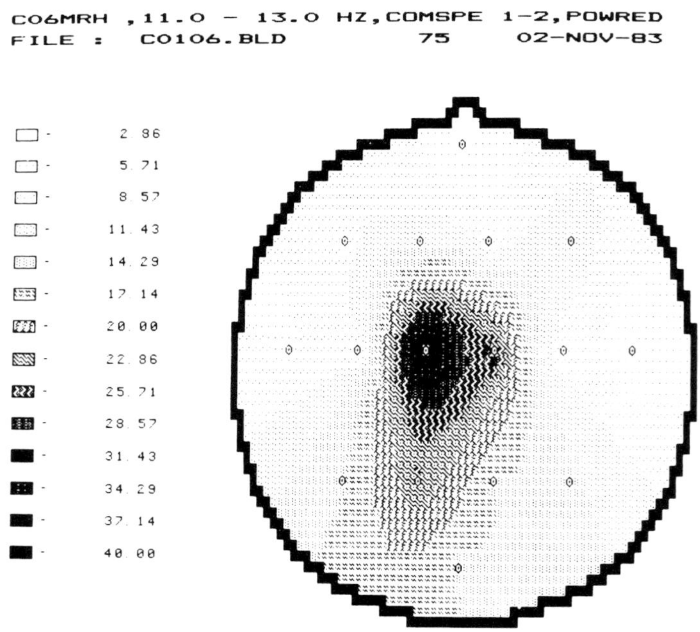
CO6MRH ,11.0 – 13.0 HZ,COMSPE 1-2,POWRED
FILE : CO106.BLD 75 02-NOV-83
2.86
5.71
8.57
11.43
14.29
17.14
20.00
22.86
25.71
28.57
31.43
34.29
37.14
40.00

b

left hand, spontaneous speech, and verbal image identification. In each case, the region of maximum ERD is different, and corresponds to the predicted anatomical locus activated in each condition.

The ease with which such statistical comparisons can be graphed is one of the more powerful features of the EEG mapping method. Since the procedure is totally noninvasive, a normative data base can be collected relatively easily for any parameters of interest. A given subject's data can then be displayed, not in the raw form, but in the form of a z-score representing the degree of deviation of the individual's activity from the appropriate normative group. For example, figure 9a illustrates the voltage distribution, in a group of normal readers, of a component of an auditory ERP at a latency of 364 ms during an auditory phonemic discrimination task [Duffy and McAnulty, 1985]. Figure 9b shows the same response from a single dyslexic individual. While there are obvious differences, it is not so obvious *where* (i. e. at what anatomic location) the differences are meaningful, since the variance at each point is not shown. At first glance, the maximum difference might seem to be in the right frontal region. However, figure 9c shows the same individual's response graphed as a z-score compared to the normative group; the area of maximum difference is now clearly seen to be in the left posterior region. Such displays add a degree of clarity to the presentation of multi-channel EEG or ERP data that far surpasses the traditional display of multiple tracings of raw data or averaged waveforms.

Of course, the validity of such statistical comparisons depends on a number of factors, including the choice of appropriate parameters to measure and display, and the screening criteria used to define normative or clinical groups (see John et al. [1980], Ahn et al. [1980], and Yingling et al. [1986] for an illustration of some of the issues encountered in application of statistical analysis of the EEG to the specific problem of learning disabilities). However, these concerns are the same for any clinical use of electrophysiological data, and are only brought into sharper focus when the data are made more accessible by graphic techniques.

Fig. 7. a Distribution of alpha activity at rest with eyes closed, showing classical occipital maximum. *b* Distribution of *change* in alpha power (event-related desynchronization, or ERD) in same subject during motor activity with right hand. Even though actual alpha power is still highest in the occipital region, the ERD is greatest over the contralateral motor cortex. From Pfurtscheller et al. [1984].

If these issues are given appropriate concern, the use of mapping techniques such as those described here can greatly facilitate the comprehensibility and utility of EEG and ERP data. In fact, there has been a rapid growth in the availability of commercial systems to produce such maps. In contrast to the high cost of X-ray CT, MRI, or PET, computerized brain mapping machines are relatively inexpensive, costing in the same range as existing multi-channel EEG and ERP equipment. Although no such software packages are yet commercially available, the technique is simple enough that in principle it could be implemented on an IBM PC or similar microcomputer which could be interfaced to existing EEG machines.

When measured against the ideal criteria of table I, EEG mapping techniques score both very high and very low. The major limitation is that the brain is not imaged directly, but only through its electrical activity as recorded at the scalp. Such recordings presumably represent primarily cortical activity, with a limited (and unknown) contribution from subcortical structures. Furthermore, the currents generated by the EEG spread widely across the scalp, and their exact distribution is a function of the geometrical orientation of the pyramidal cell generators with respect to the recording electrodes. Therefore, the special resolution is very crude in comparison with any of the techniques based on projection-reconstruction imaging.

On the other hand, these methods offer a number of unique advantages for functional analysis of brain activity. The temporal resolution is unsurpassed, since no other method comes close to resolving distinct events separated by only milliseconds. Analysis of rapid sequences of such images may offer new insights into the dynamics of cortical information flow as yet unavailable with any other technique. EEG mapping techniques are totally noninvasive and therefore can be used in any desired clinical or normal population, from neonates to the elderly, with no concern for risk from repeated studies. Within-subject designs such as pre-post treatment effects, drug effects, etc., can all be evaluated easily and economically. For these reasons, it is likely that spatio-temporal maps of a variety of brain electrical parameters will become more widely used in both research and clinical practice within the next few years.

To conclude, it is evident that no single imaging modality is, or is ever likely to become, the single 'ideal' method. The choice of a method must therefore be guided by a number of considerations, including whether the emphasis is placed on obtaining anatomical or functional information,

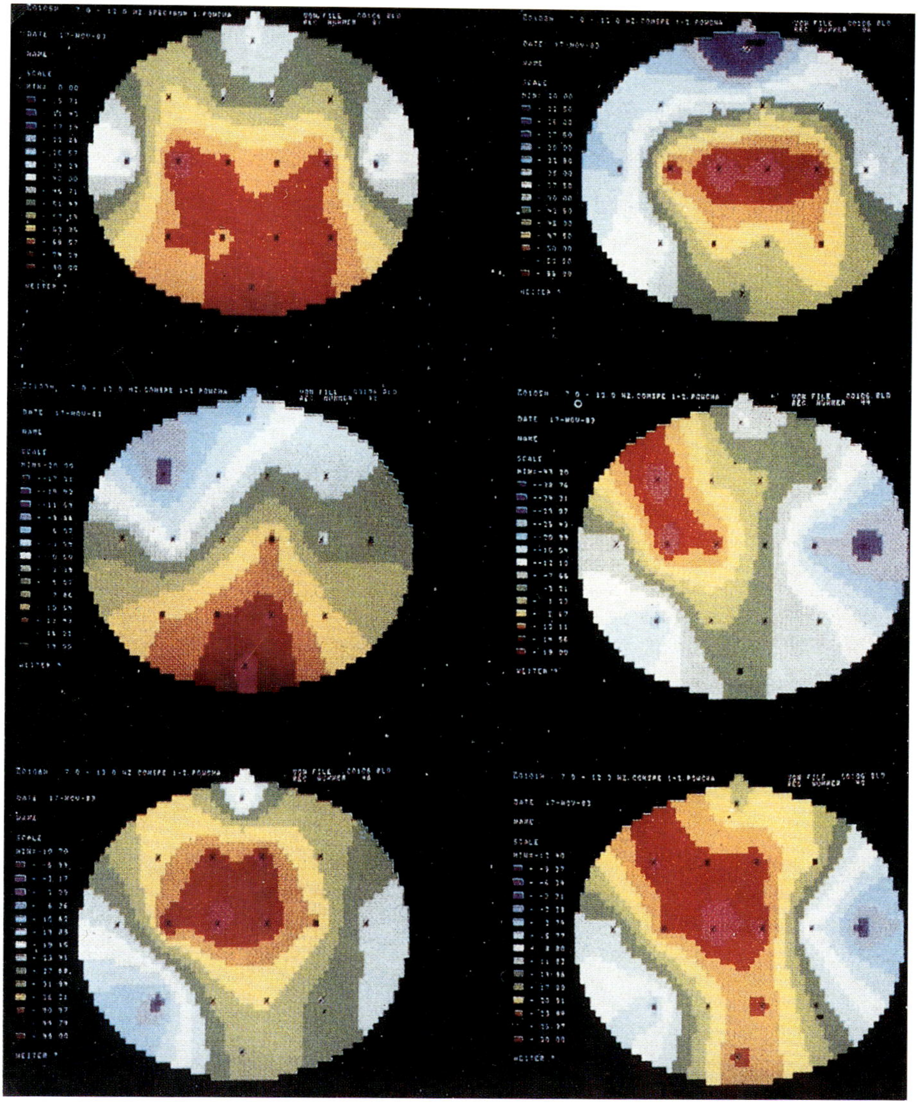

Fig. 8. EEG maps showing alpha at rest (upper left) and phasic alpha power changes (ERD) during different behavioral conditions: voluntary left hand movements (upper right); 1/s photic stimulation (middle left); spontaneous speech (middle right); spontaneous counting (lower left); and verbal image identification (lower right). Warmer colors represent higher alpha activity in the EEG map and maximal power decrease in the ERD maps. From Pfurtscheller et al. [1984].

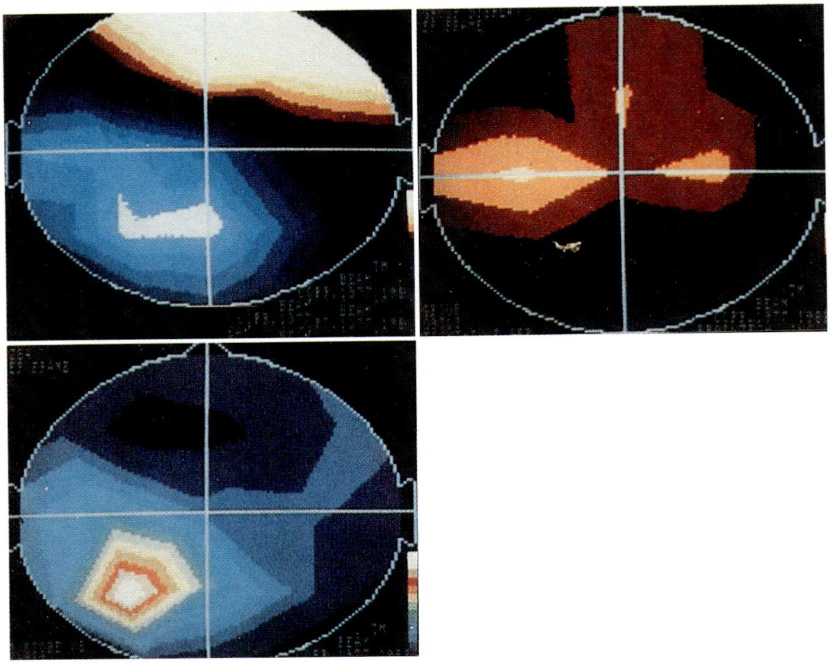

a b c

Fig. 9. a Brain electrical activity mapping (BEAM) showing a single 11-year-old dyslexic child's auditory evoked response at 364 ms latency during discrimination of the words 'tight' versus 'tyke'. *b* BEAM map of the 'tight-tyke' AER at the same latency in a nondyslexic control group. *c* Significance probability mapping (SPM) showing the z-statistic of the dyslexic child's deviance from the control group mean. Higher z-scores are represented by warmer colors; note the maximum statistical deviance is in the left posterior region, despite the apparent right frontal difference seen when comparing the upper two maps. From Duffy and McAnulty [1985].

whether cortical or subcortical information is desired, what the relevant time course is and, last but not least, the availability, invasiveness, and expense of the various techniques. Clearly, this is an area in which rapid technological advances are being made. It is likely that new techniques will be introduced which will expand still further the kinds of information that can be obtained regarding the structure and function of the living brain. Future historians of neuroscience will undoubtedly look back on the present era as representing a revolution in methodology for studying the human brain. Whether it will also be viewed as a conceptual revolution in our understanding of brain-behavior relationships will depend on the creativity and rigor with which these powerful new tools are applied.

References

Ahn, H.; Prichep, L.; John, E.R.; Baird, H.; Trepetin, M.; Kaye, H.: Developmental equations reflect brain dysfunctions. Science *210:* 1250–1262 (1980).

Duffy, F.H.; Burchfiel, J.L.; Lombroso, C.T.: Brain electrical activity mapping (BEAM): a method for extending the clinical utility of EEG and evoked potential data. Ann. Neurol. *5:* 309–321 (1979).

Duffy, F.H.; McAnulty, G.B.: Brain electrical activity mapping (BEAM): the search for physiological signature of dyslexia; in Duffy, Geschwind, Dyslexia: a neuroscientific approach to clinical evaluation, pp. 105–122 (Little, Brown, Boston 1985).

Harper, A.M.; Glass, H.I.; Steven, J.L.; Granat, A.H.: The measurement of local blood flow in the cerebral cortex from the clearance of $Xenon^{133}$. J. Neurol. Neurosurg. Psychiat. *27:* 255–258 (1964).

Ingvar, D.H.; Conqvist, S.; Ekberg, R.; Risberg, J.; Hoedt-Rasmussen, K.: Normal values of regional cerebral blood flow in man, including flow and weight estimates of gray and white matter. Acta neur. scand. *14:* suppl., pp. 72–78 (1965).

John, E.R.; Ahn, H.; Prichep, L.; Trepetin, M.; Brown, D.; Kaye, H.: Developmental equations for the electroencephalogram. Science *210:* 1255–1258 (1980).

Lassen, N.A.: Measurement of regional cerebral blood flow in humans with single-photon-emitting radioisotopes; in Sokoloff, Brain imaging and brain function. Research Publications, ARNMD, vol. 63, pp. 9–20 (Raven Press, New York 1985).

Lassen, N.A.; Ingvar, D.H.: The blood flow of the cerebral cortex determined by radioactive $Krypton^{85}$. Experientia *77:* 42 (1961).

Lassen, N.A.; Ingvar, D.H.; Skinhoj, E.: Brain function and blood flow. Sci. Am. *239:* 62–71 (1978).

Morgan, C.J.; Hendee, W.R.; Introduction to magnetic resonance imaging (Multi-Media Publishing, Denver 1984).

Morgan, C.L.: Basic principles of computed tomography (University Park Press, Baltimore 1983).

Oldendorf, W.H.: The quest for an image of brain: computerized tomography in the perspective of past and future imaging methods (Raven Press, New York 1980).

Pfurtscheller, G.; Ladurner, G.; Maresch, H.; Vollmer, R.: Brain electrical activity mapping in normal and ischemic brain; in Pfurtscheller et al., Brain ischemia: quantitative EEG and imaging techniques. Prog. Brain Res., vol. 62, pp. 287–302 (Elsevier, Amsterdam 1984).

Phelps, M.E; Mazziotta, J.C.: Positron emission tomography: human brain function and biochemistry. Science *228:* 799–809 (1985).

Yingling, C.D.; Brandt-Zawadski, M.N.; Cann, C.E.; McMurdo, K.: Behavioral activation of cortical and subcortical structures imaged with Xenon-enhanced CT scan. J. clin. exp. Neuropsychol. *7:* 632 (1985).

Yingling, C.D.; Galin, D.; Fein, G.; Peltzman, D.; Davenport, L.: Neurometrics does not detect 'pure' dyslexics. Electroenceph. clin. Neurophysiol. *63:* 426–430 (1986).

Charles D. Yingling, PhD, Langley Porter Psychiatric Institute and Department of Neurological Surgery, University of California, San Francisco, CA 94143 (USA)

Mueller (ed.): Neurology and Psychiatry: A Meeting of Minds,
pp. 105–153 (Karger, Basel 1989)

Positron Emission Tomography Scanning: Principles and Applications

John C. Mazziotta[1]

Department of Neurology, Division of Biophysics and Nuclear Medicine, Department of Radiological Sciences, UCLA School of Medicine, Laboratory of Nuclear Medicine, Los Angeles, Calif., USA

The recent development of positron emission tomography (PET)[2] has provided a new technique for the analytic, noninvasive measurement of local cerebral functions in humans. Investigations of cerebral function over the course of the last century have used electrophysiological, neuropsychological, and radiological approaches. While the results of these studies have been impressive and have vastly improved our understanding of normal and abnormal cerebral function, remarkably little is known about the local biochemistry and physiology of human cerebral substructures. The available information has been gained from extrapolation of animal studies to human – a strategy that is most limited in the study of human disease states. PET has provided previously unavailable insights into these local functional relationships.

PET can no longer be considered a new discipline. It has been applied to the study of normal subjects as well as patients with all of the major neurological and psychiatric disorders. These studies have demonstrated, for the first time, local cerebral responses to physiological stimuli in normal subjects and patients. The purpose of this chapter is to describe the basic principles of PET, the applications of this technology to the study of human brain function, its limitations and its future prospects.

Attempts to study human cerebral physiology, biochemistry and hemodynamics are not new. In the 1940s Kety and Schmidt [1948] measured

[1] Special thanks to all of the investigators using PET who most graciously provided information and illustrations. Special thanks to Lee Griswold for art work and to Maureen Chang for preparing and editing the manuscript. Adapted in part from Mazziotta [1985].

[2] For further definitions and explanations, see Glossary (p. 150).

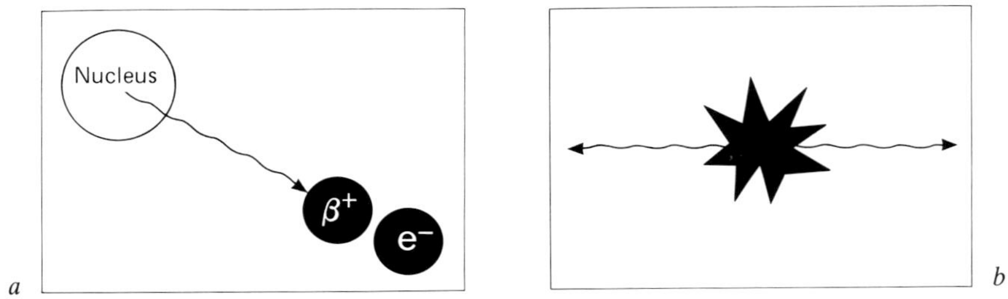

Fig. 1. The process of positron emission and annihilation. *a* Positrons are positively charged electrons that are emitted from certain unstable nuclei. These particles travel for a limited distance following their emission from a nucleus and combine with an electron at or near the point where they come to rest. *b* The combination of a positron and an electron results in annihilation; that is, the mass of the positron and the electron are converted into electromagnetic radiation in the form of two high-energy photons emitted in opposite directions. From Mazziotta [1985].

arteriovenous differences for various compounds across the brain, and when combined with information about cerebral blood flow (CBF), these measurements provided accurate determinations of global (i. e. the entire brain) blood flow, glucose and oxygen utilization. Efforts to obtain more regional information were developed in Scandinavia, where xenon-131 was used with external probes to determine CBF regionally in the brain. These studies provided the first information about human cortical responses to various physiologic stimuli and their alterations in disease states. Tomographic approaches to investigate cerebral function occurred independently and culminated in emission tomography. Positron imaging was first suggested in 1951 by Wrenn and colleagues as well as Brownell and Sweet. In the course of the last 35 years, developments in computer, electronic and cyclotron technology have advanced this discipline to the point where high-resolution, analytical measurements of biochemical, physiological and hemodynamic processes can now be made locally and in three dimensions using PET.

Positron Emitting Isotopes: What They Are and Why They Are Used

It is the unique physical properties of positron decay that allow for accurate and quantifiable imaging with PET. Positrons are positively charged electrons which are emitted from certain unstable nuclei as they decay to a more stable state (fig. 1, table I). When a positron is emitted from

Table I. A few positron-emitting isotopes that have been used in compounds designed for PET studies

Positron-emitting isotope	Half-life, min
^{11}C	20.3
^{13}N	10.0
^{15}O	1.8
^{18}F	109.0
^{68}Ga	68.3
^{75}Br	102.0
^{77}Kr	72.0
^{82}Rb	1.3

an unstable nucleus it travels a finite distance known as the positron range (actually this is a distribution of distances) before it encounters and combines with an electron. The distance traveled is related to the energy of the emitted positron particle and therefore is different for each positron-emitting isotope. When a positron combines with an electron they annihilate. That is, the masses of the electron and positron are converted to electromagnetic radiation and produce a pair of high-energy (511 keV) annihilation photons. A unique feature of this event is the fact that the two annihilation photons are emitted in essentially opposite directions. PET devices take advantage of this unique form of radiation as will be discussed below.

Table I indicates a few of the positron-emitting isotopes that have been used thus far in studies with PET. Note that some of the positron-emitting isotopes listed in table I are isotopes of natural elements of the body. The use of radioisotopes of the primary natural elements of the body (oxygen, nitrogen and carbon) allows for the labeling of various substrates, substrate analogs and drugs without disturbing their biochemical behavior. Some of the labeled compounds used for PET are analogous to those commonly used in animal studies. For example, ^{14}C which is not detectable externally, is substituded with the positron-emitting isotope ^{11}C. There is no positron-emitting isotope of hydrogen, but ^{18}F is used as a substitute for hydrogen because of its strong carbon-fluoride bond and because its similar size allows it to behave with minimal biochemical differences from the natural substance. The use of positron-emitting isotopes of natural elements in the body is in contrast to more typical nuclear medicine radiopharmaceuticals which employ iodine or technetium and result in tracers that are less likely to behave in a physiological manner in biological systems.

Examination of the half-lives of the isotopes listed in table I indicate another aspect of their use. Because the half-lives are all short, the radiation dose to the patient is low, but a cyclotron for the production of these compounds must be available at or near the site of the PET imaging. The cost and complexity of such installations must be balanced against the unique capabilites that PET technologies have and will provide in the study of human biological systems.

Coincidence Detection

As was noted above, when a positron and an electron combine and annihilate the result is the emission of two photons 180° apart. This allows for the use of an electronic form of photon collimation by recording simultaneous (within 10–20 ns) arrival of these photons in detectors on opposite sides of the head (fig. 2a). This is referred to as annihilation coincidence detection. Annihilation coincidence detection provides uniform and high spatial resolution, high detection efficiency for the events, and simultaneous collection of linear and angular data. This contrasts with the conventional use of heavy lead collimators, in which spatial resolution for the detection of radioactivity varies significantly with the distance between the detector and the source of the radioactivity. Annihilation coincidence detection provides an exact or near exact method for photon attenuation and can be designed to minimize the acceptance of scattered radiation (photons deflected into the path of a detector), a factor which reduces the quality and quantifiability of data obtained with other techniques. The use of annihilation coincidence detection establishes the origin of the recorded radiation to well-defined regions between opposing detectors. It rejects radiation that originates above and below the tomographic plane of interest (fig. 2a). Using these methods only a thin (1–2 cm) slice of tissue is sampled with relatively uniform resolution across the slice. The data from each set of detectors are collected over time at many positions and angles around the cross section of the brain.

As can be noted in figure 2a, positron annihilation events that are recorded by PET detector systems occur along a line (or a plane in three dimensions) between the two detectors. It is theoretically possible to determine where along this line the event took place if the differences in

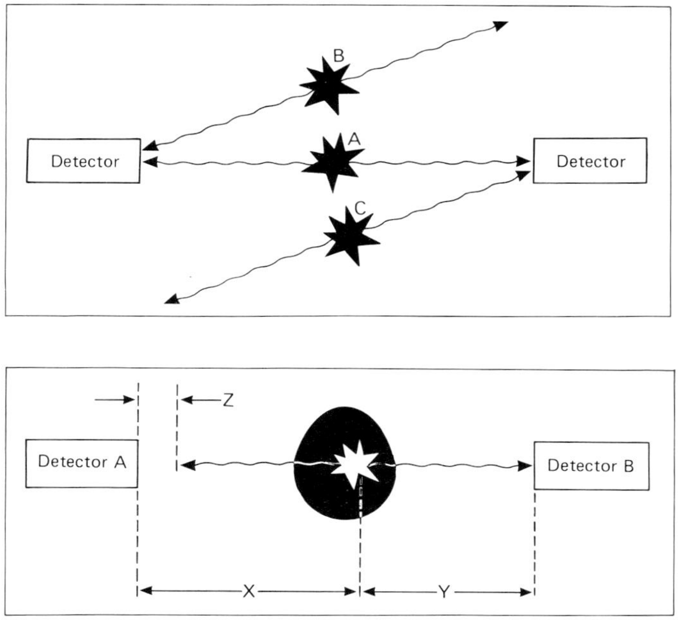

a

b

Fig. 2. PET detection schemes for identifying annihilation events. *a* This figure illustrates 3 separate annihilation events (A–C). Event A occurs in the plane between two electronically linked detectors. Since the simultaneously and oppositely emitted annihilation photons each strike the electronically linked detectors, the event at A is recorded. Events that occur above or below the plane of interest (B, C) have annihilation photons that only strike one detector. These events are discarded. This process, known as annihilation coincidence detection, rejects events that occur above and below the plane of interest and allows for relatively uniform spatial resolution within the plane of section and elimination of extraneous radioactive events that occur outside the plane of interest. *b* Time of flight principles. Annihilation events that do not occur equidistant from the two detectors will result in annihilation photons arriving at the linked detectors at different times. In this example, distance x is greater than y and x–y = z. The difference in arrival time of the two photons is equal to the time it takes the speed of light to transverse distance z. For objects the size of the human brain (10–15 cm diameter) these times are in the range of 500 ps (10^{-12} s). From Mazziotta [1985].

arrival times of the two photons can be accurately measured by the detector pair (fig. 2b). This approach, called time of flight detection, requires detectors and electronics with extremely high timing accuracy since the difference in arrival times even from the edge of a structure the size of the brain is equal to the time it takes light to travel twice this short distance. Typical times are in the range of 500 ps (10^{-12} s).

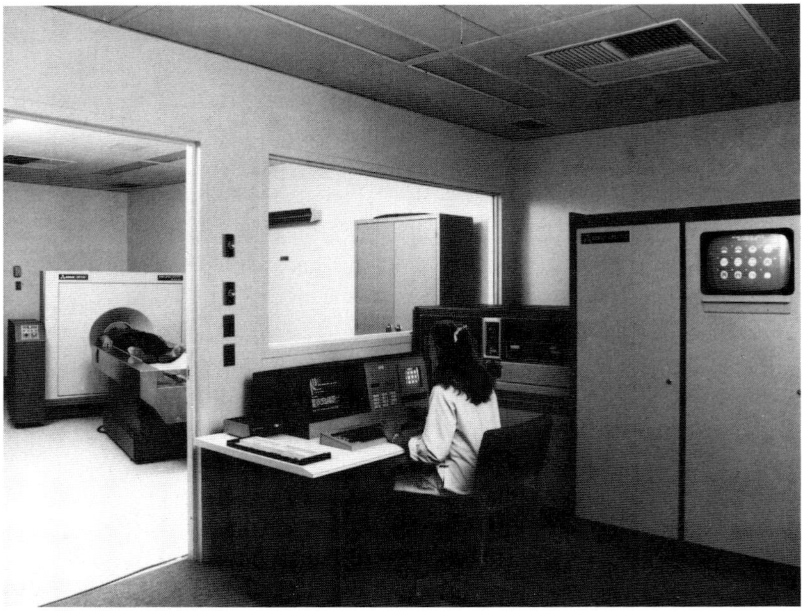

Fig. 3. The NeuroECAT PET device (CTI, Knoxville, Tenn.) in operation at UCLA. Note the patient lying on the scanner bed and the patient's head in the gantry which contains the detection system. The operator is seated at the console and directs and supervises the computer-based acquisition and reconstruction of data which is then displayed in black and white or color TV monitors. From Phelps et al. [1983].

Tomographs

The principles described above for a single pair of detectors is simply extrapolated in three dimensions for the design of a clinically applicable tomograph. Circumferential arrays of detector pairs are constructed such that each set of detectors collects data from one plane of section through the brain. By stacking multiple rings of these detectors one against the other, multiple planes of information can be obtained simultaneously. Devices are presently in use that collect 9 simultaneous planes of data and proposed instruments may be capable of collecting 20 or more planes simultaneously. The advantage of multiple simultaneous planes is that for a single radioisotope administration a more complete sample of the brain can be obtained.

Data from all sets of detectors are collected over times at many linear positions and angles around the cross-section of the brain. At this point the collected radioactivity count rate profiles resemble data collected using all forms of computed tomographic (CT) systems (e.g. X-ray, NMR, etc.). The data are then processed in a mathematically similar fashion to that used in X-ray CT scanning to reconstruct two-dimensional maps of tissue radioactivity concentrations in the brain slice. Lastly, the image is corrected for attenuation of the emitted radioactivity that occurs as it passes through the cranial structures.

Final image resolution is dependent on a number of factors. These factors include the size of crystals used to detect the activity, the spacing of these detectors, the number of radioactive events that comprise a given image and a number of other factors. As PET instruments improve, the positron range itself will be the ultimate limiting factor. This theoretical limit of resolution is in the range of a few millimeters. However, the present practical limit of resolution, dictated mainly by financial factors in the construction of these devices, is in the range of 3–4 mm.

A typical PET device includes a gantry with the detector system, a bed that is adjustable for positioning the patient, a computer to monitor and store acquired data as well as reconstruct the final images and display monitors for their presentation (fig. 3).

Labeled Compounds

A partial list of the more pertinent labeled compounds synthesized and considered for use in human subjects is shown in table II. The actual synthesis of these compounds is a complex task. The resultant product must have a high specific activity (ratio of the radiolabeled compound to the total compound), a high chemical yield and purity and utilize techniques that are rapid enough to accommodate the short half-lives of positron-emitting isotopes. While there are positron-emitting isotopes of gallium, rubidium, bromine, phosphorous, iron, copper and many others, in this chapter studies will be described using radioisotopes of oxygen, nitrogen, carbon and fluorine.

The appropriate selection of the labeled compound and the sensitivity of PET devices allow for the measurement of very low (picomolar) concentrations of radioisotopes in the brain. This radioassay detection senstitivity is unequaled in noninvasive imaging techniques and allows for the measurement of tissue concentrations in the range of those found for neurotransmitters and drugs.

Table II. Partial list of compounds labeled with positron-emitting radionuclides

Cerebral blood flow
$H_2{}^{15}O$, $C^{15}O_2$, ^{77}Kr, CH_3-^{18}F-antipyrine, ^{11}C-alcohols, ^{18}F-ethanol
Cerebral blood volume
^{11}CO, $C^{15}O$, ^{68}Ga-EDTA [a]
Cerebral tissue pH
^{11}C-DMO, $^{11}CO_2$
Transport and metabolism
Oxygen
$^{15}O_2$
Glucose, glucose analogs and metabolites
(^{18}F)2-Deoxy-2-fluoro-*D*-glucose,
2-(^{11}C)-Deoxy-*D*-glucose, ^{11}C-*D*-glucose,
3-(^{11}C)-O-Methy-*D*-glucose
^{11}C-Lactate, pyruvate, acetate, succinate, oxaloacetate
Amino acids: ^{13}N-labeled
L-(^{13}N)-Glutamate, α- and ω-glutamine, alanine, aspartate, leucine, valine, isoleucine, methionine
Amino acids: ^{11}C-labeled
L-(^{11}C)-Aspartate, leucine, glutamate, valine, *D*-,*L*-(^{11}C)-alanine, leucine, tryptophan, 1-aminocyclopentane carboxylic acid, 1-aminocyclobutane carboxylic acid
Free fatty acids
^{11}C-Palmitic acid, oleic acid, heptadecanoic acid, β-methyl-heptadecanoic acid

Tracer Kinetics

To measure local cerebral physiologic processes after the intravenous injection or inhalation of positron-labeled compounds, appropriate mathematical tracer kinetic models, based on the principles of tracer and competitive enzyme kinetics, are needed. Models exist for the measurement of local rates of blood flow, membrane transport, metabolism, protein synthesis, blood volume, pH and receptor binding.

The tracer kinetic models provide a framework that describes the kinetics of the process under study and the mathematical equations for calculating the rates of these processes. Such models reduce complex biological systems into a few compartments (fig. 4–6) and attempt to estimate the rates of processes in those compartments by utilizing information about the delivery of the labeled compound into the compartments (by

Table II (cont.)

Molecular diffusion
^{68}Ga-EDTA, ^{82}Rb
Protein synthesis
L-[1-^{11}C]-Leucine, methionine, phenylalanine, (^{11}C-methyl)-*L*-methionine
Neurotransmitter systems and drugs
Dopaminergic
^{18}F-, ^{11}C-Spiperone, ^{75}Br-, ^{76}Br-*p*-bromo-spiperone, ^{18}F-haloperidol, ^{11}C-pimozide, ^{11}C-methylspiperone, ^{11}C-*L*-dopa, [6-^{18}F]-fluoro-*L*-dopa
Benzodiazepine
^{11}C-Flunitrazepam, diazepam, ^{18}F-valium
Cholinergic
^{11}C-Imipramine, QNB [b]
Opiate
^{11}C-Etorphine, N-methyl-^{11}C-morphine, heroin, ^{11}C-carfentanil
Adrenergic
^{11}C-Norepinephrine, propanolol
Anticonvulsants
^{11}C-Valproate, diphenylhydantoin

[a] Ethylenediaminetetra-acetic acid.
[b] Quinuclidinyl benzilate.

serially sampling blood from the patient) and the delivery, accumulation and clearance of the radiolabeled compound in the tissue (by serially imaging the brain).

An example of the kinetic modeling approach is shown in figure 5 for the glucose analog, 2-fluoro-deoxyglucose (FDG). ^{14}C-labeled deoxyglucose was initially used by Sokoloff et al. [1977] in animal experiments using autoradiography to develop the tracer kinetic method for determining cerebral glucose utilization. This deoxyglucose analog competes with glucose for membrane transport sites and for hexokinase to be phosphorylated to the end product deoxyglucose-6-PO_4. Unlike natural glucose-6-PO_4, deoxyglucose-6-PO_4 is not a substrate for further metabolism and is therefore essentially trapped in the cell. The use of deoxyglucose represents an approach, with a substrate analog, to isolate a segment (transport and phosphorylation) of a complex reaction sequence and to permit accurate

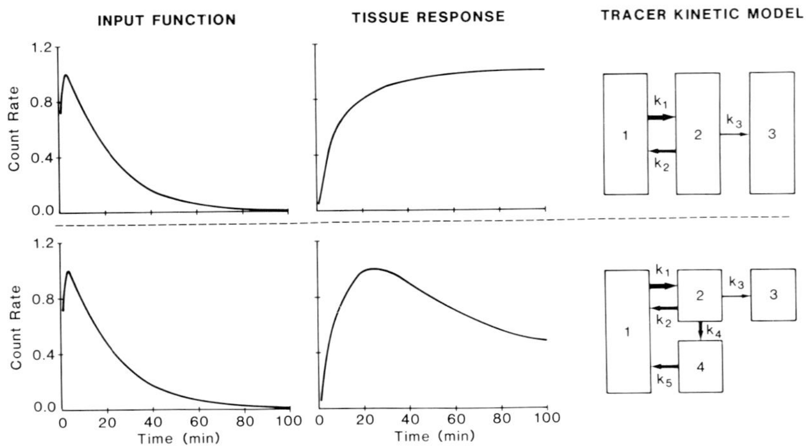

Fig. 4. Examples of typical tissue response curves when the input function is the same and the models are different (top and bottom). Thickness of arrows illustrates relative fluxes of tracer in different pathways for which the rates are described by rate constants (k). From Phelps et al. [1982].

estimates of the rates of these processes. The labeling of deoxyglucose with ^{18}F provided a positron-emitting form of this glucose analog for its application in human subjects with PET. Once a tracer kinetic model has been validated, the operational equations of the model can be incorporated into the tomograph computer and can be used to directly convert the tomographic images into parametric maps of the physiologic process of interest in the appropriate units (in this case, micromoles of glucose used per minute per gram of tissue).

CBF can be measured with PET by a variety of techniques. One approach is to have the subject continuously inhale ^{15}O-labeled carbon dioxide (fig. 6) until the concentration of the radioisotope reaches a dynamic equilibrium in the brain. This point occurs when the delivered radioactivity from the lung equals that due to the physical decay of the isotope and its biological clearance. ^{15}O tissue concentrations obtained with this method are nonlinearly related to blood flow. The effect can be corrected to provide measurements of absolute flow in the brain. After blood flow is measured by this method, local cerebral metabolic rate for oxygen utilization ($LCMRO_2$) can be determined by the continuous

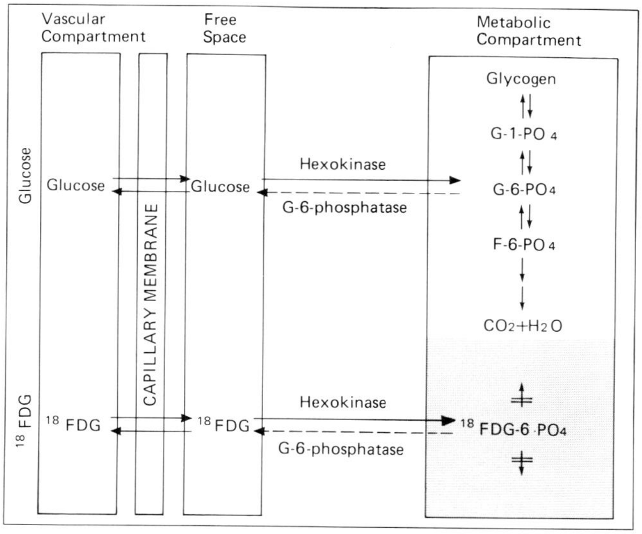

Fig. 5. Model for the glucose analog 2-fluoro-2-deoxyglucose (FDG) labeled with the positron-emitting isotope ^{18}F. The illustration shows the competition of FDG with glucose for forward and reserve transport, hexokinase for phosphorylation, and glucose-6-phosphatase (G-6-P) for dephosphorylation. Dashed lines indicate that the latter process is slow. Because FDG-6-PO_4 is not a substrate for subsequent glycolytic reactions or glycogen formation, it is essentially trapped in the cell. The glucose analog is a biochemical trick to isolate transport and hexokinase-mediated phosphorylation steps of glycolysis. The accumulation of the end product of the reaction (FDG-6-PO_4) in tissue permits the use of a relatively simple mathematical model and study method. Because in steady state the rate of phosphorylation is equal to the glycolytic rate from exogeneous glucose (assuming negligible glycogen formation), FDG provides a measure of the latter process. From Phelps et al. [1983].

inhalation of ^{15}O-labeled O_2. Images obtained during the continuous inhalation of ^{15}O-labeled O_2 are corrected for the blood flow component (i. e. ^{15}O-O_2 is metabolized to ^{15}O-H_2O which in turn is redelivered to the brain in proportion to blood flow), by dividing the ^{15}O-O_2 image by the ^{15}O-CO_2 image. This ratio image is proportional to the oxygen extraction fraction (OEF) or the arteriovenous oxygen difference divided by the arterial oxygen concentration. When this ratio image of OEF is multiplied by the blood flow and the arterial oxygen concentration, local cerebral metabolic rates for oxygen utilization are obtained.

A wide range of tracer kinetic strategies has been employed to measure the biochemical, physiological and hemodynamic variables listed in

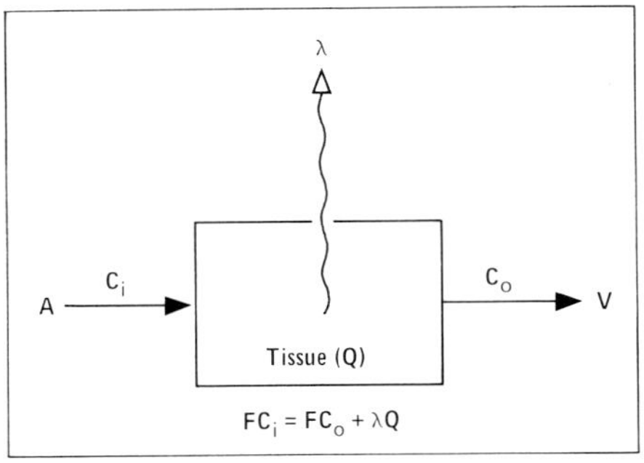

Fig. 6. Trace kinetic model for the continuous inhalation, steady-state method of determining CBF. The tracer is transported to and removed from the region by blood flow, F. The concentration of the tracer in arterial blood (A) is denoted by C_i and the total amount of tracer in the region by Q. The administered tracer has a radioactivity decay constant (λ) equal to 0.693/half-life. The clearance of the tracer by the venous system (V) of the brain is denoted by C_o. At equilibrium, the rate at which the tracer is added to the compartment (FC_i) is equal to the rate of biological clearance (FC_o) plus the rate of physical decay (λQ). From Mazziotta [1985].

table II. The reader is referred to the various review articles listed in the reference list at the end of this chapter for details of these approaches.

Making a PET Measurement

All the methods and approaches described above are combined to perform a human PET study (fig. 7). If a study of glucose metabolism is required, the ^{18}F is produced by the on-site cyclotron and FDG synthesized in the radiopharmaceutical laboratory. An appropriate dose (5–10 mCi) is obtained and injected intravenously into the subject. Serial blood samples are drawn to monitor the arterial input function described above and in figure 4. At the appropriate time, 30–40 min for the deoxyglucose method, tomographic imaging commences. Cross-sectional tomographic images of radioisotope concentrations of FDG are reconstructed and corrected for attenuation. These images, combined with the arterial input function for FDG and values for natural serum glucose, are used with the operation equation of the tracer kinetic model for deoxyglucose to convert the radioisotope concentration images into images of cerebral glucose metabolism. Anatomical regions of interest are then drawn on the resultant images and local metabolic rate values for glucose are obtained for given brain

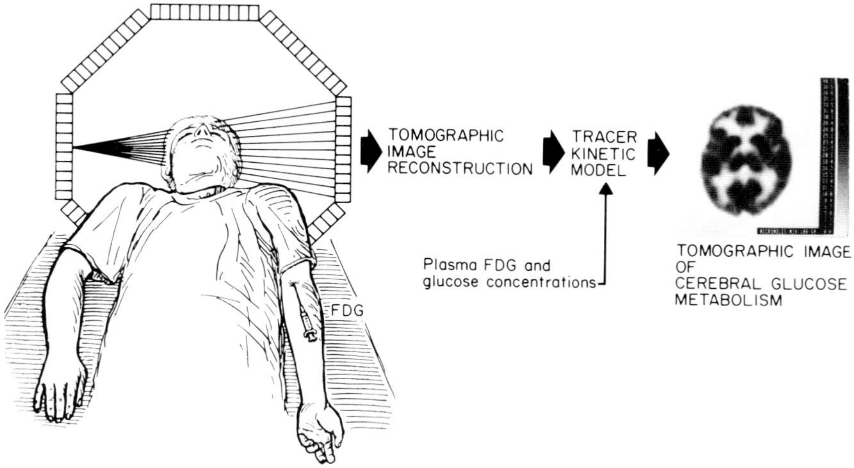

Fig. 7. The sequence of events involved in the PET measurement of local cerebral metabolic rate for glucose with FDG. About 40 min after intravenous injection of FDG, tomographic data are collected and cross-sectional images are reconstructed of the ^{18}F tissue activity distribution. Plasma FDG and glucose concentration are entered into the computer of the tomograph that also contains the operational equation of the FDG tracer kinetic model. Images are converted to local cerebral metabolic rate for glucose in units of $\mu mol \cdot min^{-1} \cdot g$ $tissue^{-1}$. Tomographic images are displayed on television screens with a gray scale in proportion to local cerebral metabolic rate for glucose (black being the highest) and numerical values are shown beside the scale. Lines drawn through the head show that a single detector on the patient's right side can seek out annihilation coincidences occurring in the multiple detectors on the other side of the head. From Phelps et al. [1983].

structures. While illustrated for the measurement of glucose metabolism with FDG, the same principles apply to all tracer kinetic measurments with PET.

Types of Studies Obtainable

Figure 8 illustrates a typical study of a normal subject with FDG to determine cerebral glucose metabolism. As can be seen, such images provide a high degree of spatial resolution resulting in good anatomical detail of cerebral structures.

To characterize the local function of the brain there are numerous variables that one would like to measure, depending upon the problem

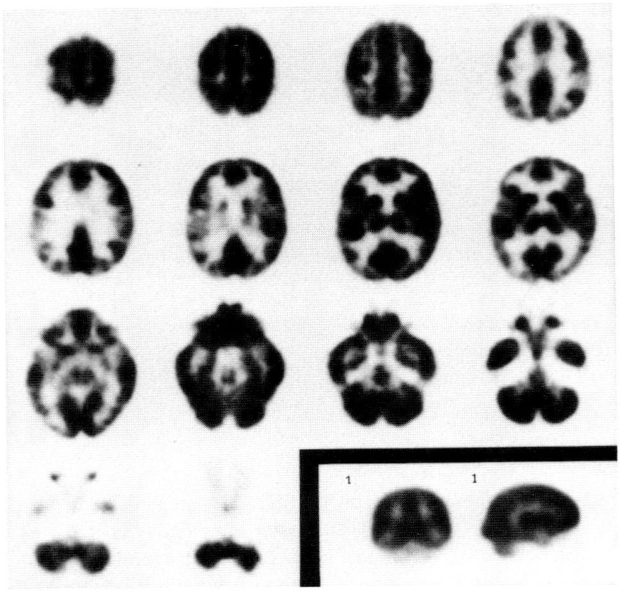

Fig. 8. Complete set of FDG-PET images from a normal subject, demonstrating LCMRGlc. These images were obtained at 8-mm intervals parallel to the canthomeatal plane with the NeuroECAT (fig. 3) system (image spatial resolution of 8.4 × 8.4 × 12.5 mm). The two images in the lower right corner are anterior-posterior and lateral two-dimensional views (rectilinear studies) of the same subject obtained prior to the tomographic examination. The NeuroECAT provides identification of the position of the tomographic planes, and superimposes their location on the rectilinear images. These features and the tilting capability of the gantry allow for orienting the head in the true axial plane and selecting appropriate tomographic levels. Gray scale is in units of $\mu mol \cdot min^{-1} \cdot g^{-1}$ with black representing the highest value. At this spatial resolution, the folds in the cortical ribbon are clearly delineated, as are the subcortical structures including the thalamus, caudate, and the lenticular nuclei (putamen-globus pallidus complex). Both the posterior and anterior limbs of the internal capsule are visualized. Substructures of the posterior fossa are visible and include the brainstem and the substructures of the cerebellum, such as the cerebellar cortex, vermis, and dentate nuclei. From Phelps et al. [1982].

under study. The primary variables of interest studied thus far with PET include local cerebral blood flow (LCBF), oxygen ($LCMRO_2$) and glucose (LCMRGlc) metabolism, since they normally form the supply/demand basis of local function in the brain. That is to say, under normal conditions glucose and oxygen metabolism are related by a constant stoichiometric (i.e. the numerical relationship between chemical processes) relationship

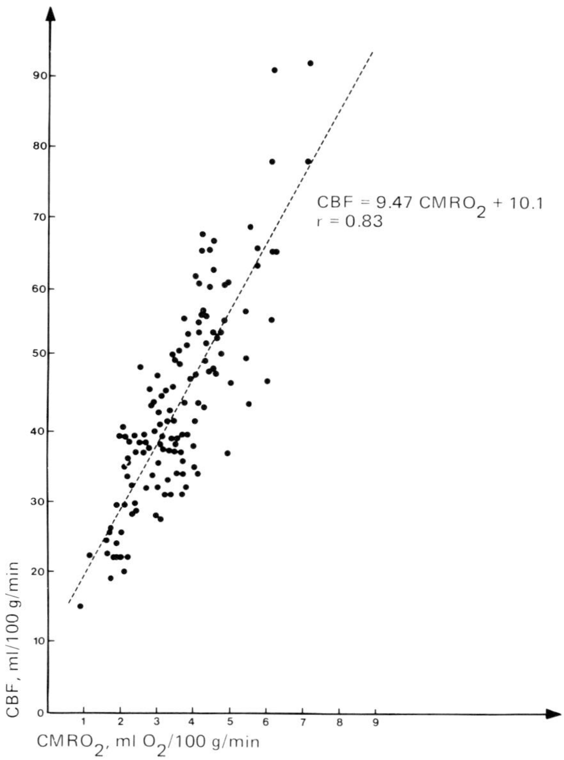

Fig. 9. Plot of local CBF versus $CMRO_2$ in 131 brain regions in 19 control studies, showing the constant relationship between CBF and $CMRO^2$ across a wide range of values. From Baron [1983].

and blood flow is determined by metabolic demand (i.e. metabolic regulation of flow or flow-metabolism coupling). This relationship is found to be true on a local level using PET to measure CBF and $CMRO_2$ in normocapnic and normotensive young volunteers (fig. 9). A similar type coupling has been found between blood flow and glucose metabolism in young normal individuals. This confirms in humans the expected flow-glucose metabolic coupling which has been demonstrated in rats using autoradiography. While these expected stoichiometric relationships in normals have been consistently found with PET, these relationships are altered in human disease processes.

The tight coupling between flow, oxygen and glucose metabolism represents an important normal interrelationship of the brain which is subject to derangement in pathologic states. As will be seen below, in the discussion on pathological states, combined measurement of these variables is a sensitive indicator of pathophysiological alterations in brain function. The local interrelationships between flow, metabolism, protein synthesis, tissue pH and other PET-measurable variables are yet to be defined but are expected to add further dimensions to the understanding of the complex interrelationships that produce cerebral biochemical and hemodynamic homeostasis.

Normal Subjects Studied during Sensory and Motor Stimulation

There are a number of reasons for performing behavioral activation studies in normal populations with PET. First, sensory, motor and cognitive studies with PET are able to map the cortical and subcortical extent of specific cerebral processes using truly physiological tasks and appropriate stimulation paradigms. Such studies allow, for the the first time in humans, local three-dimensional examination of the functional organization of the brain in response to such stimuli.

Second, through a comprehensive investigation of such tasks in normal populations, sets of paradigms will be developed which predictably activate cortical and subcortical brain regions. These paradigms can then be used in patient populations to unmask more subtle alterations in metabolism, flow or other physiological variables that might go undetected in simple resting PET imaging sessions. The use of such provocative behavioral stimuli, and potentially the use of pharmacological stimuli as well, can enhance the diagnostic specificity and anatomical localization of functional lesions in patients with various forms of neuropathology.

Third, stimulation paradigms can be used to study the recovery of brain function following cerebral injury. Such studies should not only provide insights into the fundamental processes of cerebral reorganization after injury, but can also potentially provide guidelines for the pathophysiologically oriented rehabilitation of such brain-injured individuals.

Studies of the human visual system have been performed with PET to measure glucose metabolism (fig. 10–12) and CBF. These studies provided the first local information on the human visual system's stimulus-metabolic

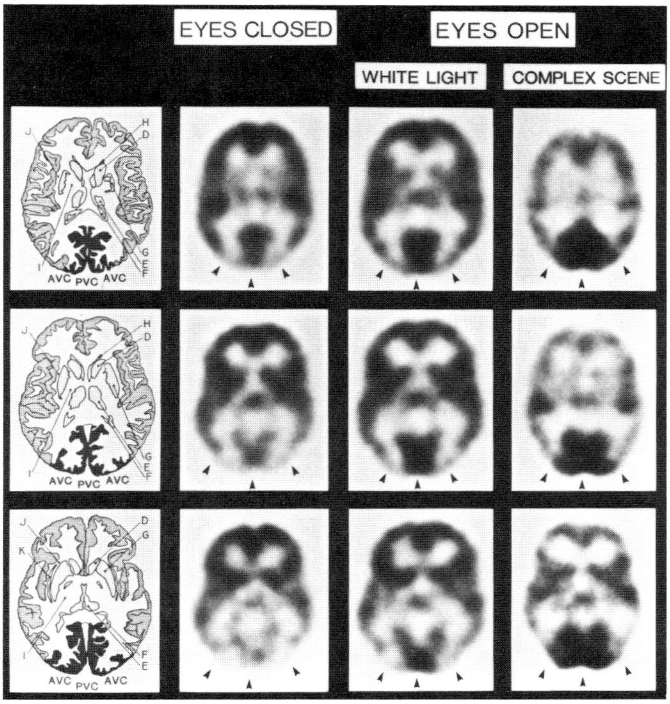

Fig. 10. Example of the use of PET and FDG to measure stimulated responses of the human visual cortex. Top and bottom rows of images are 3.6 and 4.4 and above the orbitomeatal plane, respectively. In an 'eyes closed' study the subject is blindfolded. In the 'eyes open' study, the subject is observing a plain white light source (570 lux), while in the 'complex scene', the subject is viewing an outdoor scene. The primary visual cortex (PVC) is seen in the midline of the occipital lobes (arrows) and the associative visual cortex (AVC) on the dorsolateral surface of the occipital lobes (arrows), bilaterally. Note increased LCMRGlc from eyes closed to open with major response in PVC while in the complex scene there is not only a further increase of LCMRGlc of PVC but spread of activity involving the AVC. From Phelps et al. [1981b].

response characteristics. This characterization includes: (1) glucose metabolism varies in magnitude and spatial distribution with the stimulus complexity; (2) equal cortical functional inputs from each eye are received by both visual cortices; (3) predictable retinal-cortical topographic representations can be identified, and (4) CBF varies (i.e. increases, peaks and declines) as a function of stimulus frequency.

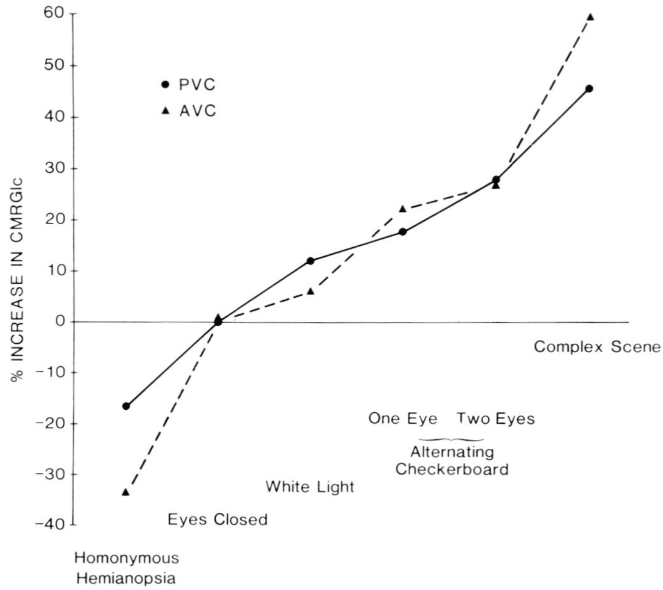

Fig. 11. Graph of percent change in LCMRGlc as a function of visual input. Zero line represents the normal eyes-closed (ears open) control state. Notice the progressive increase in glucose utilization and functional activity of the visual cortex with increasing complexity of visual stimulation. Lesions in the lateral geniculate and/or optic radiations (i.e. not in the visual cortex), which produce homonymous hemianopsia, cause relative decreases in the activity of the visual cortex below the values obtained in the eyes-closed state of normal individuals. Note also that the higher order, associative visual cortex (AVC) increases at a greater rate as scene complexity increases when compared to the primary visual cortex (PVC). Data for each segmental increase are significant ($p<0.05$ for white light to one-eye, and one-eye to two-eye checkerboard stimulation; $p<0.01$ for the others for the PVC; and $p<0.01$ for AVC), except for the AVC between one- and two-eye stimulations, which are not significantly different. From Phelps et al. [1981b].

In studies of patients with lesions of the visual pathway (optic radiations, thalamus, optic nerve) but in whom the visual cortex itself was structurally intact (by X-ray CT), functional LCMRGlc deficits in the visual cortex have been demonstrated. A subject with a seizure focus in his visual cortex was studied with PET. Clinically he had a left half field defect interictally and reduced glucose metabolism in the contralateral right visual cortex (fig. 12). Ictally, visual hallucinations occurred and large increases (1.7–2.5 times the contralateral side) in glucose metabolism of the affected

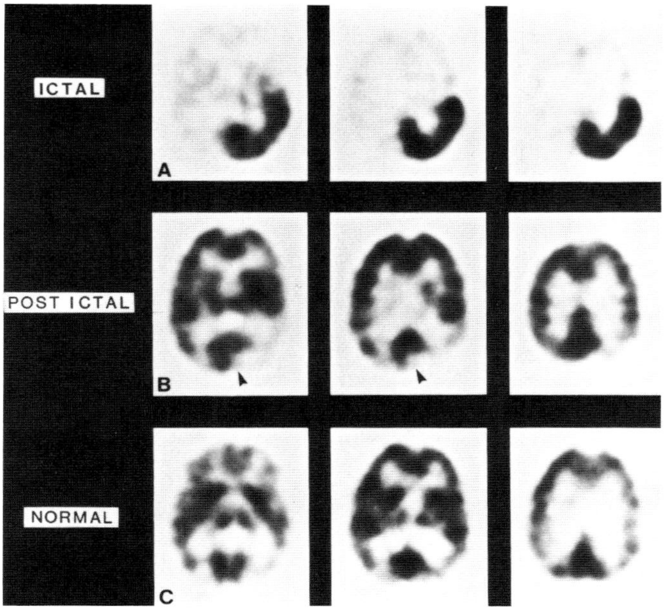

Fig. 12. Selected tomographic sections from three FDG-PET scans of a patient with complex partial seizures and a lesion in the right occipital lobe (same patient as in fig. 15e). Seizures began with visual hallucinations in the left superior quadrant, followed by loss of consciousness and automatisms. Ictal EEG discharges originated in the right occipital lobe and quickly spread to the temporal lobe. *a* The ictal scan demonstrates hypermetabolism in the right occipital and temporal lobes, with profound hypometabolism in the remainder of the brain. *b* One month following an episode of partial status epilepticus there was persistent hypometabolism of the right occipital and temporal lobes, including the calcarine cortex (arrows); a pattern that is metabolically reversed from that seen in *a*. During this time the patient had a left homonymous hemianopsia (i.e. loss of vision in left visual field). *c* This scan was obtained one year following the scan in *b*. The patient remained seizure free. Minimal hypometabolism is still seen at the right occipitotemporal junction and the right visual cortex is now normal. This corresponded to the clinical resolution of the left visual field deficit. X-ray CT was normal. These studies demonstrate a prolonged focal postictal hypometabolism, associated with a clinical deficit, both of which were reversible. In addition, this study serves as an example of changing LCMRGlc that corresponds to behavioral changes with no alterations in the X-ray CT study. From Engel et al. [1983b].

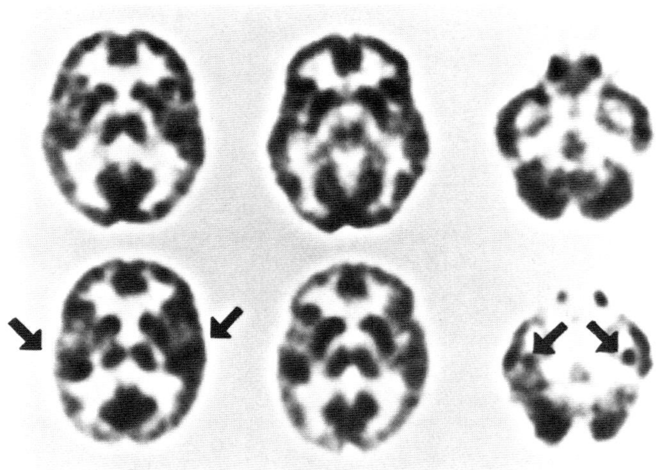

Fig. 13. Two sets of images from 2 normal subjects studied with FDG to determine glucose metabolism in a control (top row) and auditory-stimulated state (bottom row). The top row of images was obtained from a subject with no auditory stimulation. The bottom row was obtained from a second subject listening to a factual story monaurally. Note the activation of the primary auditory cortex situated bilaterally in the posterior transverse, temporal cortical zone. The left-right asymmetries closely parallel known anatomical asymmetries for these areas in the human brain (i.e. the region on the left is larger, wedge-shaped, and more posterior than its counterpart on the right). Note also the lowest hippocampus during the verbal task: The subject was instructed to remember specific phrases of the auditory stimulus material (a Sherlock Holmes story) and told that he would be paid in proportion to his performance on an examination following the stimulation task. From Mazziotta et al. [1982].

visual cortex were found for the same areas which were hypometabolic interictally (fig. 12). These and other studies have demonstrated excellent clinical-PET correlations of visual pathway lesions both within and outside the visual cortex.

The human auditory system has been examined with PET and these studies indicate a correlation between the distribution of glucose utilization and the content of the stimulus and, in some cases, the strategy used by the subject to solve the task. While complex patterns of responses to auditory stimuli were observed, verbal stimuli caused asymmetric increases in glucose utilization in the left hemisphere in right-handed individuals. Nonverbal stimuli, such as chords, activated primarily right hemisphere areas particularly in the inferior frontal, parietal, and superior temporal regions. In subjects who listened to sequences of notes and were asked to determine whether notes in one sequence differed from those in another, the pattern of glucose utilization correlated with the strategy used by the subject. Individuals who used specific visual imagery and analytic strategies ('visualizing' frequency histograms or musical scales in their minds) had predominantly left hemisphere asymmetries and increases in glucose utilization in the posterior temporal region. Subjects who did not use a visual strategy to solve the task but rather used mental 'resigning' of the notes had activations in the inferior parietal regions of the right hemisphere. In addition, subjects who were asked to recall specific aspects of auditory stimuli had activations of the mesial temporal lobe (hippocampus, parahippocampus) that were never seen in situations where auditory perception without memory tasks were required (fig. 13).

Somatosensory and motor task paradigms have also been performed with PET and have demonstrated the wide range and complexity of functional responses that the human brain generates in processing and interpreting such information.

Through a comprehensive investigation of tasks such as these in normal populations, sets of paradigms will be developed which predictively activate cortical and subcortical brain regions. These paradigms can then be used in patient populations to unmask more subtle alterations in physiological variables that might go undetected in simple resting PET studies. The use of such provocative behavioral, and potentially pharmacological, stimuli can enhance the diagnostic specificity and anatomical localization of functional lesions thus far disclosed by PET in patients with various forms of neuropathology. Studies designed to examine the uniquely human characteristics of language, cognition and emotion are in the process of development at the present time.

Patient Studies

As will be seen in the sections that follow, the ability to make funtional measurements of physiologic, biochemical and hemodynamic processes allows for an earlier and significantly more comprehensive perspective on pathological processes that affect the brain than can be obtained from structural information above. All neuropathologic states affect or are caused by changes in cerebral biochemistry. In general, subtle alterations in these processes preceded structural changes which are detectable by more

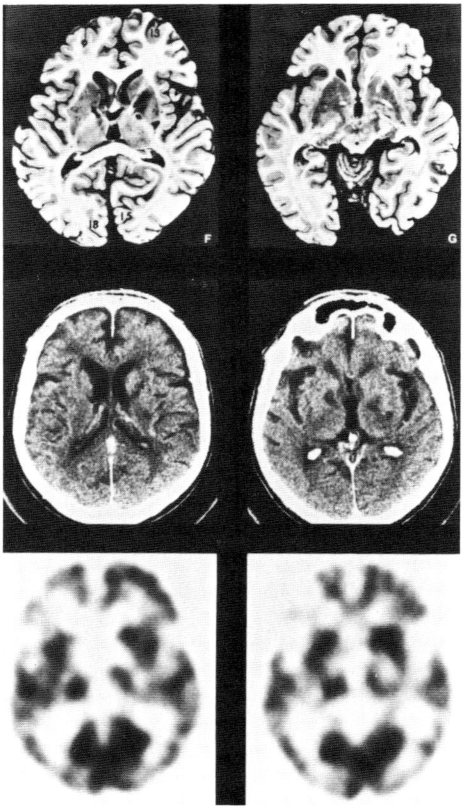

Fig. 14. Structural versus functional anatomy. Images obtained with 3 different methods from a patient with multiple infarct dementia. Patient had X-ray CT (center row) and PET studies of glucose utilization with FDG (bottom row) on the same day. Seven days later patient died of nonneurological causes and gross and microscopic evaluation of the brain (top row) was performed. Both forms of stuctural imaging (X-ray CT and postmortem) and the metabolic study with PET demonstrated multiple small infarctions of deep structures of the brain (striatum, thalamus and internal capsule). Neither structural imaging techniques demonstrated abnormalities of the cortex. PET, however, demonstrated widespread abnormalities of frontal cortex particularly on the left. These distant effects probably represent disruption of afferent and efferent fiber systems between the frontal cortical areas and subcortical zones, most likely resulting from small subcortical infarcts seen structurally and metabolically. From Metter et al. [1985].

conventional radiological approaches. The measurement of the biochemical process, therefore, should allow for earlier detection of these processes and a better understanding of their fundamental mechanisms.

Examples already demonstrate the ability of PET to identify functional abnormalities that are greater in anatomic extent and are seen earlier than structural abnormalities imaged with CT or MRI (fig. 14). In general, functional lesions identified with PET are greater in extent and magnitude than those seen structurally with techniques such as X-ray CT. This more comprehensive view of cerebral pathophysiology, when correlated with behavioral determinations of the patient's signs and symptoms, should provide a better understanding of structure-function relationships in the brain in both health and disease.

Seizure Disorders

PET has been employed to define the three-dimensional distribution and magnitude of local abnormalities in CBF and metabolism in patients with epilepsy. These measurements have been obtained in both ictal and interictal states to examine partial and generalized seizures in combination with surface and depth EEG, pathological and clinical data. The results provide evidence that PET and EEG identify different aspects of cerebral function and can be used in combination to complement one another and to examine the neuroanatomical basis of human and experimental epileptic disorders. Thus far, these studies have realized two important goals: (1) to identify interictal, ictal and postictal patterns of metabolic anatomy in epileptic conditions that could aid in clinical diagnosis and perhaps reveal which structures are responsible for specific epileptiform events, and (2) to improve the accuracy of localization of the epileptogenic lesion in patients with intractable partial epilepsy who are candidates for surgical therapy.

Patients with partial epilepsy whose seizures originate in the temporal lobe have been studied most extensively with PET and FDG to determine cerebral glucose metabolism. Approximately 70% of these patients have demonstrated one or more zones of hypometabolism on interictal scans (fig. 15). The site, size and shape of the hypometabolic region varies from patient to patient. Typically this zone of hypometabolism is large, encompassing the entire temporal lobe (lateral as well as medial) (fig. 15) and may include areas of the frontal and parietal cortex as well. Similar patterns have also been described for $LCMRO_2$ and CBF determinations.

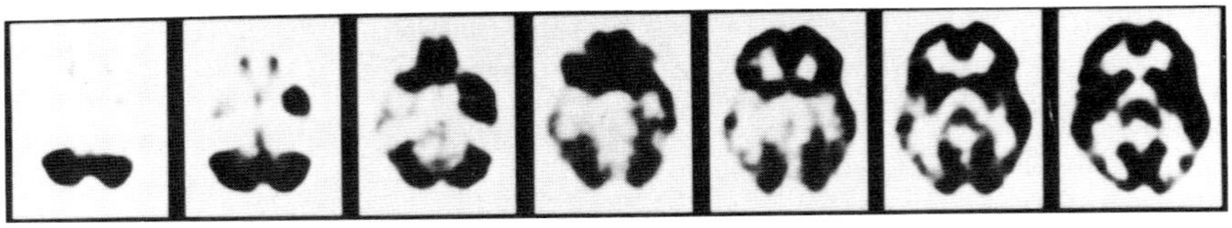

Fig. 15. Seven consecutive transverse interictal FDG-PET images from a patient with complex partial seizures that began electrographically in the left mesial temporal lobe. X-ray CT scan was normal. This image set demonstrates hypometabolism of the entire left temporal lobe which can be seen on every plane that passes through this structure. To be significant, focal hypometabolism must be present on two or more adjacent planes to rule out artifacts due to angulation errors in the plane of section, or normal variation in anatomy. The patient underwent a left anterior temporal lobectomy and was found to have hippocampal sclerosis. From Engel et al. [1983a].

Interictal hypometabolism associated with partial epilepsy has been studied in relation to electrophysiological (EEG) data. Thus far, no correlation has been found between the frequency of interictal spikes and the degree of hypometabolism found in the PET images. While quantitation of these electrophysiological measures has largely failed to correlate with quantitative abnormalities of glucose metabolism, anatomical localization criteria determined by the two techniques demonstrates good and complementary results. These results indicate that both PET and EEG are good localizers of epileptic activity and should be considered complementary rather than redundant. PET can aid in the localization process when the EEG findings are inconsistent, thus allowing patients access to surgery who might have otherwise been disqualified. The EEG can be utilized to verify the epileptogenic nature of a PET-identified zone of hypometabolism.

The correlation between hypometabolic zones of glucose metabolism demonstrated by PET and pathologic lesions identified in surgically resected brain specimens has been excellent. In the first 25 patients thus far reported following both studies, lesions were identified in 19 by histologic examination. There was an excellent correlation between the site of the hypometabolism and the presence of a pathologic abnormality in the surgical specimens. Of interest is the fact that the hypometabolic zone identified in the PET images was consistently larger than the lesions identified in the surgical specimens. This discrepancy may be due to ultrastructural abnormalities (e.g. decreased cell processes or synaptic densities) not identified in typical light microscopic examination of the

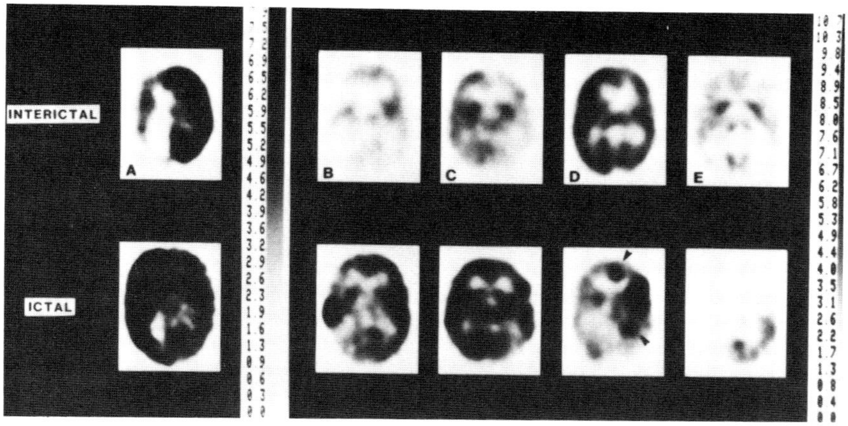

Fig. 16. Representative planes of section of interictal (top row) and ictal (bottom row) FDG scans from five patients with partial seizures. Scales in this and figure 17 indicate the calculated local cerebral metabolic rate for glucose in $mg \cdot min^{-1} \cdot 100 g^{-1}$. Scans *B–E* are all displayed using the same scale, chosen to best illustrate values for maximal ictal activation. Scan *A* is scaled differently as a result of the limited photographic range available to illustrate the data. X-ray CT scans were abnormal for patient *A*, who had left-hemisphere atrophy, and patient *E*, who had a small right occipital glioma. *A* Ictal activation of the entire left hemisphere occurred with nine seizures that originated electrically in the left parietal area and clinically spread to involve both sides of the body, the right side more than the left. *B* Selective ictal hypermetabolism of the left perisylvian area occurred within a larger zone that had been hypometabolic interictally. Seven seizures occurred during the ictal state that were confined electrographically to left temporal and central electrodes and behaviorally to the right arm and face. A second ictal scan (not shown) in this patient demonstrated the same pattern. *C* Hypermetabolism of the entire brain – prominent in the right precentral area, which was hypometabolic interictally – accompanied epilepsia partialis continua involving the left leg and arm. The ictal EEG contained no localizing abnormalities. *D* Seven complex partial seizures manifested by twitching of the left side of the mouth and head, and eye turning to the left were associated with increased metabolic activity in right temporal and frontal structures, including discrete activation of hippocampus and cingulate cortex (arrows) and decreased metabolic activity elswhere. *E* Three seizures that originated in the right occiput and spread into the right temporal lobe. These episodes began with visual auras in the left visual field progressing to complex partial symptomatology. This was associated with hypermetabolism of the right occipital and temporal lobes and hypometabolism elsewhere (see fig. 12 for details). From Engel et al. [1982].

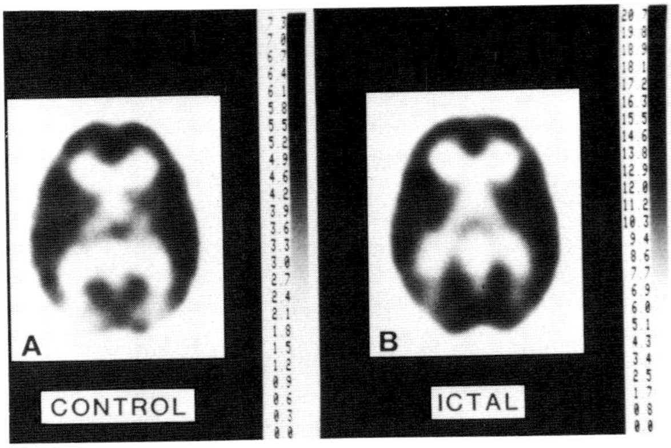

Fig. 17. Representative sections from two FDG scans of a patient with petit mal absences. *A* Control study obtained several months following successful treatment, during 10 min of hyperventilation when no absences occured. *B* Ictal study obtained before treatment was instituted, during 10min of hyperventilation when absences were frequent. Note that the gray scales (as in fig. 15 in $mg \cdot min^{-1} \cdot 100g^{-1}$) are different for the two studies and that, although the patterns are identical, the ictal study demonstrates a global threefold increase in estimated metabolic rate. From Engel et al. [1982].

tissue. Studies are presently under way with electron microscopy to determine if this is the case. Failure to demonstrate such an abnormality would mean that the lesion size discrepancy is due to functional causes. It seems likely that this is at least in part true. The fact that hypometabolic zones are capable of substantial hypermetabolism during ictal PET studies (fig. 12, 16) and that they may be reversible following nonablative surgical procedures, provides inferential evidence for the functional hypothesis.

Ictal studies have been performed with FDG and PET. However, the deoxyglucose method requires steady-state conditions for the accurate determination of absolute metabolic rates. For this reason, the standard technique can only be used in a qualified fashion in conditions where large transient changes in glucose utilization occur for time periods substantially less than 40 min. Despite these problems, patterns of cerebral metabolic anatomy have been obtained using these techniques. As demonstrated in figure 16, ictal studies of glucose metabolism in patients during seizures demonstrate relative increases in metabolism compared to both the interictal state in the same patient and to control values in normal populations. The pattern and distribution is quite varied. These can include patterns that are either global, hemispheric, multifocal, lobar or focal (fig. 16).

The great individual variability in the metabolic patterns of ictal phenomena, combined with methodological problems of the deoxyglucose method, makes it unlikely that FDG-PET studies of partial seizures can be reliably used to localize the site of an epileptogenic lesion. Present strategies employ only the use of the interictal sudies for determination of the seizure focus and as a criterion for selection of candidates for surgical therapy.

In contrast to partial seizures where focal brain regions have demonstrated ictal and interictal glucose metabolic changes, generalized seizures (petit mal and electroshock-induced generalized tonic clonic convulsions) show global, generalized changes in glucose metabolism (fig. 17).

Future PET studies in patients with epilepsy will undoubtedly include the addition of behavioral or pharmacological stimuli to serve as provocative maneuvers. Additionally, a number of agents relevant to studies of patients with epilepsy have already been labeled with positron-emitting isotopes. The list of such compounds includes: ^{11}C-flunitrazepan, ^{11}C-pimozide, ^{18}F-spiperone, ^{11}C-methylspiperone, ^{11}C-carfentanil, ^{11}C-valproic acid and ^{11}C-diphenylhydantoin (see table II). Such compounds provide the opportunity to study local neurochemistry in epileptic foci as well as in distant sites in patients with seizure disorders.

Cerebrovascular Disease

To understand the complex interrelationships that occur during cerebral ischemia and stroke one needs to examine the interactions between blood flow, metabolism and other physiological variables as a function of the site of injury, the time course of the injury and the etiology of the ischemia. PET has already demonstrated its ability to provide this sort of information. Knowledge of these pathophysiological states for specific stroke syndromes in individual patients, both as a function of time and in relation to clinical phenomena pertaining to outcome, provides the best opportunity for understanding the mechanisms that underly stroke. Most importantly, such data are critical to the design of specific therapies for the amelioration of irreversible cerebral injury due to perfusion insufficiencies.

Initial PET studies using ^{15}O-labeled compounds to measure CBF, oxygen utilization and extraction were performed at relatively late times ($\geq$3 days) after the stroke ictus. A number of generalizations can be made about these initial studies. First, all demonstrated a reduction in oxygen

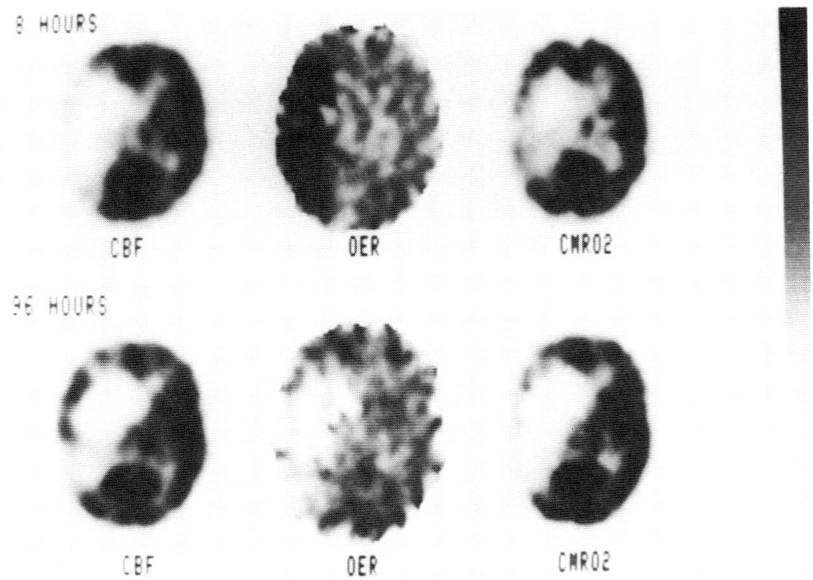

Fig. 18. Critical perfusion and luxury perfusion. The figure demonstrates the transition from a high oxygen extraction (OER) in the lesion early (8h) after the onset of symptoms from ischemia to low oxygen extraction accompanied by low oxygen consumption ($CMRO_2$) at a later (96h) stage in the same patient. Note the greater severity of the changes in the sucortical structures supplied by deep penetrating end arteries. There was no clinical change between the measurements. From Frackowiak and Wise [1983].

utilization in tissue that was ultimately to demonstrate completed infarction by diminished attenuation values on X-ray CT. Second, perfusion was typically in excess of oxygen requirements for the tissue and resulted in uniformly decreased oxygen extraction fractions in these late cases. Third, CBF was typically in excess of metabolic needs and was quite variable. Flow values were found to be high, low and normal in the area of ultimate infarction. In addition, the pattern of flow abnormalities was heterogeneous within the area of ultimate infarction.

These studies, performed at late times, suggested that oxygen utilization and extraction fractions were more reliable predictors of ultimate tissue outcome than blood flow and that a threshold value for tissue viability could be determined. An initial threshold value of 58 μmol $O_2 \cdot min^{-1} \cdot 100\,g^{-1}$ for oxygen utilization was found to predict a poor clinical outcome and presumed nonviabilitiy of tissue. Low oxygen utilization with severly reduced oxygen extraction is representative of cell death. The high variability of flow values has been attributed by various investigators, depending on the time course of its appearance, to derangements in vascular autoregulation, capillary hyperplasia and post-infarct reperfusion.

An important observation was made in patients studied at times earlier than 3 days after the stroke ictus. This observation was an increased oxygen extraction or 'critical' perfusion (fig. 18). In patients studied less than 12h after the onset of symptoms, all but one had increased oxygen extraction fractions. Twelve of 14 patients studied at 24 h or more after symptoms, however, had decreased oxygen extraction fractions (fig. 18). In follow-up studies, 8 of 9 patients had decreases in oxygen extraction fractions between the first and second study. The typical time for this transition was between 12 and 24 h after the onset of symptoms. The change in extraction fraction was more commonly due to an increase in blood flow but in some cases was attributed to a combined decrease in flow and oxygen utilization, the reduction of the latter process being greater. Such studies demonstrate that: (1) luxury perfusion (blood flow in excess of metabolic needs) can occur with high, low or normal absolute values of CBF; (2) increases in oxygen extraction are relatively short in duration; (3) changes in oxidative metabolism are reversible (no improvement in oxygen utilization was ever observed), and (4) the drop in oxygen extraction fraction with time may reflect tissue reperfusion, further decreases in oxygen utilization, or both.

All of the patients in the studies described above had persistent symptoms and ultimately had completed infarctions. More recent studies have examined patients with less severe cerebral ischemia to determine a relationship between blood volume, oxygen utilization and blood flow. In these patients, a change in the normal flow-volume ratio occurred. While normal individuals, on average, have a value of 10.2 ± 0.9 for this ratio, patients with carotid occlusions have reductions in the ratio and a mean value of 6.9 ± 1.4 for the hemisphere ipsilateral to the occlusion (fig. 19). It was observed that the oxygen extraction fraction would start to decrease when this ratio dropped below the value of 5.5.

Combining all these data one arrives at a hypothetical temporal sequence of flow, blood volume, oxygen extraction and utilization relationships. Initially, when perfusion pressure to the brain is reduced the patient remains symptom-free due to compensatory mechanisms (vasodilatation) (fig. 19). Oxygen extraction and utilization remain normal. Further reductions in cerebral perfusion initiate a secondary reserve mechanism, that of

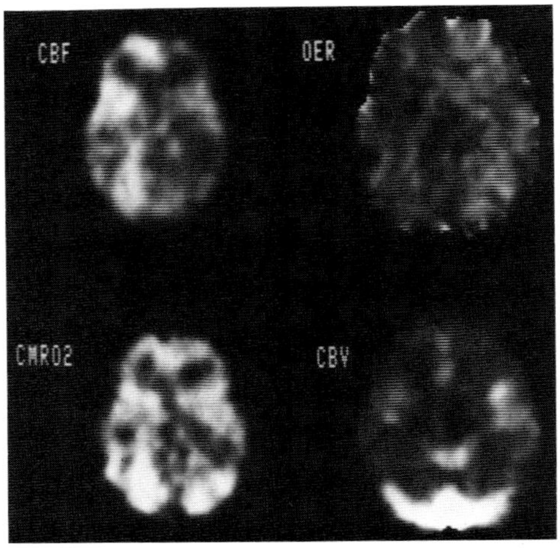

Fig. 19. Chronically diminished perfusion reserve in this patient with a unilateral complete carotid occlusion. The ipsilateral (right) hemisphere shows a lower bood flow (–26%) but a higher oxygen extraction (+30%) and a similar oxygen consumption (–2%) compared with the contralateral side. This is accompanied by an increase in the cerebral blood volume (CBV) of the affected side (+24%), indicating compensatory vasodilation. From Frackowiak and Wise [1983].

further desaturation of arterial blood with a resultant increase in oxygen extraction fraction (fig. 18). Initial data indicate that this should occur when the flow/volume ratio is reduced below 5.5. At this point local increases in blood volume and extraction fraction with reduced flow and normal oxygen utilization have been found. Further reductions in brain perfusion exceed the reserve systems of the brain to meet metabolic demands, oxygen utilization drops and then symptoms begin. This condition, which fulfills the criteria for ischemia, will occur in proportion to the severity and duration of the perfusion limitation. Imaging during this period reveals increased oxygen extraction fractions and decreased oxygen utilization. If the severity and duration of these events is such that irreversible tissue damage occurs, the oxygen extraction fraction will drop, typically at around 24 h after the initial insult, and blood flow assumes the more variable pattern described above. At this point oxygen utilization and extraction are low and their site predicts the ultimate structural tissue damage that will be identified with X-ray CT. While still speculative, the presently available PET data make this a plausible working hypothesis for the sequence of pathophysiological events which occur as a consequence of progressive cerebral perfusion reductions. As discussed below, the addition of information about glucose utilization, pH and other variables are needed to further understand the full pathophysiological temporal sequence of events that occur to produce ischemic brain infarction. One should keep in mind that cerebrovascular disease is not a single entity in terms of its nature or time course. Therefore, many different descriptions of these heterogeneous pathophysiological events will undoubtedly emerge with further PET investigations.

Such data can be used to classify patients into treatment categories. Patients with low blood flow and mild reductions in oxygen utilization would represent individuals with viable but ischemic tissue who might benefit from increased perfusion. Such candidates would be selected for endarterectomy or extracranial-intracranial bypass procedures (fig. 20). Patients with intermediate reductions in oxygen utilization, having viable though metabolically damaged brain tissue, might benefit from maneuvers designed to minimize cerebral metabolic demands. On the other hand, patients with profound decreases in oxygen utilization and extraction fractions, below threshold values for viability, would only be candidates for more conservative therapy. Following classification, follow-up PET studies could monitor the effects of these attempted interventions (fig. 20).

Cerebral Neoplasms

Considerable data are available about the metabolism of cerebral tumors as measured with PET. These studies have added to the anatomical data on human primary cerebral neoplasms obtained from cerebral angiography, pneumoencephalography, and X-ray CT. Anatomically based radiological techniques have provided substantial information about cerebral gliomas but can be inconclusive in the detection of early tumors, discrimination of tumor from edema, histologic grading of tumors and in differentiating tumor recurrence from radiation necrosis. Prompted by a positive correlation between the degree of malignancy and glycolysis, PET studies at the National Institutes of Health in the USA have studied this relationship in human gliomas using FDG and PET to measure cerebral glucose metabolic rates.

When tumor tissue makes a transition from well-differentiated slow-growing conditions to poorly differentiated and rapid growing states, glycolytic rates increase. This change in glycolytic rate is associated with

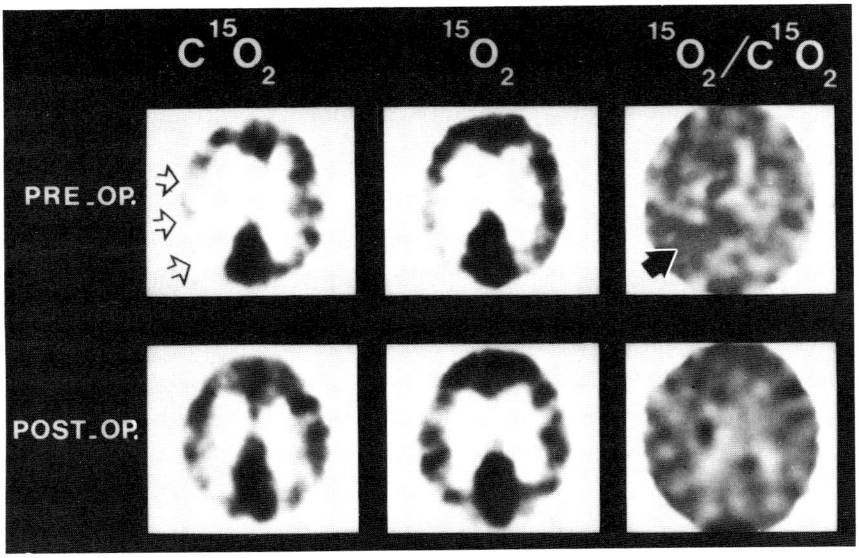

a

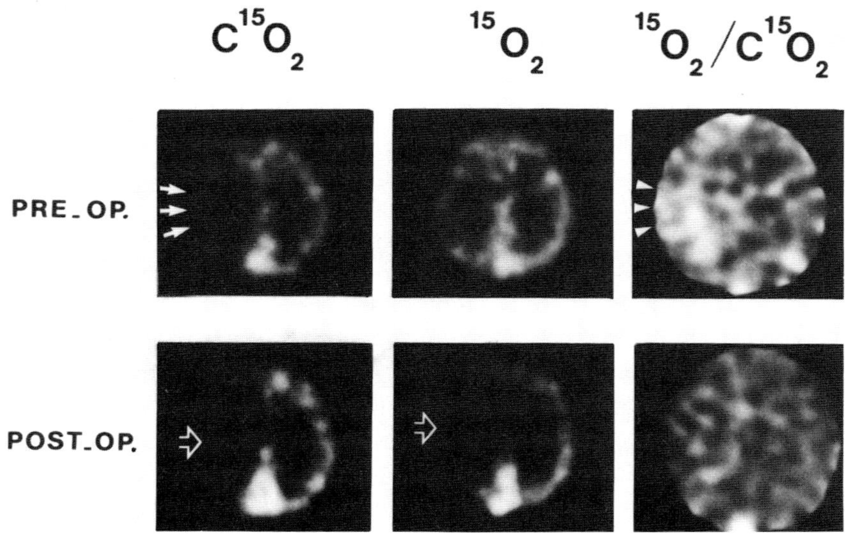

b

Fig. 20. CBF, cerebral metabolic rate for oxygen and oxygen extraction in 2 patients studied before and after extracranial-intercranial (EC-IC) bypass. *a* Preoperative studies in a patient with a left internal carotid occlusion and focal transient ischemic attacks. Preoperative PET study showed diminished CBF in a region corresponding to the patient's clinical symptoms. There was a mild decrease in oxygen metabolism and an increased oxygen extraction fraction consistent with viable though jeopardized tissue. After bypass surgery (postoperative) all variables measured by PET returned to normal and the transient ischemic

a shift away from oxidative metabolism and towards the glycolytic pathway, even though oxygen availability is adequate. This hypothesis predicted that human PET studies would find evidence of high glucose metabolism in the core of tumors which were poorly differentiated and rapidly growing. This hypothesis was substantiated and a remarkable correlation between metabolic rate and histologic rate of gliomas has been found. The most consistent finding is the appearance of 'hot spots' of hypermetabolism in virtually all grade three and four gliomas. These areas of hypermetabolism have only rarely been identified in low-grade tumors (I, II). In fact, investigators performing these studies are so confident that hypermetabolic regions are only associated with high-grade gliomas that they are awaiting autopsy confirmation of the few possible false-positive low-grade (hypermetabolic) tumor cases. In contrast to the high glucose utilization rates associated with high-grade gliomas, these same patients demonstrate decreases in oxygen extraction fractions and oxygen utilization. These changes occur despite normal blood flow. This discrepancy between flow and oxygen metabolism reflected the marked reduction in oxygen utilization that had been predicted.

Combining all these studies, one concludes that cerebral gliomas have heightened glucose utilization rates despite reduced oxygen utilization. This shift away from oxidative metabolism confirms the prediction of the experimental data which indicated that fast-growing tumors had augmentation of the glycolytic pathway despite adequate oxygen availability. Such data are important in the selection of appropriate radiation or chemotherapeutic regimens for the treatment of such tumors. The use of PET to monitor the effects of these therapeutic modalities while measuring tumor stoichiometry should play a significant role in the future management and understanding of these disorders.

^{11}C-labeled methionine has also been used to evaluate cerebral gliomas. In low-grade tumors with reduced glucose metabolism and limited blood-brain barrier abnormalities, methionine incorporation was increased compared to normal brain. Autopsy confirmation studies in such patients

---

attacks stopped. *b* Patient with identical clinical and angiographic findings as in *a* with decreased blood flow, mild decrease in oxygen utilization and increased oxygen extraction fraction preoperatively. Following EC-IC bypass, patient had a persistent neurologic deficit. Both blood flow and oxygen utilization are reduced further than in the preoperative study. These findings were indicative of infarction. Postoperative angiogram revealed nonpatency of the bypass. From Baron et al. [1981].

has demonstrated that tumor infiltration is consistent with the methionine distributions. Amino acid uptake has also been used to identify (for biopsy placement) the site of low-grade gliomas that have minimal changes in blood-brain barrier permeability or glucose utilization.

An important clinical problem is the differentiation of recurrent tumor from radiation necrosis. Both are attended by a deterioration in clinical status and both may have may similar appearance on X-ray CT imaging. This issue has been studied with combined X-ray CT and PET-FDG measurements. The results indicate that while X-ray CT could not differentiate between the two entities, glucose metabolism was consistently low in areas of radiation necrosis and high in patients with recurrent tumor. This was consistent with experimental data demonstrating that tumor glycolysis decreased following radiation exposure in the range typically given for clinical tumor therapy.

Degenerative Disorders

Conventional neurologic imaging techniques have failed to provide specific insights into the mechanisms underlying dementing processes. Functional PET studies offer new hope in this realm. While most reports thus far concentrate on Alzheimer's disease, data are also available for multi-infarct dementia, Huntington's disease and some uncommon dementing processes.

The data thus far available from PET demonstrate a positive correlation between the severity of dementia and the reductions in glucose or oxygen metabolism in the brain. The PET data may also help to separate patient groups where organic dementias may be clinically confused with pseudodementia (i.e. depression with psychomotor retardation in elderly patients) (fig. 21). This is in contrast to X-ray CT data of brain structure in which consistency is lacking between behavioral disability and X-ray CT measurements of cerebral atrophy. Structural measurements of brain atrophy from X-ray CT in demented patients overlap substantially with atrophy seen in elderly but otherwise normal aged individuals.

CBF, oxygen and glucose utilization have been studied in Alzheimer's disease although no study to date has measured all three variables in the same patient group. These data have demonstrated an inverse relationship between global metabolic rate and the severity of the dementing process. Local abnormalities have been most severe in parietal and temporal cortex, intermediate for frontal cortex and least severe in primary visual, motor,

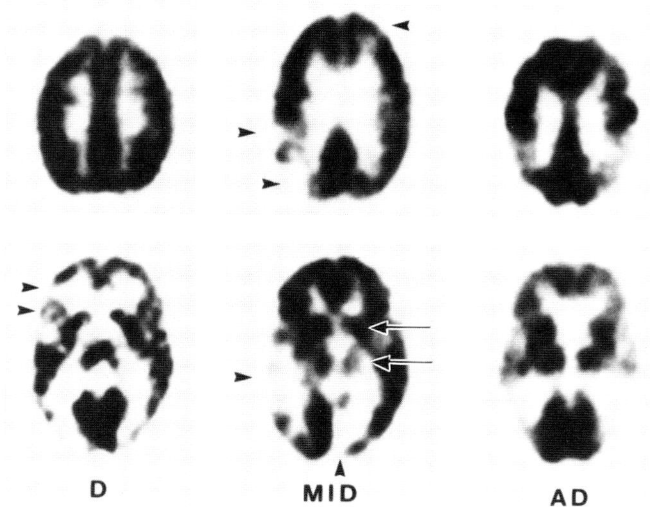

Fig. 21. Differential diagnosis and pathophysiology with PET. Three elderly patients (one in each column) with abnormal glucose utilization. Column D images are from a patient with chronic depression (pseudodementia) who demonstrated decreased glucose utilization (left/right 0.91 + 0.08 versus 1.00 ± 0.05 in controls) of the left inferior frontal cortex (arrows) but was otherwise normal. Images in the column labeled MID are from a patient with multiple infarct dementia demonstrating multiple focal areas of cortical and subcortical decreased glucose utilization (from 17 to 48%) resulting from direct and remote effects of small cerebral infarctions. The column labeled AD is from a patient with moderately severe presumed Alzheimer's disease. Note the extremely low glucose utilization of the posterior parietal (47% decrease), inferior frontal (28% decrease) (bottom image) and temporal cortex (25% decrease) with relative sparing of the primary visual, sensory-motor cortical and subcortical zones (about 12% decrease). Alzheimer's disease patients have also shown an average decrease of global supratentorial glucose utilization (33%), compared to age-matched normal control subjects, with the major abnormalities occurring in neocortical zones. This study demonstrates the differential diagnostic capability of PET to separate patients with processes affecting mental abilities based on pathophysiological patterns observed in the functional images. From Kuhl [1984].

and sensory cortical areas and subcortical zones (fig. 21). The metabolic rates in demented patients are consistently lower than those found in age-matched normal populations.

In appears that there are metabolic correlations with the symptom and sign complex presented by the patient having presumed Alzheimer's disease. Patients have been studied with specific constructional abnormalities, language abnormalities and pure memory disorders. In groups with abnormal spatial and constructional test scores, maximal glucose utilization decreases were found in right cortex (relative to the left side) whereas in patients with specific language abnormalities, the metabolic decrements were more profound in the left frontal-temporal-parietal region. In patients with pure memory abnormalities there was no evidence of left-right metabolic asymmetries. In such patients it has been concluded that focal abnormalities could be identified in the metabolic images which were correlated with predominant clinical symptoms.

Overall, studies of Alzheimer's disease patients with PET have demonstrated global reductions in metabolic rate with maximal bilateral focal metabolic abnormalities in temporal-parietal regions followed by frontal cortical abnormalities and relative sparing of primary sensory-motor cortical and subcortical zones. Patients with multiple infarct dementia have been studied with PET and FDG to measure glucose metabolism and X-ray CT. In one study, 39 cerebral abnormalities were found through the combined use of PET and X-ray CT. In lesions identified by both imaging modalities, metabolic rate reductions averaged 48%. In lesions identified by PET but missed by X-ray CT (n = 24), average metabolic rate reductions were only 17%. Five lesions were detected by X-ray CT but not identified in glucose utilization images. All of these lesions occurred in the white matter and it is uncertain whether they could have been detected with PET using image display parameters more suitable for the visualization of white matter.

The large discrepancy between the number of lesions detected by X-ray CT and PET probably reflects the functional imaging capacity of the latter modality. It is likely that small focal infarcts detected by X-ray CT produce metabolic suppression at distant sites (fig. 14). The distant functional lesions have no stuctural counterpart and therefore would only be demonstrated by PET and not by X-ray CT. In this manner a single structural abnormality evidenced on X-ray CT could have multiple areas of metabolic suppression seen with PET as a result of the multiple efferent projections emanating from the structural abnormality. Better definition of this hypothesis awaits further documentation with combined X-ray CT and PET studies in patients with multiple infarct dementia.

Patients with Huntington's disease have been examined with PET to determine cerebral glucose utilization (fig. 22). In symptomatic patients (age range 17–71 years) who had disease durations of from 1 to 15 years, measures of glucose metabolism as well as X-ray CT indices of atrophy have been examined. These data were compared with age-matched controls.

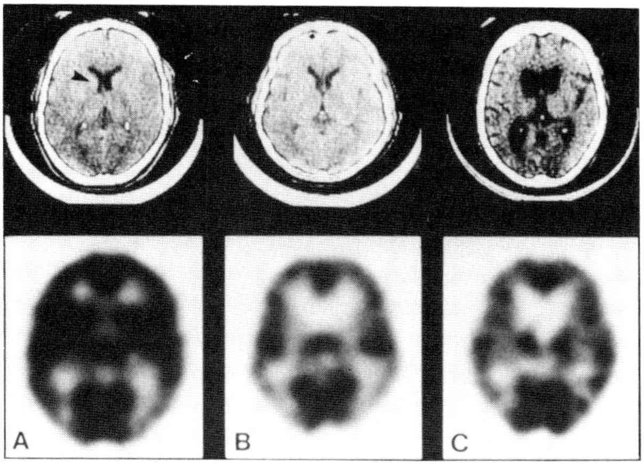

Fig. 22. Atrophy and local cerebral glucose metabolism in Huntington's disease demonstrated by X-ray CT and PET images. All PET images were obtained using FDG for measurement of LCMRGlc. *A* Normal individual demonstrating the structural and metabolic appearance of the normal caudate nucleus and putamen (arrow). *B* Patient with early clinical Huntington's disease, demonstrating the normal structural appearance of the caudate nucleus on X-ray CT but profound hypometabolism of caudate and putamen bilaterally in the PET image. *C* Subject with late Huntington's disease, demonstrating both structural (cortical and subcortical atrophy) and functional abnormalities of the caudate and putamen, bilaterally. Such studies demonstrate that the functional (as measured by LCMRGlc) abnormalities of the basal ganglia in patients with early Huntington's disease precede structural cell loss sufficient to produce changes in the X-ray CT. From Kuhl et al. [1981].

Structurally X-ray CT demonstrated caudate atrophy that paralleled the duration of the disease. Patients with early disease had no X-ray CT abnormalities. However, affected patients had profound caudate hypometabolism for glucose which in cases of longer duration included the putamen as well. Even in those cases with early clinical findings and little or no structural changes on X-ray CT, clear evidence of caudate hypometabolism for glucose was demonstrated (fig. 22). The severity of the choreoathetosis did not correlate with mean cortical or global glucose utilization. In these studies, metabolic dysfunction preceded gross X-ray CT indications of cell loss.

In patients at risk for Huntington's disease, again studied with FDG and PET, X-ray CT scans were consistently normal but metabolic data suggested the possibility that the caudate may be hypometabolic in some asymptomatic at-risk subjects (fig. 23). The data from this at-risk group

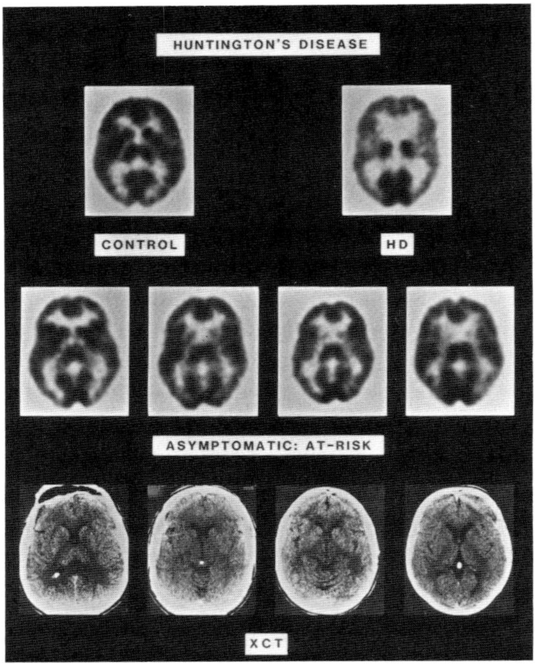

Fig. 23. Subjects at risk for Huntington's disease (HD). Comparison of at-risk subjects with normal controls and symptomatic HD patients. Top row demonstrates a control image at the left and a symptomatic Huntington's patient at the right. Notice the gross hypometabolism in the caudate and lenticular nuclei in the symptomatic patient versus control. Middle and lower rows: Four clinically asymptomatic individuals who are at risk for HD. Bottom row demonstrates their normal X-ray CT studies. Middle row indicates that graded changes can be observed in these patients in the region of the caudate nucleus. The left-most image of the middle row indicates that most of these patients have caudate metabolism indistinguishable from control subjects. However, reductions in caudate metabolism can be mild (left center), moderate (right center), or severe (far right). From Mazziotta et al. [1987].

overlapped with that from normal control populations substantially but the range of variability was nearly twice as large in the at-risk group when metabolic indices of the caudate were compared. Of the 15 at-risk patients originally reported, 3 of the 4 with the most abnormal caudate glucose utilization have now developed symptoms of Huntington's disease. The results of this study may be indicative of metabolic alterations in Huntington's disease that are occurring and can be detected with PET, but are still within the compensatory capacity of the brain in terms of the lack of recognized signs or symptoms. Such a finding would be in keeping with the introductory comments of this chapter where it was proposed that biochemical lesions would provide the earliest opportunity for detecting abnormalities in cerebral disorders.

Psychiatric Disorders

Few cerebral disorders are better suited for study with PET than psychiatric diseases. Despite detailed investigations, no other imaging technique has provided specific insights into the etiology or anatomical locations associated with the many and varied psychiatric syndromes. Many studies have indicated that there are underlying biochemical mechanisms that are affected in these syndromes and result in abnormal states of behavior. The response of patients with these disorders to drug manipulations that correlate with changes in mood and behavior support the pervasive biochemical evidence relating psychological and behavior abnormalities with biochemical mechanims. Nevertheless, techniques used to study these perturbations have done little to specify which neuroanatomical stuctures are involved or the temporal relationship of mood and behavior to biochemical changes in the brain.

Initial PET studies of psychiatric disease focused on small groups of patients. These initial studies used PET and FDG to examine schizophrenic patients. Conflicting information emerged. Most studies indicated a relative decrease in frontal cortex glucose utilization in these patient groups. In addition, there is some evidence that these metabolic rates increased following treatment. The findings, however, could not be confirmed in studies utilizing oxygen-15-labeled compounds to determine cerebral oxygen utilization and blood flow in schizophrenic groups.

Studies have also been performed in patients with affective disorders, including both unipolar depression and bipolar manic-depressive illness (fig. 24). Subjects in these studies were drug-free and the results demonstrated that bipolar depressed patients had global supratentorial glucose metabolic rates which were significantly lower than those found in patients with unipolar depression, hypomania and normal control populations. In rapid cycling (24- to 48-hour cycles) bipolar patients the same pattern was observed during the depressive phase. The same patients, when later studied in hypomanic phases of the illness, showed glucose utilization rates that were not different from normals. Although the major changes seen

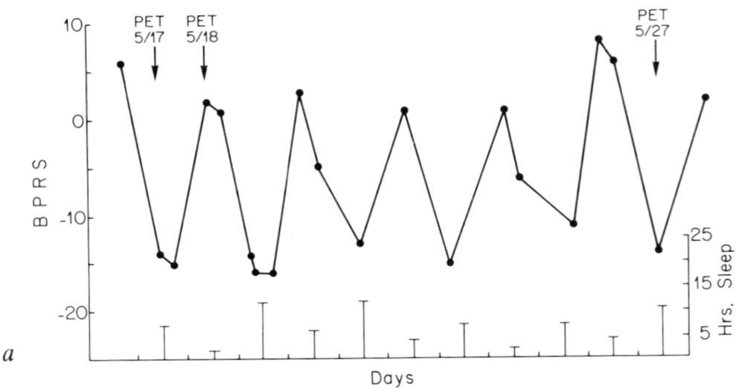

a

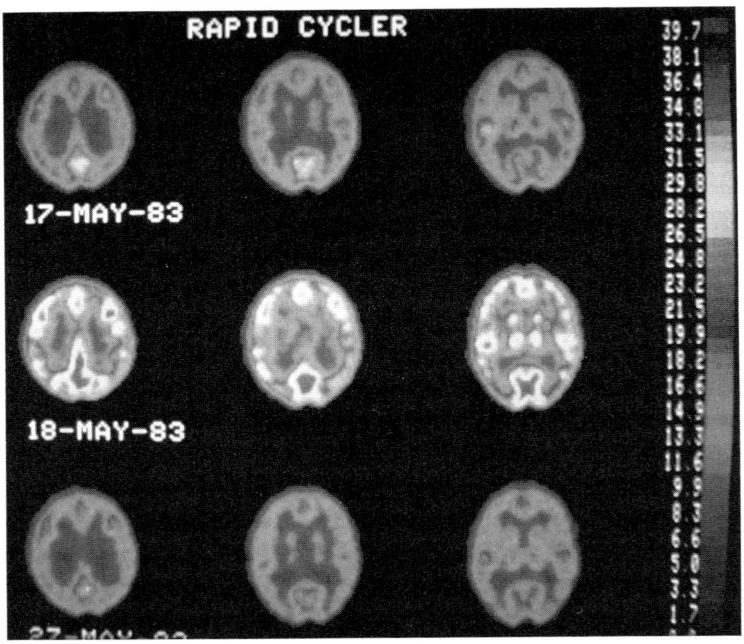

b

Fig. 24. Affective disorders. *a* Graph of the mood fluctuations of a rapid cycling bipolar (manic-depressive) affective disorder patient. The patient cycled between mood states every 24–28h. Brief psychiatric rating scale (BPRS) on the left indicating relative mania (positive values) and relative depression (negative values). Sleep cycles varied in parallel with mood swings. Three studies of cerebral glucose utilization with PET were obtained, two during depressive states and one during hypomania. *b* Glucose utilization images of the rapid cycling bipolar patient described in *a*. Scale to right is glucose utilization rates $\mu mol \cdot min^{-1} \cdot 100 g^{-1}$. Studies on 5-17-83 and 5-27-83 were performed when the patient was in depressed state while

were global, the largest differences occurred in frontal and the anterior cingulate cortices (fig. 24). Patients with unipolar mood disorders (depression) studied in drug-free states demonstrated global supratentorial glucose metabolic rates that were not different from normal controls. However, these patients did exhibit significantly depressed values of glucose utilization in the striata bilaterally. This reduced striatal metabolism recovered to normal levels in patients who became euthymic spontaneously or by drug therapy.

The results of these studies indicate that PET has the ability to demonstrate functional changes in cerebral biochemistry associated with behavioral disorders. The complex behaviors involved, the difficulties in characterizing those behaviors, and the diagnostic difficulties in obtaining both patient and control groups, make these studies formidable endeavors. The use of stimulation paradigms (behavioral or pharmacological) may enhance the specificity and accuracy of such work in the future. In addition, the use of positron-labeled ligands and drugs will provide an additional dimension in the analysis and investigation of these complex and heterogeneous disorders.

Neurotransmitter Systems

The neuropharmacology of the human brain can be examined with PET through the use of two different strategies. In the first, pharmacological doses of drugs can be administered to normal subjects and patients with cerebral disorders and their effect on processes such as blood flow and metabolism can be examined to determine the anatomical sites where drug-induced alterations in biochemical processes occur. Alternately, the drug itself can be labeled with a positron-emitting isotope and its pharmacokinetic behavior can be examined directly in vivo under conditions where the

---

the study on 5-18-83 was during a hypomanic state. Global supratentorial reductions in glucose utilization (relative to the scan obtained during hypomania) can be seen for the two studies obtained in the depressed state. The global increase in glucose utilization from supratentorial levels from depression to hypomania was about 40%. The calculated values of LCMRGlc in the two depressed states agreed within 5%. The global glucose utilization rate in the hypomanic state is not significantly different from that of age-matched normals. These studies demonstrate the ability of PET to provide pathophysiological insights into abnormal behavior that occurs as a manifestation of psychiatric disorders. From Baxter et al. [1985].

drug was present in tracer amounts or in concentrations where the pharmacological effects are produced. Either way, biochemical assays can be performed to examine the pharmacological effects of specific agents on behavior, symptoms and the structure-function relationships in the human brain and to identify neurochemical systems involved in specific cerebral disorders. The anatomical sites of these effects can be correlated with neurochemical systems associated with such sites in the brain as determined through in vitro studies of human tissue and animal studies of these systems.

The selection of a positron-labeled agent for the study of neurotransmitter processes requires that a number of conditions be satisfied: (1) high specific activity of the labeled agent; (2) good blood-brain barrier permeability and extraction; (3) limited metabolism of the agent and/or metabolites that do not cross the blood-brain barrier; (4) the agent should be specific for a class of neurotransmitter receptors; (5) rapid clearance from nonspecific binding sites in the brain, and (6) high affinity for the receptor system of interest.

The emphasis on the development of appropriate PET compounds has led to the capacity, in the dopaminergic system, to examine both the presynaptic and postsynaptic components of neurotransmitter-receptor system. In such studies, ^{18}F-*L*-dopa was used to examine the presynaptic distribution of stored neurotransmitter via the positron-labeled precursor compound. The postsynaptic receptor distribution has been examined using the positron-labeled ligands ^{11}C-methylspiperone and ^{18}F-fluoroethylspiperone. These studies allow for the detailed evaluation of receptor systems and alterations in these systems produced in disease states. Additional studies have also been performed with ^{11}C-carfentanil to determine the distribution of opiate receptors. Using this compound the specific distribution of the appropriate subclass of opiate receptors (μ) was identified in PET images obtained 30–60 min following the intravenous administration of the compound. It was also demonstrated that binding of the labeled compound could be blocked by the antagonist compound naloxone. Approximately 90% of the specific opiate receptor binding in the thalamus and basal ganglia was displaced by this manipulation.

Such studies indicate the specificity of ligand binding-PET evaluations and the types of strategies that can be uses to evaluate the kinetic behavior of such compounds. Human studies have also been performed with carbon-11-labeled diphenylhydantoin, pimozide, valproic acid, chlorpromazine and with a benzodiazepine receptor binding agent. These labeled ligands provide the opportunity to study directly and in vivo receptor-ligand kinetics as well as the pharmacokinetics of anticonvulsants and other drugs in the brain of normal individuals and in patients with various neurological and psychiatric disorders.

The ability to observe in vivo drug pharmacokinetics can be used in identifying the responsiveness of different patient groups to specific pharmacologically active agents. For example, consider a presumed clinically homogeneous population of patients in whom a specific drug is effective in alleviating symptoms in approximately 15%. Such a therapy would be considered relatively ineffective for the population as a whole. However, for the 15% that responded, the therapy was quite effective. Conventional techniques may not be sensitive enough to identify subpopulations with specific pharmacological sensitivities to different agents. PET studies with either of the two strategies outlined above could provide additional diagnostic information that could potentially distinguish such subgroups and allow for more specific and pathophysiologically appropriate therapies to be employed.

Future Prospects

Numerous university and commercial efforts are underway to reduce the complexity of PET technology. Technetium-operated and PET-devoted cyclotron installations have been described and are in the process of development. Such installations would reduce the cost of the equipment both in terms of the initial expenditure and in terms of overheads for sophisticated operating staffs. This reduction in cost and complexity should result in a wider distribution of PET installations and could potentially make such technology available to nonuniversity-based centers.

Technological advances in instrumentation have progressed at a rapid rate (fig. 25). Image resolution has improved from 30mm to the range of 5mm in the last 10 years. Newer instrumentation provides not only improved anatomical delineation but increased quantitative accuracy in the analytic measurements that are obtained in PET studies. Further advances in PET imaging technology should allow the theoretical limits of resolution to be approached in the very near future.

The development of appropriate tracer kinetic methods and labeled compounds will progressively increase the number and types of biochemical and physiological processes that can be determined with PET. The development of new compounds and the validation of models for their use

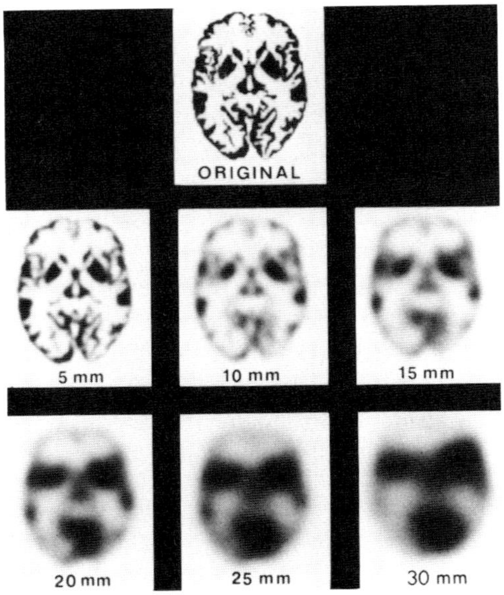

Fig. 25. Simulation of reconstructed images of a cross-section of the human brain showing the effect of PET resolution. A brain slice was digitized, gray and white matter structures given relative concentration values in a ratio of 4:1 (shown as the original at the top), profiles were then generated at multiple angles to simulate PET data, and images were reconstructed at different PET spatial resolutions (values shown below each image). Most actual images shown in this monograph would correspond to those in the 10 to 20 mm range. Systems are now being designed that will equal the 5-mm example. From Mazziotta et al. [1981b].

is a complex, time-consuming and difficult process. At present, emphasis is placed on the development of ligands and precursors for studies of neurotransmitter systems. The ability to make such measurements should be unique to PET since the requirement for measuring picomolar to nanomolar concentrations will be required for such investigations. Automated systems for the synthesis of compounds will again reduce cost and complexity.

As was noted above, the use of behavioral and pharmacological stimulation paradigms should increase the specificity and anatomical accuracy of measurements thus far obtained in patient populations with PET. These studies will undoubtedly expand in the very near future and provide stimulation paradigms that can be used as probes in patient populations. Thus, much in the same way that a cardiologist would use physical exercise to reveal latent abnormalities in coronary perfusion, so too can the neuroscientist use sensory, motor and cognitive tasks to stress regional brain reserve and identify latent abnormalities, the limits of compensatory mechanisms and the means used by the brain to recover or maintain function in the face of injury.

Since PET and autoradiography share a common feature, the tracer kinetic method, objective and valid comparisons between animal models and human conditions can now be made. Results obtained with either PET or autoradiography can be scrutinized for similarities and differences. The PET methods can be used to validate or refute animal models of specific human disorders. The selected models can then be used to explore these human conditions in experimental paradigms that either are too invasive or logistically too complex to perform in patients.

Undoubtedly all of these directions will be followed in the upcoming years. At present some 60 PET installations are operational in the world. It is anticipated that this number will increase substantially in the coming few years. Even if a wider dissemination of PET technology is not realized, the principles underlying normal cerebral function and abnormal cerebral states that can be identified with PET will provide unique and previously unavailable information that can be applied in general terms to all patients with these disorders.

Glossary

Annihilation coincidence detection
The electronic scheme of linking radiation detectors in pairs to accept only photons that arrive at approximately the same time on opposite sides of the head

Attenuation
The absorption or deflection of photons

Collimation
The barrier that allows for selective viewing of only a portion of the environment

CT
Computed tomography; prefix indicates specific modality (e. g. X-ray CT)

LCMRGlc
Local cerebral metabolic rate for glucose utilization

$LCMRO_2$
Local cerebral metabolic rate for oxygen utilization

LOEF
Local oxygen extraction fraction (also referred to as oxygen extraction ratio, OER)

PET
Positron emission tomography (also known als positron CT)

Positron
A positively charged electron emitted from certain unstable nuclei

Positron range
Distance traveled by a positron prior to its combining with an electron

Respiratory quotient
Ratio of carbon dioxide production to oxygen utilization

Specific activity
Ratio of the pure specifically labeled compound to the total compound

Steady state
A state of a dynamic system that is not changing with time

Stoichiometry
Numerical relationships in chemical processes

Tracer
A measurable indicator that is introduced in a small amount to follow dynamic processes of a transport/reaction system; usually the tracer is structurally related to the natural substance involved in the dynamic process or has similar transport properties

Tracer kinetic modeling
The use of mathematical description/formulation to incorporate a priori information about the behavior of a tracer in a dynamic system in order to facilitate the extraction of useful information from the kinetics of tracer in tissue

References

Ackerman, R.H.; Correia, J.A.; Alpert, N.A.; et al.: Positron imaging in ischemic stroke disease using compounds labeled with oxygen-15. Archs Neurol. *38:* 537–543 (1981).

Baron, J.C.: The interrelationships of cerebral blood flow and cerebral metabolism and its study with positron emission tomography in man; in Reba, Goodenough, Davidson, Diagnostic imaging in medicine, pp. 407–435 (Martinus Nijhoff,m Boston 1983).

Baron, J.C.; Bousser, M.H.; Rey, A.; et al.: Reversal of focal 'misery-perfusion syndrome' by extra-intracranial arterial bypass in hemodynamic cerebral ischemia. Stroke *12:* 454–459 (1981).

Baxter, L.R.; Phelps, M.E.; Mazziotta, J.C.; Schwartz, J.M.; Gerner, R.H.; Selin, C.E.; Sumida, R.M.: Cerebral metabolic rate for glucose in mood disorders studied with PET and (F-18)-fluorodeoxyglucose (FDG). Archs gen. Psychiat. *42:* 441–447 (1985).

DiChiro, G.; DeLaPaz, R.L.; Brooks, R.A.; et al.: Glucose utilization of cerebral gliomas measured by [^{18}F]fluorodeoxyglucose and positron emission tomography. Neurology *32:* 1323–1329 (1982).

Engel, J., Jr.; Brown, W.J.; Kuhl, D.E.; Phelps, M.E.; Mazziotta, J.C.; Crandall, P.H.: Pathological findings underlying focal temporal lobe hypometabolism in partial epilepsy. Ann. Neurol. *12:* 518–528 (1982).

Engel, J., Jr.; Crandall, P.H.; Rausch, R.: Surgical treatment of the partial epilepsies; in Rosenberg, Grossman; et al., The clinical neurosciences, vol. 2, pp. 1349–1380 (Churchill Livingston, New York 1983a).

Engel, J., Jr.; Kuhl, D.E.; Phelps, M.E.: Patterns of human local cerebral glucose metabolism during epileptic seizures. Science *218:* 64–66 (1982).

Engel, J., Jr.; Kuhl, D.E.; Phelps, M.E.; Rausch, R.; Nuwer, M: Local cerebral metabolism during partial seizures. Neurology *33:* 400–413 (1983b).

Foster, N.L.; Chase, T.N.; Fedio, P.; et al.: Alzheimer's disease: focal cortical changes shown by positron emission tomography. Neurology *33:* 961–965 (1983).

Frackowiak, R.; Lenzi, G.; Jones, T.; et al.: Quantitative measurement of regional cerebral blood flow and oxygen metabolism in man using ^{15}O and positron emission tomography: theory, procedure and normal values. J. Comput. assist. Tomogr. *4:* 727–736 (1980).

Frackowiak, R.S.; Pozzilli, C.; Legg, N.J.; et al.: Regional cerebral oxygen supply and utilization in dementia. Brain *104:* 753–778 (1981).

Frackowiak, R.S.; Wise, R.J.: Positron tomography in ischemic cerebrovascular disease. Neurol. Clin. *1:* 183–200 (1983).

Garnett, E.S.; Firnau, G.; Nahmias, C.: Dopamine visualized in the basal ganglia of living man. Nature *305:* 137–138 (1983).

Greenberg, J.; Reivich, M.; Alavi, A.; et al.: Metabolic mapping of functional activity in human subjects with the [^{18}F] fluorodeoxyglucose technique. Science *212:* 678–680 (1981).

Greitz, T.; Ingvar, D.; Widen, L. (eds.): Positron emission tomography (Raven Press, New York 1985).

Heiss, W.D.; Phelps, M.E. (eds.): Positron emission tomography of the brain (Springer, New York 1983).

Jones, T.; Chesler, D.A.; Ter-Pogossian, M.M.: The continuous inhalation of oxygen-15 for assessing regional oxygen extraction in the brain of man. Br. J. Radiol. *49:* 339–343 (1976).

Kety, S.S.; Schmidt, C.E.: The nitrous oxide method for the quantitative determination of cerebral blood flow in man: theory, procedure and normal values. J. clin. Invest. *27:* 476–483 (1948).

Kuhl, D.E.: Imaging local brain function with emission computed tomography. Radiology *150:* 625–631 (1984).

Kuhl, D.E.; Phelps, M.E.; Kowell, A.P.; Metter, E.J.; Selin, C.; Winter, J.: Mapping local metabolism and perfusion in normal and ischemic brain by emission computed tomography of ^{18}FDG and $^{13}NH_3$. Ann. Neurol. *8:* 47–60 (1980).

Kuhl, D.E.; Phelps, M.E.; Markham, C.; et al.: Local cerebral glucose metabolism in Huntington's disease determined by emission computed tomography of ^{18}F-fluorodeoxyglucose. J. cereb. Bld Flow Met. *1:* suppl. 1, pp. S459–S460 (1981).

Kuhl, D.E.; Phelps, M.E.; Markham, C.H.; et al.: Cerebral metabolism and atrophy in Huntington's disease determined by ^{18}FDG and computed tomography scan. Ann. Neurol. *12:* 425–434 (1982).

Lassen, N.A.; Perl, W.: Tracer kinetic methods in medical physiology (Raven Press, New York 1979).

Martin, W.R.; Raichle, M.E.: Cerebellar blood flow and metabolism in cerebral hemisphere infarction. Ann. Neurol. *14:* 168–176 (1983).

Mazziotta, J.C.; Phelps, M.E.; Carson, R.E.; et al.: Tomographic mapping of human cerebral metabolism; auditory stimulation. Neurology *32:* 921–937 (1982).

Mazziotta, J.C.; Phelps, M.E.; Miller, J.; et al.: Tomographic mapping of human cerebral metabolism: normal unstimulated state. Neurology *31:* 503–516 (1981a).

Mazziotta, J.C.: PET scanning: principles and applications. Disc. Neurosci. *2:* 9–47 (1985).

Mazziotta, J.C.; Phelps, M.E.; Pahl, J.; Huang, S.C.; Baxter, L.R.; Riege, W.; Hoffman, J.; Kuhl, E.; Lanto, A.; Wapenski, J.; Markham, C.H.: Cerebral glucose utilization reductions in clinically asymptomatic subjects at risk for Huntington's disease. New Engl. J. Med. *316:* 357–362 (1987).

Mazziotta, J.C.; Phelps, M.E.; Plummer, D.; et al.: Quantitation in positron computed tomography. 5. Physical-anatomical factors. J. Comput. assist. Tomogr. *5:* 734–743 (1981b).

Metter, E.J.; Mazziotta, J.C.; Itabashi, H.; Mankovich, N.J.; Kuhl, D.E.; Phelps, M.E.: Comparison of X-ray CT, glucose metabolism and post-mortem data in a patient with multiple cerebral infarctions. Neurology *35:* 1695–1701 (1985).

Mintum, M.A.; Raichle, M.E.; Kilbourne, M.R.; Wooten, G.F.; Welch, M.J.: A quantitative model for the in vivo assessment of drug binding sites with positron emission tomography. Ann. Neurol. *15:* 217–227 (1984).

Patronas, N.J.; DiChiro, G.; Brooks, R.A.; et al.: Work in progress: [^{18}F]fluorodeoxyglucose and positron emission tomography in the evaluation of radiation necrosis of the brain. Radiology *144:* 885–889 (1982).

Phelps, M.E.; Huang, S.C.; Hoffman, E.J.; Selin, C.; Sokoloff, L.; Kuhl, D.E.: Tomographic measurement of local cerebral glucose metabolic rate in humans with (F-18)2-fluoro-2-deoxyglucose: validation of method. Ann. Neurol. *6:* 371–388 (1979).

Phelps, M.E.; Huang, S.C.; Hoffman, E.J.; Plummer, D.; Carson, R.: An analysis of signal amplification using small detectors in positron emission tomography. J. Comput. assist. Tomogr. *6:* 551–565 (1981a).

Phelps, M.E.; Mazziotta, J.C.; Huang, S.C.: Study of cerebral function with positron computed tomography. J. cerebr. Blood Flow Metab. *2:* 113–162 (1982).

Phelps, M.E.; Mazziotta, J.C.; Kuhl, D.E.; et al.: Tomographic mapping of human cerebral metabolism: visual stimulation and deprivation. Neurology *31:* 517–529 (1981b).

Phelps, M.E.; Mazziotta, J.C.; Schelbert, H.J. (eds.): The tracer kinetic study of cerebral and myocardial function: positron emission tomography and autoradiography (Raven Press, New York 1985).

Phelps, M.E.; Schelbert, H.R.; Mazziotta, J.C.: Positron computed tomography for studies of myocardial and cerebral function. Ann. intern. Med. *98:* 339–359 (1983).

Raichle, M.E.: Positron emission tomography. Ann. Rev. Neurosci. *6:* 249–267 (1983).

Sedval, G.; Farde, L.; Persson, A.; Wiesel, F.A.: Imaging of neurotransmitter receptors in the living human brain. (Archs gen. Psychiat. *43:* 995–1005 (1986).

Sokoloff, L.; Reivich, M.; Kennedy, C.; DesRosiers, M.H.; Patlak, C.S.; Pettigrew, K.D.; Sakurada, O.; Shinohara, M.: The [^{14}C]deoxyglucose method for the measurement of local cerebral glucose utilization: theory, procedure and normal values in the conscious and anesthetized albino rat. J. Neurochem. *28:* 897–916 (1977).

Syrota, A.; Castaing, M.; Rougemont, D.; et al.: Tissue acid base balance and oxygen metabolism in human cerebral infarction studied with PET. Ann. Neurol. *14:* 419–428 (1983).

Ter-Pogossian, M.M.: Physical aspects of emission computed tomography; in Newton, Potts, Radiology of the skull and brain: technical aspects of computed tomography, pp. 4372–4388 (Mosby, St Louis 1981).

Ter-Pogossian, M.M.; Phelps, M.E.; Brownell, G.L.; Cox, J.R., Jr.; Davis, D.O.; Evans, R.G. (eds.): Reconstruction tomography in diagnostic radiology and nuclear medicine (University Park Press, Baltimore 1977).

Wagner, H.N.; Burns, H.D.; Dunnals, R.F.; Wong, D.F.; Langstrom, B.; Dueffler, T.; Frost, J.J.; LRavert, H.T.; Links, J.M.; Rosenbloom, S.B.; Lukas, S.E.; Kramer, A.V.; Kuhar, M.J.: Imaging dopamine receptors in the human brain by positron tomography. Science *22:* 1264–1266 (1983).

Walker, M.D.: Research issues in positron emission tomography. Ann. Neurol. *15:* suppl., pp. S1–S204 (1984).

Wise, R.J.; Bernardi, S.; Frackowiak, R.S.; Legg, N.J.; Jones, T.: Serial observations in the pathophysiology of acute stroke. Brain *106:* 197–222 (1983).

John C. Mazziotta, MD, PhD, Department of Neurology, Division of Biophysics and Nuclear Medicine, UCLA School of Medicine, Los Angeles, CA 90024 (USA)

Neurobehavioral Syndromes

Mueller (ed.): Neurology and Psychiatry: A Meeting of Minds,
pp. 156–174 (Karger, Basel 1989)

Neuropsychiatry and Tourette's

Oliver W. Sacks
Department of Neurology, Albert Einstein College of Medicine, New York, N.Y., USA

I want to edge into my subject indirectly and personally, by recalling my own education as a neurologist, and how this served – or failed to serve – me in later years, when I encountered the realities of various syndromes and afflictions, in particular, *encephalitis lethargica* and Tourette's syndrome[1], a syndrome of multiple convulsive tics. As a resident in neurology, I 'rotated' through psychiatry, just as psychiatric residents 'rotated' through neurology. These short rotations did nothing for us in terms of bringing about any unity of the two. One gained a little extraneous psychiatric knowledge, or a little extraneous neurological knowledge, but no real sense that the two were, or could be, related. I even think it encouraged, rather than prevented, some dissociation between neurological and psychiatric orientations, between body and mind, a dissociation which common experience, life itself, contradicts at every point.

When I emerged from residency to encounter the full reality of patients, I often found I had to be as much a psychiatrist as a neurologist. I felt this strongly when seeing patients with migraine, whose moods and feelings, attitudes and perceptions, could alter pari passu with their neurophysiologies: these patients showed me the absolute continuity of body and mind. But it was another affliction that was my real education, my education, that is, as a neuropsychiatrist. This was the encephalitis lethargica, the great sleeping sickness that affected nearly 5 million between 1918 and 1927. The moment of truth, or revelation, or 'conversion' for me was when I encountered some eighty-odd postencephalitic patients

[1] Properly speaking, 'Gilles de la Tourette syndrome', but for brevity's sake, often 'Tourette's syndrome' or just 'Tourette's'.

at a hospital in New York. These patients had a myriad of disorders both 'neurologic' and 'psychiatric': Parkinsonism, myoclonus, chorea, tics, strange compulsions, phobias, obsessions, gusts of passion. A 'pure' neurologist or a 'pure' psychiatrist with such patients would be utterly lost. The neurological, the psychiatric, *had* to be conjoined. One had to be as observant and knowledgeable about the psychological, the psychodynamic, as about the physiological, the neurodynamic.

What I found for myself here was no more than a repetition of what had been found in the 1920s, when the epidemic encephalitis burst upon the world. And of all the pioneer observers of that time, I found Smith Ely Jelliffe and his writings [Jelliffe, 1927, 1932] the most penetrating and the most faithful to experience. Jelliffe was both a neurologist *and* an analyst[2], equally 'Sherringtonian' and 'Freudian' in outlook, as indeed one has to be if one is to observe such patients, for *they* are equally Sherringtonian and Freudian. Thus, Jelliffe felt impelled to write in 1927:

> In the monumental strides made by neuropsychiatry in the past ten years, no single advance has approached in importance that made through the study of epidemic encephalitis... An entirely new orientation has been made imperative.

This 'new orientation' of which Jelliffe spoke, and of which he himself was a notable exemplar, did not involve merely combining neurological and psychiatric knowledge (as every neurologist and psychiatrist does to some extent), but *conjoining* them, seeing them as inseparable, seeing how psychiatric phenomena might emerge from the physiological, or how, conversely, they might be transformed into it – and, thus, how both approaches had to be used, together, if one were to understand oculogyric crises, respiratory disorders, tics. Thus, although the respiratory disorders could in part be explained as the consequence of excitatory lesions in the respiratory systems of the upper and lower brainstem, they had also to be seen as 'respiratory behavior'. This 'new orientation', it must be stressed, was thus something quite beyond the 'old' neuropsychiatry – and also, to my mind, quite different from what we now call behavioral neurology or biological psychiatry (though both of these also stemmed from experience with postencephalitic patients, from observation of dramatic behavioral disorders with a clear organic basis). And the difference lies in a sense of process, the dynamics, both neural and psychic, of the disorders.

[2] It is of interest that Jelliffe could not be *accepted* as both, and tended to be seen by neurologists as an 'analyst', and by analysts as a 'neurologist'. The notion of a *neuropsychiatrist,* apparently, was anathema to both.

When I gave my postencephalitic patients *L*-dopa they 'awakened', and their 'awakenings' were simultaneously physical and mental: motor, intellectual, perceptual, affective, all at once and inseparably [Sacks, 1974]. I have to say that such a global awakening or animation was in contradiction to our concepts of neuroanatomy at the time (1969), a neuroanatomy that (as Prof. Nauta has reminded us at this conference) was essentially compartmentalized in character, seeing the motor, the intellectual and the affective in quite separate and noncommunicating compartments of the brain. The anatomist in me, subservient to this notion, said, 'This can't be. Such an "awakening" should not happen' – but clearly it *was* happening, and common experience, furthermore, said it should. After some conflict, I deferred to my experience, and saw and described these awakenings as global, even though this meant abjuring various anatomical and physiological suppositions. Sooner or later, I thought, anatomy would catch up to reality.

One of the great delights of the last two decades is to have been present at a creative revolution, to have seen just such a 'new' anatomy (and new orientation) emerge at the hands of Nauta and others. He has shown us, in innumerable ways, how the motor and affective and intellective parts of the brain are inseparably entwined and integrated at every point, so that, though separate, they *act* as a unity [Nauta, this volume]. I bring up this point because all of us who first saw the effects of *L*-dopa found ourselves in a situation of conflict, and many of us dealt with this by distorting or reducing or denying our own experience. We spoke of the motor effects of *L*-dopa as *the* effects and anything else (if we admitted it at all) as incidental, adventitious, mere 'side' effects – neurologizing them, so to speak, out of existence.

But we could not perceive these 'awakenings' in their totality without a neuropsychiatric, or Jelliffian, perspective. And if this was so for the initial 'awakening', how much more so was it of the later effects, the excitation not merely of motor excesses, but of perceptual, intellectual and affective excesses. Parkinsonism itself is not 'purely' motor – there is, for example, in many akinetic patients, a corresponding 'stickiness' of mind or bradyphrenia, the thought stream as slow and sluggish as the motor stream. The thought stream, the stream of consciousness, speeded up in these patients with *L*-dopa, often speeding too far, into a veritable tachyphrenia, with thoughts and associations almost too fast to follow. Again, there is not merely motor, but perceptual inertia in Parkinsonism: a perspective drawing of a cube or a staircase, for example, which the normal mind perceives first this way and then that, in alternating perceptual configurations or hypotheses, may be absolutely frozen in one configuration for the Parkinsonian; it will unfreeze as he 'awakens' and may then thrust in the opposite direction, with a near-delirium of perceptual hypotheses alternating many times a second. Again there may be, at least in post-encephalitic patients, an apathy as profound as the lack or impoverishment of movement. This too is reversed by *L*-dopa, and they may then be thrust into the other direction, into a state of heightened, excessive and (so to speak) convulsive emotion.

This amplification, often sudden and convulsive, affecting motor, intellectual, perceptual and affective life, might produce a peculiar hyperanimation, very similar to that of Tourette's syndrome. It was indeed in such a context, with these overenergized patients, that I first saw and spoke of 'Tourettism' – two years before I actually saw a patient with 'Tourette's syndrome' [Sacks, 1982]. I need to stress that this was my own path to Tourette's syndrome – it was, from the start, a neuropsychiatric path, and one brought about by observation of postencephalitic patients and syndromes. Thus, I was neither tempted to 'neurologize' nor 'psychiatrize' Tourette's – tendencies which have been all too common in this century.

Tourette's syndrome was described a century ago by Georges Gilles de la Tourette[3], a singularly imaginative and gifted pupil of Charcot (like his contemporaries Babinski and Freud) [Gilles de la Tourette, 1885; Goetz and Klawans, 1982] (fig. 1, 2). The atmosphere around Charcot and of Paris at that time was one of rare imaginativeness and excitement – an atmosphere in which natural history, clinical naturalism, flourished as it had never done before, and in a most heightened, and sometimes dramatic, form. Such an atmosphere was a prerequisite for the perception and delineation of such a syndrome. The compartmentalizing and conceptualizing of medicine characteristic of medicine today had only just started on its huge and arduous journey, and a free and untrammeled (at times almost novelistic) naturalism was still open to the clinical minds of the time. If Tourette, like so many of the superspecialists of our own time, had thought narrowly in terms of 'motor disorders', he could have described the movements, but nothing else of what we now call Tourette's syndrome. Fortunately, he was able to describe the echolalia, the coprolalia, the imitations, the impulsions, all of the complex 'mental' aspects of the

[3] A vivid account of Tourette's short but often dramatic life (he was shot in 1893 by a deluded patient) has recently been provided by A.J. Lees [1986].

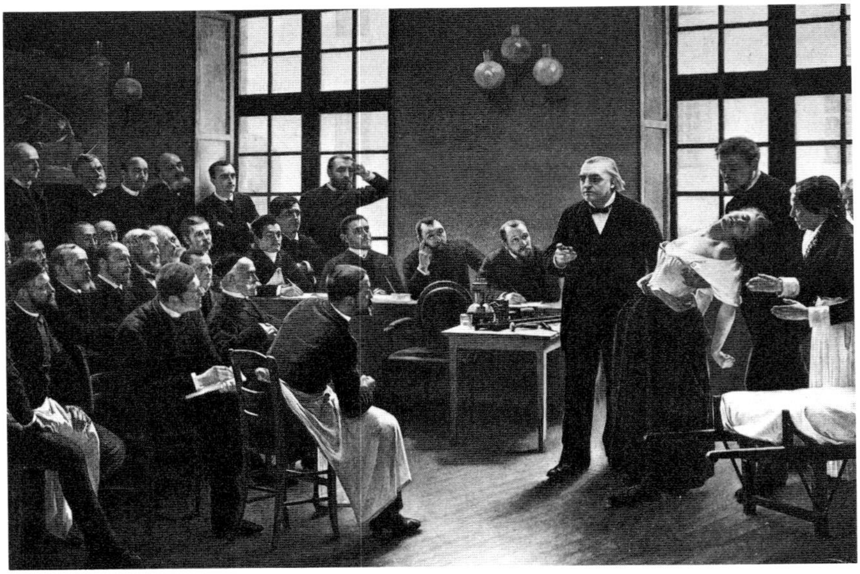

Fig. 1. A clinical lecture by Jean M. Charcot at the Salpetrière. Tourette is to be seen in the center foreground wearing an apron. Courtesy of The Bettmann Archive.

syndrome. He described it, in short, as a neuropsychiatric syndrome, although no such portentous word would have occurred to him in this context. He simply considered himself a clinical naturalist, describing whatever he saw with an open, unbiased, undivided fullness. Tourette sketched the outlines of his syndrome; others were to add detail, flesh it out. Tourette made it possible to see the syndrome, by first seeing it – there always has to be someone who sees something first, and thereby makes it possible for everyone else to see what they had failed to see before. Following his description in 1885, new cases were seen and described by the score, often with a wonderful richness which was beyond anything which had hitherto existed in clinical medicine, and which was all too soon to vanish completely.

This was a time when medical descriptions were full of a precision, delicacy and (not least) humor, a time when naturalism (or what we now call phenomenology) had not yet collapsed under the advances of science. It was, by the same token, a time in which patients and physicians still spoke the same language – and thus it was possible for both to collaborate,

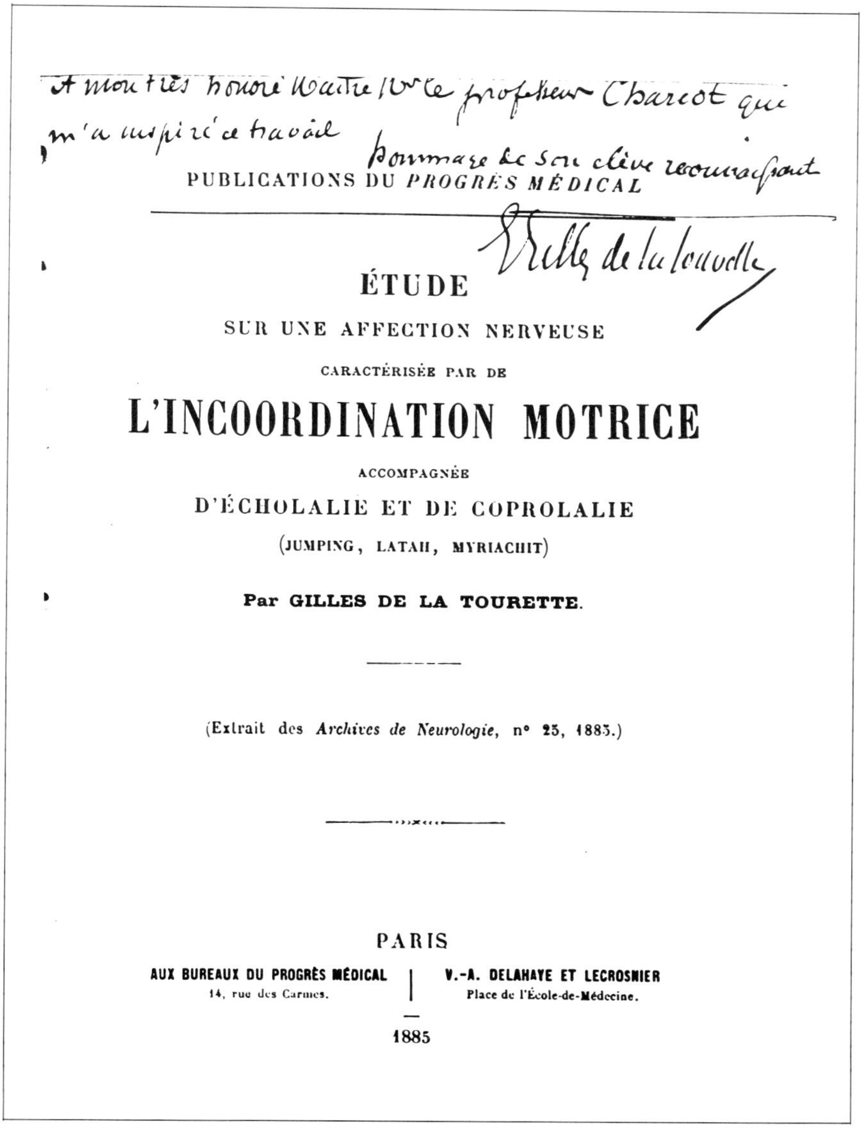

A mon très honoré Maître Mr le professeur Charcot qui m'a inspiré ce travail
hommage de son élève reconnaissant

PUBLICATIONS DU *PROGRÈS MÉDICAL*

Gilles de la Tourette

ÉTUDE

SUR UNE AFFECTION NERVEUSE

CARACTÉRISÉE PAR DE

L'INCOORDINATION MOTRICE

ACCOMPAGNÉE

D'ÉCHOLALIE ET DE COPROLALIE

(JUMPING, LATAH, MYRIACHIT)

Par GILLES DE LA TOURETTE.

(Extrait des *Archives de Neurologie*, n° 25, 1885.)

PARIS

AUX BUREAUX DU PROGRÈS MÉDICAL | V.-A. DELAHAYE ET LECROSNIER
14, rue des Carmes. | Place de l'École-de-Médecine.

1885

Fig. 2. A rare reprint of Gilles de la Tourette's 1885 memoir, this copy inscribed to its 'inspirer' Charcot.

producing between them a perfect balance of description and comment. I want here to quote from one of the finest examples of such a collaboration I know, the anonymous *Confessions of a Ticqueur,* interlarded with the comments of his physicians, Meige and Feindel [1907]. The ticqueur, O., introduces himself – at least, the tic or Tourette part of himself (we can judge later how deeply, and in what ways, this is related to, or has interacted with, his 'real', or non-Tourette, self):

> I have always been conscious of a predilection for *imitation*[4]. A curious gesture or bizarre attitude affected by anyone was the immediate signal for an attempt on my part at its reproduction, and is still. Similarly with words or phrase, pronunciation or intonation, I was quick to mimic any peculiarity.
>
> When I was thirteen years old I remember seeing a man with a droll grimace of eyes and mouth, and from that moment I gave myself no respite until I could imitate it accurately.... for several months I kept repeating the old gentleman's grimace involuntarily. I had, in short, begun to tic.

Many other tics had such a historical origin or precipitation, given, of course, the constitutional predilection. His physicians – who, as naturalists, paid due regard to every detail; and, like psychoanalysts, often discovered significance in trifles – thus note the origin of an adolescent sniffing tic:

> He happened to be out one day for a walk with his sister during a snowstorm, and a flake entering his nostril made him sniff and sneeze half a dozen times. Long after the snow had ceased falling and the tickling sensation had vanished he repeated the performance, till it passed into a sniffing tic that continued some months...

Countless other tics, succeeding one another in kaleidoscopic patterns, are described with their origins by both patient and physician, accompanied by comments and interpretations not imposed, but emergent:

> A large number of my head and face movements (continues the patient) owe their origin to the annoyance caused me by my seeing the tip of my nose or my moustache from time to time. The former organ appears to make a sort of screen in front of me, to avoid which I turn or raise my head: I can now see the object I am facing, but, at the same time, naturally, I see my nose again at the side, whence one more tilt of the head, and so on. I am well aware of how nonsensical all this is; but it fails to deter me from my desire of playing at hide-and-seek with my nose... Similarly with my pince-nez: no sooner have I put it on than I long to alter its position in innumerable ways. I must needs push it down or raise it up, must set it further on or

[4] Imitation may become positively frenzied in that special and most severe form of Tourette's I have called 'super-Tourette's' – I describe this in a short sketch, *The Possessed* [Sacks, 1985a]. One sees here every level of imitation from the echoic to the parodic, the mimic, the pantomimic. The very physiology of Tourette's seems to dispose to hypermimia and histrionism – as is also seen in dopa-activated Parkinsonism and chorea.

further off... or attempt to displace it by tossing my head. Instead of looking tranquilly through the glasses, my eye is continually attracted to the rim, some point on which I try to focus or get into a line with the object at which I am gazing. I want to see the object and the pince-nez at the same time; as soon as I no longer see the former I wish to see it again, and similarly with the latter. My tics upset my pince-nez, and I have to invent another tic to get it back into place. The absurdity of this vicious circle does not escape my observation, and I know I am its author, yet that cannot prevent my becoming its victim.

In this same passage, the patient speaks about the relation of the ticcing, the ticqueur, to himself:

There seem to be two persons in me: the one that tics, the son of the one that does not, is an *enfant terrible,* a source of great anxiety to his parents, who become a slave to his caprices. I am at once the actor and the spectator; and the worst of it is, the exuberance of the one is not to be thwarted by the just recriminations of the other.

This description always reminds me of a patient of mine with Tourette's whose self-recriminations took the form of loud exhortations and objurgations – in particular, 'verboten!' – whenever tics and 'forbidden' impulses threatened to overwhelm him: the responses of the ego to the caprices and compulsions of his 'Tourette-self'[5].

This combination of fortuitous circumstances with forced reaction (neuropsychologists speak here of 'stimulus-slavery' and 'stimulus-bound behavior') is characteristic of frontal-lobe syndromes, as it is of early childhood, and *all* states of insufficient selectivity and inhibition, not just Tourette's – although it may take a particularly elaborate form in Tourette's, where there is full consciousness of what is happening, combined with impotence to stop it. Thus, the ticqueur, O., continues:

One day as I was moving my head I felt a 'crack' in my neck, and forthwith concluded that I had dislocated something. It was my concern, thereafter, to twist my head in a thousand different ways, and with ever-increasing violence, until at length the rediscovery of the sensation afforded me a genuine sense of satisfaction, speedily clouded by the fear of having done myself some harm... I cannot withstand the allurement or banish the sentiment of unrest.

Meige and Feindel comment here on 'the fundamental importance of the psychical element that precedes the motor reaction, with the secondary

[5] Or – should we say? – of his (Tourettized) super-ego to the impulses of his (Tourettized) id. It subsequently became apparent that 'verboten!', ejaculated with convulsive, tic-like force and speed, was uttered in the voice of his father: in short, *the introjection of the father as tic.* Such complex 'personal' vocalizations, which are especially common in super-Tourette's, may have a role similar to the hallucinatory voices in psychosis. Melanie Klein speaks of such introjections as 'internal objects' – but in Tourette's they may be exteriorized, ecphorized, as pantomimes and tics.

psychical reaction in its turn, the impulse to seek a familiar sensation...', etc. This needs to be stressed, especially in view of the current tendency to see tics as wholly motor, with no emotional or psychic component whatever. Yet it may give the psychic too large a place in the pathogeny of tics, for there are, as we shall see, many forms of ticcing in which a psychic component, though present, is clearly secondary, and has been added to some primary motor urge or impulse *in order to give it sense.* This elaboration and accretion of meaning was often very clear in my postencephalitic patients who found themselves 'Tourettized' by *L*-dopa, as in the case of the patient Miriam H.:

> An entirely novel symptom which had developed on the increased dose of *L*-dopa was a *tic,* a lightning-quick movement of the right hand to the face, occurring about twenty times an hour. When I questioned Miss H. about this symptom, shortly after its inauguration, she replied that it was 'a nonsense-movement', which had no purpose that she was aware of, and which she did not wish to make: 'I feel a tension building up in my hand', she said, 'and after a time it gets too much, and then I *have* to move it.' Within three days of its appearance, however, this tic had become associated with an intention and a use: it had become a mannerism, and was now used by Miss H. to adjust the position of her spectacles [Sacks, 1974].

But whether primary or secondary, reason or rationalization, it is these psychic aspects which confer a sort of absurd 'significance' on the tics and relate them to the life and psychic economy of the ticqueur. This is admirably formulated by Meige and Feindel: 'In this way factitious wants come into being which may be described as a sort of *parasitic function*... of which the patient is alike the creator and the dupe.' The relation of the 'host', the real-self, to the 'parasitic' tic-self is further shown by the sudden 'debauches' both forced upon and indulged by the ticqueur, the conflict between the real self's will and that of the Tourette's, a conflict which also has elements of collusion and compromise:

> In O.'s case the inhibitory influence of the will is abundantly manifest. Should he find himself in the company of one from whom he would fain conceal his tics, he is able to repress them completely for an hour or two... Nevertheless, the desire to let himself go obtrudes itself again, and if he can refrain no longer he will invent and pretext for leaving the room, abandoning himself in his moment of solitude to a veritable debauch of absurd gesticulations, a wild muscular carnival, from which he returns comforted, to resume sedately the thread of the interrupted dialogue.

The element of farce, as well as force, is very evident here, and brings to mind what I have quite recently had occasion to observe in a score or more Tourette's patients whom I have seen personally, where Tourettic tension, suddenly released, may erupt in an explosion of obscenities and profanities, bizarre animal and cartoon imitations, or mock assaults on inviting objects in the environment.

There may be an element of sadism, besides absurdity, in such 'debauches', and in other patients the affective and erotic elements of their Tourettic debauches are overwhelming. Sudden sniffing, usually of clothes or people, may occur – a sexualized olfactory compulsion associated with a convulsive hyperosmia or osmophilia[6]. I have seen patients suddenly fall upon soft objects, such as overstuffed cushions, or parts of their own bodies, such as their arms or knees – stroking, squeezing, hitting, and kissing them, muttering coprolaliac endearments and imprecations. With one patient, baked onions at mealtimes always elicited a similar reaction. Another once reacted in this way to a moth[7]. *Anything* may apparently precipitate – or in ethological terms, 'release' – such behaviors; *anything* may become the object of these sudden Tourettic and erotic attentions, and one sees why Arthur Shapiro, with his unrivalled experience of Tourette's, speaks of 'polymorphous perverseness' in these exceptionally severe cases[8].

There is sometimes a *provocative* quality in such Tourettic behavior. I have known several such patients who would play with fire, seeing how close they could get to open flames without hurt; others are attracted to fans, flywheels and other revolving objects – which exert a teasing fascination over Tourettes, and provoke dangerous (but exciting) test approaches. One patient has sudden impulsions to bite glasses – to 'test' them by biting – and may sometimes end up with a bloodied mouth and

[6] Such 'olfactory behavior', of an almost prehuman sort, may also be seen in some postencephalitics, and in the strange excitations sometimes elicited by amphetamines [1985 a, b].

[7] The sudden, convulsive hyperattention and hyperreaction has a dramatic *sensory* component as well (Tourette's *is* sensory, no less than affective and motor). Thus, the knees, the onion, the cushion, the moth, were suddenly seen with overwhelming intensity, filling the whole visual and attentional field with a peremptory, almost hallucinatory vividness and force. The stimulus, seemingly trivial and insignificant in itself, becomes endowed with a 'factitious' significance and force, to which neural and psychic mechanisms equally contribute – sudden limbic (or limbic-sensory) stimulation, and sudden hypercathexis, symbolism, projection, themselves mutually reinforcing and linked.

[8] A.J. Lees, in his excellent recent book on the subject [Lees, 1985] gives a wealth of further examples: 'Popular items to touch include fires, irons, hot plates, lighted cigarettes, door handles, railings, floors and fabrics with an erotic texture such as fur, velvet, satin and silk. Touching of breasts, bottoms and hair also occurs... (as well as) heads, noses, lips, rounded stones and sharp knives.'

broken glass. He also has sudden impulses to slam on the brakes – though he makes certain, first, the coast is clear. Obscene ejaculations and gestures (coprolalia, copropraxia) are common in Tourette's; thus Lees describes this in a single English patient:

> Vocalizations included 'zing', 'Tottenham', 'Sieg heil', 'mod' and 'monkey'. His repertoire of obscenities was equally extensive, with 'fuck', 'fuck off', 'fucking wanker', 'oral sex', 'Suki's crutch', 'tits', 'knickers' and 'cunnilingus' being shouted in an aggressive voice... Within a brief interview period he displayed... jerky obscene palm back V signs, striking of his chest with his arms, kissing his clothing and simulating masturbation (as well as a score of simpler, more banal tics).

Some patients will suddenly, for no obvious reason, begin kicking and banging, yelling and screaming, stamping and 'punding'[9], or they will giggle, or make faces, or posture, or curse. Many patients are prone to bizarre rituals, compulsions, obsessions – the need to touch a particular spot on the wall, to arrange or rearrange objects in different patterns *('délire de toucher');* to add or multiply numbers on license plates ('arithmomania'); to comment or interject while others are speaking *('folie pourquoi'* – one such patient known to me incessantly says 'what?' in a loud voice, so that others repeat or try to clarify their words, until they realize the 'what' is a tic); to mutter meaningless litanies and mantras *('tic d'incantation');* to suddenly bow or bend at the knees *('tic de salaam')*, or to give a little jump, or toss the head, on every fifth step[10]. It is understandable that such behavior may sometimes cause patients to be diagnosed as 'psychiatric' or 'schizophrenic', especially if they have no tics, when in fact they have only 'mental Tourette's' in the context of an otherwise harmonious personality.

Meige and Feindel also speak of the *mental* quality of such patients. They describe O.'s 'mobile and impulsive temperament', and (though he is not schizophrenic) his 'looseness of thought':

> His conversation is a tissue of disconnected thoughts and uncompleted sentences; he interrupts himself to diverge at a tangent on a new train of ideas – a method of procedure not

[9] This term has been used by neurobiologists to refer to stereotyped circling and other repetitive behaviors observed in amphetaminism.

[10] Samuel Johnson had many such compulsions or rituals, especially on entering houses, when he would twirl about or gesticulate in the doorway, then give a sudden spring, followed by a vast stride over the doorsill. He also exhibited litanic muttering, talking to himself, sudden ejaculations, echoing of others, strange vocalizations and ceaseless tics. It seems almost certain that Dr. Johnson had Tourette's.

without its charm, as it frequently results in picturesque and amusing associations. No sooner has he expressed one idea in words than another rises in his mind, a third, a fourth, each of which must be suitably clothed; but as time fails for this purpose, the consequence is a series of obscure ellipses, which are often captivating by their very unexpectedness.

This is an aspect of 'stimulus-bound behavior', except here the stimuli are internal, the patient's own fancies and thoughts. It may be difficult for such patients (as for volatile postencephalitics) to achieve so-called free association – that is, association seemingly random, which in fact circumscribes dominant affects and themes. 'Free association' may not work with such patients, for their associations may be so loosely and superficially connected and determined as to have no real center or implicit theme. When I sent a tape of such a patient to the Russian neuropsychologist A.R. Luria, he compared it to 'mental Brownian motion', and to the ever-changing images and associations of his 'Mnemonist' [Luria, 1968][11]:

There were many instances in which images that came to the surface in his mind steered him away from the subject of a conversation. At such moments his remarks would be cluttered with details and irrelevancies; he would become verbose, digress endlessly, and finally have to strain to get back to the subject of the conversation.

Is this not almost identical with Meige and Feindel's description of their loquacious ticqueur? Thoughtless reaction, superficial association, overcharged (yet 'factitious') affects and images, lie in wait, seductive, for the unwary ticqueur.

My own patient 'Witty Ticcy Ray' [Sacks, 1985b] felt there was a close analogy between his wit and his tics – he spoke of his 'ticcy witticisms' and 'witty ticcicisms', feeling both as expressions of the sudden, unexpected swerves and twists, the irruptions and interruptions, in his mental and motor stream. Similarly, when playing ping-pong, he would make (in his own words) 'sudden, nervous, *frivolous* shots' – shots so frivolous, so unexpected, as to be completely unanswerable. And with music too: he was a weekend jazz drummer of real virtuosity, famous for his sudden and wild

[11] The 'Mnemonist', studied in such detail by Luria, had tremendously enhanced, though unselective, powers of imagery and memory – so that any stimulus, inner or outer, was apt to lead to a veritable explosion of imagery. The Mnemonist, partly controlling, partly controlled by, the compelling force of his imagery, found it difficult to lead a normal, 'non-Mnemonist' life. There are striking resemblances to Tourette's here, not only in the existential conflict between automatism and autonomy (or, as Luria put it, between an 'It' and an 'I'), but in their peculiar and specific neurodynamics, with very rapid, uninhibited, unselective associative neural processes in both – expressed in the Mnemonist solely as sensory imagery and synesthesia, but in the Touretter, additionally, as 'motor images', behaviors, enactments or tics.

extemporizations, which would arise from a tic or a compulsive hitting of a drum and would instantly be made the nucleus of a wild and wonderful improvization, so that the 'sudden intruder' would be turned to brilliant advantage. Thus, the Touretter (as O. also intimates) may be active, not passive, in relation to his Tourette's, and turn it into exhibition and performance. Whether this should be seen as the ego mastering, colluding with, or deferring to, disease, remains a tantalizing ambiguity.

These fragments show something of the extraordinariness and complexity of Tourette's, how it is inseparably both physical and mental. And yet, as I intimated earlier, there have been the most persistent efforts, in this century, to 'physicalize' or 'mentalize' it, to make it one or the other, when it is so manifestly both. Charcot and his pupils were among the last of their profession with a combined vision of body and soul, 'It' and 'I', neurology and psychiatry. By the turn of the century a split had occurred, into a soulless neurology and a bodiless psychology, and with this any full understanding of Tourette's disappeared. The natural history, the clinical naturalism, of the last century has disappeared – a victim, paradoxically, of our advances in knowledge and thought, a physiological and psychiatric sophistication that was new to the world[12].

Meige and Feindel, writing in 1907, had probably not heard of Freud – and yet, as we see, some aspects of Tourette's syndrome, at least in its 'higher' forms, and in the most severe cases, have a strongly and unmistakably Freudian quality. Indeed, psychoanalytic formulations of tic and Tourette's syndrome dominated thinking on the subject from the seminal work of Ferenczi in the early 1920s[13] to the late 1950s, the formulations of

[12] This point is powerfully made in his autobiography by A.R. Luria, when he speaks of the effects on naturalism of scientific reductionism: 'Since the beginning of this century there has been enormous technical progress, which has changed the very structure of the scientific enterprise... Reductionism, the effort to reduce complex phenomena to their elementary particles, became the guiding principle of scientific efforts. In psychology it seemed that by reducing psychological events to elementary physiological rules, we could attain the ultimate explanation of human behaviour. Reductionism in the study of learning led to an emphasis on contiguity and reinforcement as the basic elements, the combination of which could explain the most complex forms of behaviour, including human conscious activity. In this atmosphere, *the rich and complex picture of human behaviour which had existed in the late nineteenth century disappeared*... (italics added).

[13] There was, even earlier, a brief golden period of liaison between neurology and psychoanalysis, now almost forgotten, before the first World War. Thus there was a fascinating exchange between neurologists and analysts, at the New York Academy of Medicine, in January 1914, regarding the conjunction of neural and psychic determinants in Tourette's.

Mahler and Rangel being particularly important [Mahler and Rangel, 1943; Mahler, 1949]. One cannot doubt the relevance and power of Mahler's thought – in particular, her conceptions of a 'motor ego'.[14] But the patients she analyzed showed little change in their Tourette's, the inevitable consequence of its being seen as purely psychiatric, and the consequent neglect of its neurological determinants. Many children, too many, with Tourette's were diagnosed as 'psychiatric' in this 40-year period, and submitted to penetrating, but ultimately fruitless, attempts at psychotherapy.

This, doubtless, was one factor in the demise of the psychogenic approach, the rise of our knowledge about neurotransmitters being the other. With dopamine deficiency in Parkinsonism being discovered in 1959, dopamine excess was at once suspected in Tourette's, and trial of anti-dopaminergic agents made within a year. 'The effect of the haloperidol treatment administered at this time (November 1960) was absolutely spectacular', Seignot [1976] wrote, adding, 'The theory held by many psychiatrists, and in particular by many psychoanalysts... would seem to be contradicted by this experiment.' This precipitated an abrupt (and perhaps excessive) reaction against psychological formulations, and an emphasis on exclusively chemical formulations and therapies, which have (on the whole) dominated approaches to Tourette's syndrome since the mid-1960s.

And, with this, there has been a loss of phenomenological fullness, of attention to the total experience and world of the Touretter. Tics have been classified, or reclassified, as 'movement disorders', to be ranked with dyskinesias, dystonias, myoclonus, chorea. Not that tics may not (as in postencephalitic patients) coexist with these – or, indeed, emerge or *evolve* from these. But the one thing which is crucial about tics – the sense of

Pierce Clark's 'Remarks' were discussed by Foster Kennedy and J.J. Putnam (the relevant papers, from the *Medical Record* of February 7 and 28, and March 14, 1914, were gathered together and reprinted by William Wood, New York). One can only hope that such exchanges – which ended seventy years ago with the divorce of neurology and psychiatry – may be rekindled in our time with a new neuropsychiatry.

[14] Margaret Mahler's life work centered on the exploration of ego development, the delineation of factors and circumstances – both interpersonal and intrapsychic – which might facilitate or retard its development. She observed, rightly, that with tics there might be fixation of, or regression to, a rather primitive ego-level (or 'motor ego'); but attributed this wholly to repressed aggression, thus taking insufficient account of the organic factors influencing ego development, of which Tourette's – with its ego-alien tics and impulsions – is so notable an example.

compulsion and intention which drives them, the idea or 'content' which informs them – has been forgotten again. And as for the peculiar mental Tourettism of Tourette's – the loose, rapidly changing associations and fancies, so beautifully described by Meige and Feindel, and present to some degree, or at times, in all Touretters – this now tends to be completely ignored. Thus, if one may say this without disrespect, the ninety-odd papers presented at the First International Tourette Symposium in 1981, while presenting a vast amount of new and exciting information, gave no feel whatever of what it was like to have Tourette's. I remember this vividly, for I went with a Touretter friend, and he said, 'I don't know what they're talking about, they're not talking about me. They don't put across what Tourette's is really like.'

What Tourette's is really like – this has been forgotten, and we can only recapture it if we listen minutely to our patients, and observe them, everything about them, with a comprehensive eye; or go back, as I have done here, to the older descriptions, where verisimilitude has not been sacrificed to narrow formulations or theories. But, clearly, we cannot merely go back. We need the new knowledge and concepts of our own time; we need, equally, to recover the full realism, the phenomenological fullness, of a past time; we need, above all, somehow to *combine* them.

I encountered precisely this phenomenon when I came to explore my first realm in medicine, migraine, and concluded that the present century had been characterized by both advances and retrogressions, a real gain of knowledge coupled with a real loss in general understanding.

Some very beautiful words, which go to the heart of what I am saying, were spoken by William James in remembering his old teacher Agassiz. Agassiz was a naturalist, not a theorist or abstractionist – 'the hours I spent with him', writes James, 'so taught me the difference between all possible abstractionists and all livers in the light of the world's concrete fullness, that I have never been able to forget it.' But already, in his own lifetime, Agassiz, his mode of mind, naturalism, was becoming obsolete:

> In the fifty years that have sped since he arrived here (James is writing in 1896)... our knowledge of Nature has penetrated into joints and recesses which his vision never pierced. The causal elements and not the totals are what we are now most passionately concerned to understand; and naked and poverty-sticken enough do the stripped-out elements and forces occasionally appear to us to be. But the truth of things is after all their living fullness, and some day, from a more commanding point of view than was possible to anyone in his generation, our descendants, enriched with all the spoils of our analytic investigations, will get round again to that higher and simpler way of looking at Nature.

When Freud came to give his lectures at Clark University, he was met by the aged and ailing William James. And James said to him 'Yours is the psychology of the future.' I find here an echo of his words on Agassiz, his sense that analysis, analytical investigations, if they are of the right kind, will not only lay out the workings of the world, but will restore, even enhance, the sense of its concrete fullness. This, indeed, is precisely what Freud does – at least in his marvelous case histories. This too is what Luria does, in *his* marvelous case histories – above all, in *The Mind of a Mnemonist.* And this is what we have to do with Tourette's – utilize the methods and models of the masters. What we need is to go beyond a naturalistic description – or picture, as we are given by Meige and Feindel – to a dynamic, analytical description combining the neurodynamic and the psychodynamic, the neuroanalytic and the psychoanalytic, such as Luria and Freud together might give us. Only by doing so, or so it seems to me, can we preserve the seemingly anarchic fullness of Tourette's, but also go beyond this and make sense of it all.

Recently, when I was exploring, as minutely but also as generally as I could, a remarkable patient with the severest Tourette's, I kept three books on my bedside table – *The Interpretation of Dreams, Wit and the Unconscious,* and *The Mind of a Mnemonist.* In Tourette's of ultimate severity, there are not only convulsions of Mnemonist-like perception and imagery, and of inner (often 'Freudian') passions and impulses, but instant exhibitions of these in tic and sign form. Thus, the external and the internal, the perceptual and the instinctual, all ticcishly transformed, burst forth in a sort of visible, public, phantasmagoria or dream. This can show us, as nothing else can, not only the surface stream of consciousness, but the deeper, unconscious associations, drives, images – the entire, but normally hidden, inner life of the patient. These externalized dream flashes and ticcy figments, of which dozens may occur in the course of a second, are largely beyond the power of the unaided senses to register or analyze, and require highspeed videotaping, with slow-motion playback and analysis of individual frames, or stroboscopic photography (fig. 3), to reveal their full character, connection and meaning[15]. Given this, Tourette's can make possible a veritable *microscopy of mind,* such as Freud and Luria dreamed of but never saw.

[15] Precisely such techniques are required to 'crack' sign language, and were used by Klima and Bellugi [1979] to show its hidden and unconscious character and grammar.

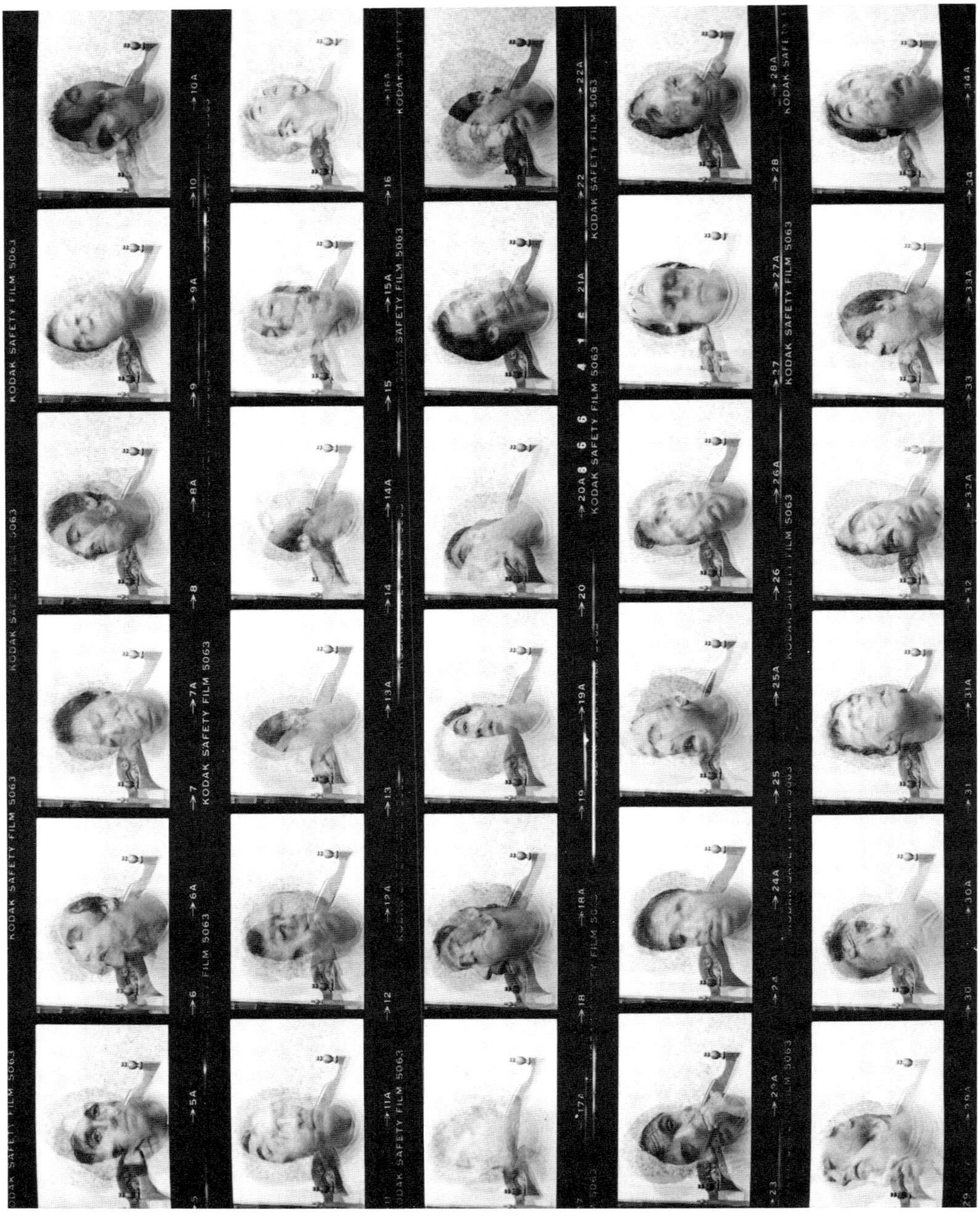
KODAK SAFETY FILM 5063

I have come full circle, and will conclude where I started. Neuropsychiatry is an old term which needs a new meaning. This new meaning has to do with the dynamics, the activities, of brain-mind – unlike biological psychiatry and behavioral neurology, which are static, diagrammatic – phrenology in new clothes.

A genuine, deep understanding of Tourette's, perhaps the most striking neuropsychiatric syndrome of all, depends on such a neuropsychiatry. And such a neuropsychiatry, in turn, can validate itself by elucidating Tourette's; such an elucidation, such a validation, are now perhaps within sight. I think that we will recapture and fully understand, in the 1980s, what Tourette half-guessed, half-hinted at when he discovered his syndrome in the 1880s.

That it should take a century to do this is not surprising[16], for we are here in realms as complex and difficult as any in physics; but, more to the point, history takes its time, must pass through stages, cannot be hurried. The three-staged movement envisaged by William James – from naive naturalism, through analysis, to a 'higher and simpler way' – would tend to take, he thought, a century or so. So, really, the timing is right, the time is ripe, for the full illumination of Tourette's by a new neuropsychiatry.

[16] But a genius may be a century ahead of his time – thus Nietzsche, in his final (1888) notes on 'Physiology and Art', made some astounding comments which apply equally (or better) to Tourette's:

'... Physiological states that are in the artist as it were moulded into a "personality"...

'The *extreme sharpness* of certain senses, so they understand a quite different sign language – and create one – the condition that seems to be a part of many nervous disorders; *extreme mobility,* that turns into an extreme urge to communicate ... a need to get rid of oneself, as it were, through signs and gestures ... an *explosive* condition. One must think of this condition as a compulsion and urge to get rid of the exuberance of inner tension through muscular activity and movements of all kinds; then as an involuntary coordination between this movement and the processes within (images, thoughts, desires) – as a kind of automatism of the whole muscular system impelled by strong stimuli from within; inability to prevent reaction; the system of inhibitions suspended, as it were...

'The *compulsion to imitate:* an extreme irritability through which a given example becomes contagious – a state is divined on the basis of signs, and immediately enacted – an image, rising up within, immediately turns into a movement of the limbs...', etc. (*The Will to Power,* section 811, March-June, 1888).

Fig. 3. The ticcish phantasmagoria of Tourette's. Photograph by Lowell Handler, 1985.

References

Gilles de la Tourette, G.: Etude sur nerveus caracterisée par de l'incoordination motrice accompagnée d'écholalie et de coprolalie. Archs Neurol. *9:* 19–42, 158–200 (1885).

Goetz, C.G.; Klawans, H.L.: Gilles de la Tourette on Tourette syndrome; in Friedhoff, Chase, Proc. 1st Int. Conf. Gilles de la Tourette Syndrome, 1981. Adv. Neurol., vol. 35, pp. 1–16 (Raven Press, New York 1982).

Jelliffe, S.E.: Postencephalitic respiratory disorders (Nervous & Mental Disease Publishing, Washington 1927).

Jelliffe, S.E.: Psychopathology of forced movements and the oculogyric crises of lethargic encephalitis (Nervous & Mental Disease Publishing, Washington 1932).

Klima, E.S.; Bellugi, U.: The signs of language (Harvard University Press, Cambridge 1979).

Lees, A.J.: Tics and related disorders (Churchill-Livingstone, New York 1985).

Lees, A.J.: Georges Gilles de la Tourette: the man and his times. Revue neurol. *142:* 808–816 (1986).

Luria, A.R.: The mind of a mnemonist (Basic Books, New York 1968).

Mahler, M.S.: Psychoanalytic evaluation of tic in psychopathology of children. Psychoanalytic study of the child (International University Press, New York 1949).

Mahler, M.S.; Rangel, L.: A psychosomatic study of 'maladie des tics' (Gilles de la Tourette disease). Psychoanal. Q. *17:* 579–603 (1943).

Meige, G.; Feindel, E.: Tics and their treatment (transl. and edited by S.A.K. Wilson from 1902 original) (Wood, New York 1907).

Nauta, W. J.H.: Reciprocal links of the corpus striatum with the cerebral cortex and limbic system: a common substrate for movement and thoughts? (this volume).

Sacks, O.W.: Awakenings (Doubleday, New York 1974).

Sacks, O.W.: Acquired Tourettism in adult life; in Friedhoff, Chase, Proc. 1st Int. Conf. Gilles de la Tourette Syndrome, 1981. Adv. Neurol., vol. 35, pp. 89–92 (Raven Press, New York 1982).

Sacks, O.W.: The possessed; in Sacks, The man who mistook his wife for a hat (Summit, New York 1985a).

Sacks, O.W.: Witty ticcy Ray; in Sacks, The man who mistook his wife for a hat, pp. 87–96 (Summit, New York 1985b).

Seignot, J.-N.: A case of Gilles de la Tourette's disease after 10 years' treatment with haloperidol; in Abuzzahab, Anderson, International Registry; Gilles de la Tourette syndrome, vol. 1, pp. 159–162 (Mason, St. Paul 1976).

Oliver W. Sacks, MD, 119 Horton Street, Bronx, NY 10464 (USA)

Mueller (ed.): Neurology and Psychiatry: A Meeting of Minds,
pp. 175–191 (Karger, Basel 1989)

Some Neurobehavioral Aspects of Closed Head Injury

Michael P. Alexander

Behavioral Neurology, Braintree Hospital, and Department of Neurology,
Boston University School of Medicine, Boston, Mass., USA

Traumatic brain injury is the most common neurologic disease in America today [Kurtze, 1982]. Even when attention is limited to severe traumatic, nonpenetrating head injury, the prevalence of post-traumatic encephalopathy is probably matched only by epilepsy, stroke, Alzheimer's disease and multiple sclerosis. When the age of the average patient and his/her life expectancy with the disorder are both considered, the relative significance of traumatic brain injury is apparent.

Despite the prevalence and despite the frequency of major cognitive or behavioral sequelae, severe traumatic brain injury has not seen much directed neurobehavioral research. There have been two major reasons for this neglect.

There is a commonly held idea that severe closed head injury (CHI) provides no insights into brain-behavior relationships because the neuropathology is 'dirty' – that is to say, unlocalizable, or diffuse or multiple or all three or worse. There is another commonly held belief that the neurobehavioral deficits following even severe CHI are subtle and often cannot be easily distinguished from explicitly psychiatric behaviors after trauma. These two assumptions about behavioral residuals of CHI have thus far only been challenged by psychometric analyses – analyses which generally consider the CHI population to be pathologically homogeneous, except for severity, and which often include a non-CHI control group to exclude psychiatric effects [Brooks et al., 1980]. These analyses have been useful to document that CHI leaves residual deficits which are not subtle, which are readily distinguished from psychiatric syndromes, and which, as a group effect, have measurably predictable evolution over time. These data are also useful in clinical assessment, prognostication and perhaps in devising treatments, but they offer no useful explanation of the structural-functional relationships which would define a science of CHI management.

The techniques for such a science are not readily at hand, but there are vantage points which offer some limited views of specific clinical-anatomical relationships in CHI. From this vantage point we will ask, 'Do those syndrome types each have unique pathologies?' and 'What are the identifiable syndrome types after CHI?'

Focal Cortical Contusions

Focal cortical contusions (FCC) can be caused by two different processes. First, a direct effect of trauma can cause FCC at a point of contact (coup) or directly across the brain from the point of contact (contre coup). The injuries are related to skull deformation and to the linear inertial movement of the brain after the skull has impacted, deformed and even rebounded [Ommaya et al., 1971]. FCC in these circumstances are often associated with skull fractures and with damage to vascular structures at the point of contact which, in turn, may cause epidural and/or subdural hematomas. Second, an indirect effect of trauma can cause FCC distant from the point of contact. These injuries are caused by inertial rotatory movement of the brain within the skull. Where relatively mobile brain surfaces (those not tightly tethered to basal penetrating vessels or to the falx) abut a very rough inner table of the skull, abrasive cortical injuries can occur. These indirect FCC are much more common than the direct, and they tend to occur in two places – orbitofrontal/frontal polar cortex and anterior temporal cortex (fig. 1, 2) [Adams, 1975]. They are also commonly bilateral although not necessarily symmetrical. The exact pathology of FCC is somewhat variable. Depending upon the degree of injury to vascular structures of the surface of the brain, there may be only abrasive disruption of gyral crests or there may be localized edema and/or hemorrhage into the FCC. The hemorrhage may track a great distance into the subjacent white matter pathways. In summary, FCC occur in some patients with CHI, and the pathophysiology is reasonably well understood.

What are the clinical phenomena? Patients with FCC may never be unconscious, and it is a reasonable presumption that the cases without unconsciousness represent nearly pure FCC. Therefore, the duration of

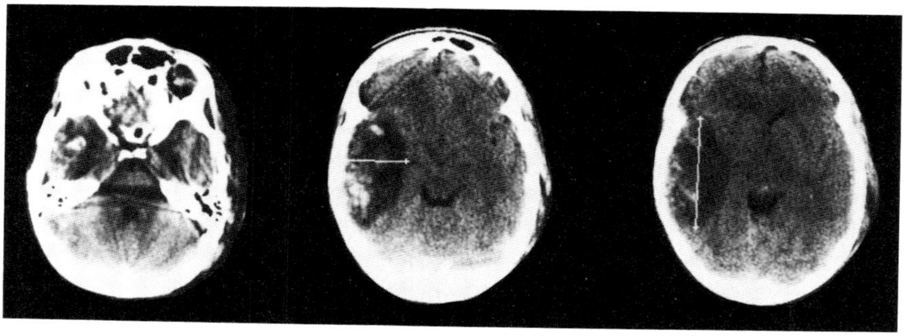

Fig. 1. Nonenhanced CT performed 4 days after injury in a 30-year-old woman who fell from a moving car while inebriated. Total duration of coma was a few hours, but the post-traumatic confusional state lasted weeks. CT demonstrates a typical hemorrhagic contusion of the temporal lobe. Note that the hemorrhage is visualized in the lowest part of the middle cranial fossa as irregular mixed densities (blood and surrounding edema). This unilateral right temporal lobe lesion produced profound affective and behavioral changes, still very apparent 4 months after injury. This case represents relatively isolated focal cortical contusion.

coma has almost no relationship to severity of FCC. The location of the FCC is very important in explicating the clinical syndrome. Direct FCC may occur anywhere in the brain, depending upon only the point of contact and the presence or absence of skull deformity and/or fracture.

The clinical phenomena will be directly predictable from the point of injury. Post-mortem [Adams, 1975] and computerized tomography (CT) studies [Clifton et al., 1980] both document that indirect FCC are almost always located on the inferior frontal surface or the anterior, inferior temporal surface. The acute effects of these FCC depend upon the site of the lesion but also upon the mass effect determined by the extent of hemorrhage beyond the cortical surface [Lobato et al., 1983]. Damage to temporal neocortex and subjacent white matter may disrupt input to hippocampus and amygdala with subsequent prominent impairments of memory and affect. If the hemorrhagic extension of FCC tracks up and back in the temporal lobe, there may be damage to pathways projecting to primary and secondary auditory cortex with subsequent language comprehension deficits. Damage to posterior inferior frontal regions may disrupt septal structures and projections to and from basal forebrain or hypothalamus with subsequent amnesia and motivational deficits [Alexander and Freedman, 1984]. Damage to more anterior inferior frontal regions may extend up into the subventricular white matter pathways including

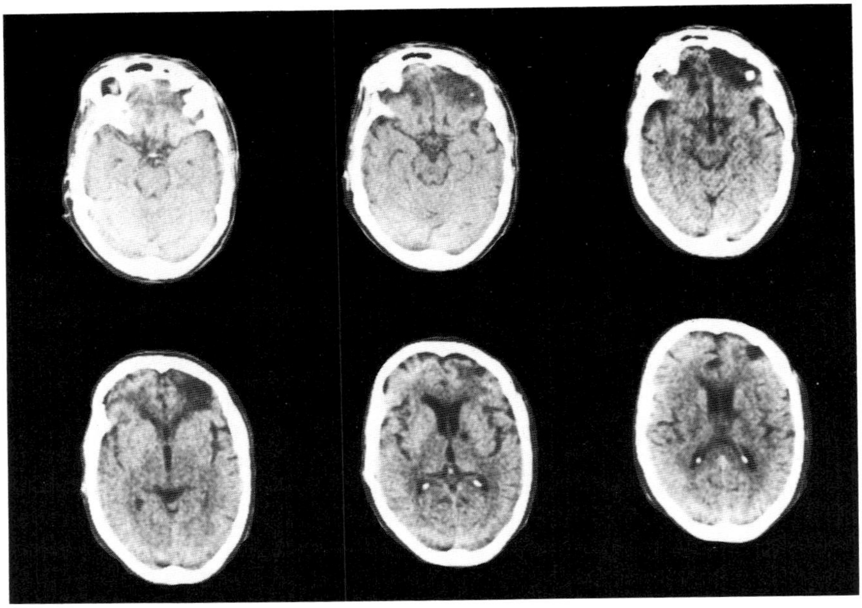

Fig. 2. Nonenhanced CT performed 3 months after injury in a 44-year-old woman who fell from a balcony. Total duration of coma was 2 weeks with a post-traumatic confusional state of over 2 months. CT demonstrates the typical residual changes of severe contusion of the orbital frontal lobes. Low density changes are noted beginning at the lowest level of the orbital regions (upper left-hand image) and these low density areas track up into the frontal white matter anterior to the frontal horns of the lateral ventricles. These bilateral frontal lesions (left greater than right) produced dramatic personality change. This case represents a combination of severe diffuse injury and severe bilateral focal cortical contusion.

dopaminergic projections to cingulum and frontal cortex with subsequent attentional and motor activation deficits [Ross and Stewart, 1981]. The late effects of these lesions depend upon the extent of tissue destruction as opposed to mass effect and displacement. These cortical regions are major neocortical limbic projection centers, and deficits in personality, motivation, and behavior are not unexpected [Nauta and Feirtag, 1986]. The subjacent white matter in these regions contains important projections of sensory association cortex to limbic system (anterior temporal) or of bidirectional limbic to neocortical (frontal) systems. Again, deficits in arousal, attention, motivation and memory are dominant. Patients with these inferior limbic neocortical lesions do not have significant deficits in language, perception, praxis or sensorimotor function. There are few other clinical settings in which previously well young people may suddenly develop bilateral limbic cortical deficits.

Diffuse Axonal Injury

The second recognized pathological process generated by CHI is diffuse axonal injury (DAI). DAI is caused by the rotatory inertial forces which are absorbed by the brain after sudden cranial deceleration. The physics and neuropathology have been established through both primate experimental and human postmortem avenues [Adams et al., 1982; Gennarelli et al., 1982]. In the postmortem studies of Adams et al. [1977, 1982], two types of lesions were observed in patients who were unconscious from the moment of injury until death. First, there were widespread, microscopic areas of axonal disruptions and, at times, small blood vessel ruptures with petechial hemorrhage. Second, there were macroscopic areas of softening, often hemorrhagic, along the corpus callosum at the lateral margins of the lateral ventricle and in the dorsolateral quadrant of the midbrain. The experimental model of Gennarelli et al. [1982] reproduced these exact lesions in nonhuman primates with a purely inertial injury. The severity of neuropathologic change was closely related to the duration of unconsciousness and to residual neurological deficits. We presume that the patient with immediate loss of consciousness but no CT evidence of focal lesion has suffered DAI in pure form.

In the last few years a number of careful CT studies have outlined the various CT findings which may reflect DAI [Lobato et al., 1983]. In these studies there has been no direct confirmation of neuropathology; we retain our presumption from the animal studies that instant loss of consciousness without major FCC is the clinical hallmark of DAI. Although CT does not demonstrate FCC, several abnormalities may be observed. Scattered punctate hemorrhages in deep white matter are a frequent finding (fig. 3). Rapid development of diffuse cerebral edema is another common finding, particularly in children. Larger localized areas of patchy hemorrhage in the periventricular white matter or in the posterior mesencephalon are uncommon but occasionally observed. Whatever the initial profile, the subsequent demonstration of enlarged ventricles is also a common finding in DAI, presumably atrophy secondary to deep damage [Meyers et al., 1983]. We have also infrequently observed larger hemorrhages in the capsular-

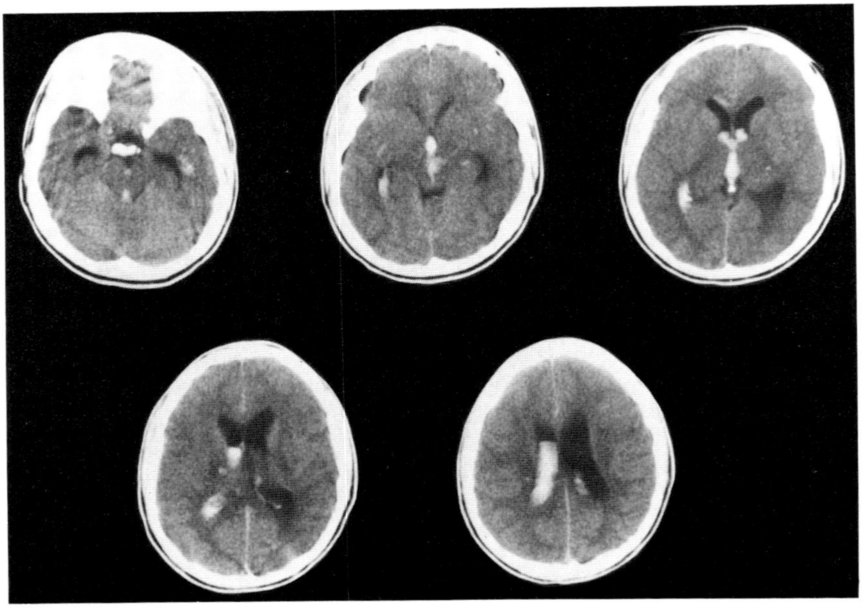

Fig. 3. Nonenhanced CT performed on the day of injury in a 16-year-old boy injured in a car accident. Total duration of coma was 3 weeks, and post-traumatic confusional state lasted a total of 2 months. CT demonstrates blood in the entire ventricular system, as well as patchy punctate blood densities in the white matter of both hemispheres – note the small hemorrhages in the right periventricular area, the anterior corpus callosum, the deep left temporal lobe, and the medial midbrain. This patient had persistent bilateral motor deficits, both corticospinal and cerebellar outflow type, and marked cognitive impairments – easily overloaded memory, slowness, and concreteness. This case represents pure diffuse axonal injury with very dramatic CT findings; many equally badly injured patients have much less striking changes on CT.

putaminal region in cases of DAI (fig. 4), perhaps due to shearing injury to the lenticulostriate penetrators. All of the above CT profiles, as well as a totally normal CT, are compatible with DAI, probably of different severities. In summary, DAI occurs in CHI as a result of a clearly identified pathophysiology.

The clinical phenomena are less definitely understood. Patients with DAI are probably always unconscious at outset. Depth of coma, as measured by a clinical instrument such as the Glasgow Coma Scale [Teasdale and Jennett, 1974] and duration of coma, are likely reflections of the severity of DAI, as they are in the primate model. Concussion is the

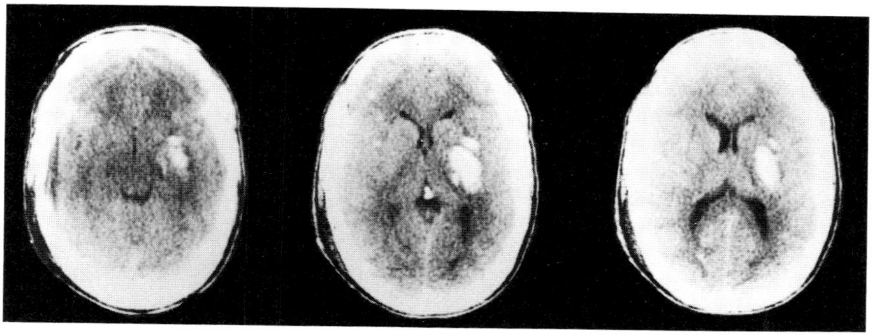

Fig. 4. Nonenhanced CT performed on the day of injury in an 18-year-old boy injured in a car accident. Duration of coma was less than 1 day; post-traumatic confusional state lasted 1 week. CT demonstrates a multilobulated hemorrhage in the left putamen. Several small punctate hemorrhages can also be seen in the deep right frontal white matter. This patient had right hemiparesis and fluent aphasia which cleared almost completely in 2 months. Moderate memory and cognitive impairments were more persistent. This case represents a form of diffuse axonal injury with a superimposed specific focal hemorrhagic component.

mildest clinically recognizable DAI [Oppenheimer, 1968]; instant death at impact, the most severe [Adams et al., 1982]. Skull fractures and intracranial, extracerebral hematomas are less frequent than FCC cases [Adams et al., 1982].

Some elements of clinical impairment can be identified as specific subsets of the DAI pathology. In the motor domain: hemiparesis greater in the leg may be secondary to the periventricular predominance of white matter damage [Gennarelli et al., 1982]. Efferent cerebellar signs are probably secondary to mesencephalic tegmentum injury involving the superior cerebellar peduncle. Oculomotor disturbances are due to posterior mesencephalic damage. In the experimental model DAI changes are most marked in parasagittal regions [Gennarelli et al., 1982]. In humans this would be a potential basis for the commonly observed prolonged mutism and hypokinesia [Botez and Barbeau, 1971]. As acute loss of consciousness is the hallmark of DAI, prolonged alteration in arousal, alertness and attention are probably the residual deficits. In mild cases this is manifested as a period of poor concentration and reduced speed of information processing – the postconcussive encephalopathy. In progressively more severe cases this is manifested as coma, moving to confusional state, moving to prolonged deficits in concentration and mental endurance.

Disturbances in language, praxis and perception are not seen except as manifestations of a confusional state.

Before concluding this section a brief summary of the behavioral neurology of minor head injury is warranted. Minor head injury is more common than severe injury [Kurtze, 1982] but the proper management of minor head injury has been much more difficult to establish. A postmortem study of humans with minor head injury (who died of some systemic injury) revealed disrupted axons in much the same manner and distribution as in the cases of severe head injury [Oppenheimer, 1968].

The changes were, of course, much less prominent. Jane et al. [1985] demonstrated DAI in monkeys subjected to mild inertial injury with brief loss of consciousness. There seems to be a direct continuum to the more severe injury induced by the techniques of Gennarelli et al. [1982].

The clinical manifestations of minor injuries are reasonably well understood [Colohan et al., 1986]. Acutely, there is a brief loss or alteration of consciousness, followed by a brief period of confusion. Over the next few hours the patient may come to feel quite normal although some residual mental slowness is apparent. As the patient returns to normal activities, symptoms of disturbed function may be more apparent. Patients commonly are impaired by headache, dizziness or equilibrium impairment, poor concentration and/or memory and easy fatigability. Poor equilibrium may be secondary to injury to the peripheral mechanisms of equilibrium (the semicircular canal) or to the eighth cranial nerve, both within the temporal bone. DAI may also involve central vestibular connections. Detailed vestibular testing will clarify the source of symptoms [Rowe and Carlson, 1980]; the prognosis is generally good. Concentration and/or memory impairment seems to be caused by direct central damage. The natural history of attentional disturbance after minor CHI has been well described by Gronwall and Wrightson [1974]. They defined a course of slow recovery to normal over 5–10 weeks. Rimel et al. [1981] have documented that cognitive deficits, emotional disturbances and secondary psychosocial and vocational problems can be propagated for a long period of time.

It often becomes very difficult to establish how much of a profile of impairment is due to direct cognitive injury and how much is due to secondary depression or anxiety. We recommend that patients with a minor CHI be treated methodically [Gronwall, 1987]. They must take a few days off from routine demands. Depending upon the nature of employment, return should be part time. Any demands upon equilibrium (scaffolding, heights etc.) may demand careful neurological assessment before return.

Activities requiring high attentional capacity (driving, vigilance tasks, etc.) will have to be part time or at least scheduled with frequent breaks. The patient must be reassured that the symptoms are direct consequences of CHI, not 'psychological', but also assured, perhaps even instructed, that they will clear over 5–10 weeks. If the patient remains symptomatic, neuropsychological and neurological evaluations should be structured to define cognitive deficits [Rimel et al., 1981; Barth et al., 1983]. If they are more severe than anticipated, it is likely that the severity of injury has been underestimated, and the natural history of recovery may be longer than expected. Assessment should also be structured to identify secondary psychological factors which may emerge if the patient has not had opportunity to recover before returning to normal activities. We believe that anxiety and depression both occur, and both are readily treated with focused psychotherapy or appropriate drugs.

Hypoxic-Ischemic Injury

The third well-recognized pathology of CHI is hypoxic-ischemic injury (HII) [Graham et al., 1979]. Two factors contribute to HII. Compression of vascular structures, by edematous brain and/or extracerebral masses (subdural or epidural hematomas), may reduce blood supply to a region of brain. Systemic injury with blood loss, shock, or systemic hypoxia may also contribute to HII. In postmortem and clinical studies, there has been evidence that both factors are often present. Increased intracranial pressure with cerebral edema and/or a large mass, especially when combined with a systemic factor reducing cerebral perfusion, may result in widespread, but patchy, even microscopic, areas of ischemic neuronal injury predominantly in the terminal arterial border zones across the frontoparietal cortex. Lateral cerebral herniation with compression of the posterior cerebral artery or arteries may produce localized infarction in the temporo-occipital region(s). Central cerebral herniation with compression of mesencephalic perforating arteries may produce localized infarction in the medial midbrain.

The clinical syndrome of *diffuse* HII is not known. Patients who survive CHI to a persistent vegetative state may have *diffuse* HII. Some survivors with profound dementia (an otherwise unusual outcome) may have suffered *diffuse* HII. Infarctions in the territories of the posterior cerebral arteries are, on the other hand, amongst the most intensively studied

Table I. Schema for classification of neuropathology associated with closed head injury

Focal cortical contusions	*Direct* (at point of injury): clinical consequences depend solely upon the exact location of the injury; location often related to the site of skull fracture or overlying subdural hematoma
	Indirect (due to inertial forces): location overwhelmingly inferior temporal and inferior frontal; clinical consequences are fairly predictable = deficits in memory, emotion and behavior
Diffuse axonal injury	*Widespread:* present in all cases; maximal in parasagittal distribution; clinical consequences are motor (akinesia, mutism, paresis) and attentional
	Small Focal: not present in all cases, but when present are maximal in the paraventricular white matter along the corpus callosum and in the dorsolateral brainstem tegmentum; clinical consequences are an exaggeration of the effect of widespread lesions plus specific brainstem signs (oculomotor and cerebellar outflow)
Hypoxic-ischemic	*Diffuse:* microscopic injuries are predominantly localized to cortical arterial borderzone regions; clinical consequences are not really known but may contribute to dementia or to persistent vegetative state
	Focal: in posterior cerebral artery territories with central visual and memory deficits

lesions in behavioral neurology. The clinical-anatomical correlations are very well established for alexia [Greenblatt, 1983], visual agnosia (Alexander and Albert 1983], amnesia [Victor et al., 1961] etc., but they are not explicitly relevant to the neurology of CHI.

These three distinct neuropathologies intersect after CHI. FCC may occur anywhere depending upon physical factors of injury but tend to be located in neocortical limbic regions. They may be shallow and thus very local, or they may extend into subjacent white matter and there have profound, if unpredictable, pathway effects. DAI produces small lesions distributed down the paramedial axis of the brain with acute and chronic consequences for motor function, behavior and attention. HII produces either scattered neuronal injury or else discrete infarction in temporo-occipital cortex (summarized in table I).

At the present time, the best biologic measure of FCC is brain imaging,

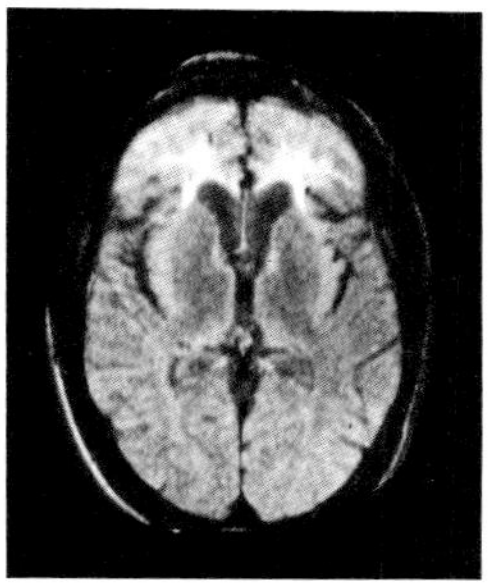

Fig. 5. MRI scan, spin echo type, performed 6 years after a severe closed head injury in a 24-year-old man. Duration of coma was 7–10 days; post-traumatic confusional state lasted 3 weeks. Acute CT was unremarkable (small subdural hygromas only), and CT done a few months prior to this MRI was entirely normal except for moderately large ventricles for age. This scan reveals areas of increased signal in the periventricular white matter of both frontal lobes. Clinical findings at the time of the scan were primarily personality alterations – irritability, tangentiality and socially inappropriate intrusiveness. These changes on MRI probably represent glial scarring in the areas of greatest diffuse axonal injury. Scans such as this suggest that MRI is the best way to quantify the pathologic anatomy of diffuse injury.

either CT [Lobato et al., 1983] or magnetic resonance imaging (MRI) [Levin et al., 1985]. MRI has the distinct advantage for this population of demonstrating inferior cortical surfaces without any obscuring bone artifact. The best measure of DAI is the constellation of clinical measures – depth of coma, duration of coma, and duration of confusion. Valid, objective clinical measures of attention may eventually be developed; MRI shows promise as a tool to demonstrate directly the distribution of DAI (fig. 5). The best measure of HII is imaging for cortical atrophy due to diffuse HII or for focal infarction secondary to HII in the posterior-cerebral artery territory. The clinical, behavioral or neuroimaging consequences of combinations of pathologies are not known with certainty and, of course, combinations of pathology are more common than any one pathology alone (table I).

The second aspect of CHI in this review is an examination of some unusual behaviors after CHI which might be directly related to combinations of lesions which no other neurological illness can produce. Two examples are illuminating – extraordinary confabulation and reduplicative paramnesias; either or both of which might serve as windows upon the neurology of delusional thinking.

Extraordinary confabulation [Stuss et al., 1978] is confabulation of preposterous and fantastical quality which is often rooted in some environmental cue around the patient, which may be repeatedly produced over a long period of time, and which the patient may come to insist is correct even when all physical evidence is arrayed against him. Patients have insisted (while in a hospital bed and hospital garb) that they were kayaking, being debriefed after a space flight and attending class in their old high school. Although usually present in patients with memory deficits, these confabulations are not based simply on memory failures. The confabulations are very different from the limited confabulations of a patient with stable but severe alcoholic Korsakoff's syndrome. The extraordinary confabulations may persist even after memory improves. Uncommon in other clinical settings, except perhaps after rupture of anterior communicating artery aneurysm, they are quite common after CHI – particularly in patients with bilateral orbitofrontal FCC and enough DAI to produce a confusional state. Extraordinary confabulations tend to appear as the confusional state is clearing. The confabulations are usually related to some event in the patient's life, and they often have a grandiose, epic quality. While not intensely invested in the confabulation, the patients nevertheless argue against all reason and fact that their recall is correct.

Reduplicative paramnesia (RP) [Weinstein and Kahn, 1955] is an inaccurate recollection based on some fragmentary but distorted recall (paramnesia) in which some person or place becomes two related people or places (reduplication). These RPs may persist after memory has recovered, and the patient will often insist that they are correct even after he has recovered well enough to reason out the truth. Transient RP of place is common after large right hemisphere lesions of any type, but persistent RP of place or person is rare. It has been described after CHI in which a particular constellation of lesions occurs – bilateral orbitofrontal FCC and enough DAI to produce a lengthy confusional state plus specifically right parietal FCC for RP of place [Benson et al., 1976] or right temporal FCC for RP of person [Alexander et al., 1978]. As in the extraordinary confabulations, RP tends to emerge as confusion is clearing. The patients may resist, argue and reason against all attempts to clarify 'their' confusion.

RP of person has a particularly compelling parallel in conventional psychiatric phenomenology – the Capgras' syndrome [Capgras and Reboul-Lachaux, 1923] or the delusion of imposters. Originally described in patients with the diagnosis of psychotic depression, but now more commonly diagnosed in patients with a diagnosis of schizophrenia, Capgras' syndrome is a restricted delusion that someone important to the patient (family member, physician, etc.) has been replaced with an imposter; only the patient can tell the difference. In RP of person, the patient also believes that someone important has been replaced but usually by a substitute who does not carry the ominous implications of an imposter. We have reported a patient with the stable and dramatic delusion that his wife and five children had been replaced by another woman and her five children who were 'almost' identical to the originals [Alexander et al., 1978]. The patient could not explain how this substitution had occurred or how others could distinguish the two families. He attributed no threatening motive to the substitution and, in fact, was pleased that two families would care about him so much. He recognized that the story did not sound believable, acknowledged that he would not believe it if someone else told him, but repeatedly asserted his conviction that it was true. This patient had bilateral orbitofrontal damage (right greater than left) and extensive right inferior temporal damage, the RP developed as he was emerging from a confusional state. The specific deficits of visual memory [Milner, 1968] and of capacity to assess familiarity secondary to right temporal injury plus the attentional, problem solving and affective deficits of orbital frontal injury appear to have combined to produce the delusional state. Very similar functional deficits associated with the major psychoses (thought disorders) can apparently lead to a similar syndrome.

These two phenomena (extraordinary confabulation and RP of person) suggest a cerebral mechanism for the development of delusions. They are the result of impaired problem solving (defective strategy formation and defective inferential reasoning) when there is simultaneously a disturbance in the ability to establish a situational context (either amnesia for the context or perceptual/familiarity impairments which mislabel the context) and also a disturbance in affective labelling of experience (either flat, apathetic acceptance of the improbable as real [CHI] or suspicious, hyperattentive rejection of the probable [psychosis]). There are few other diseases which could generate this constellation of structural lesions which reconstitute the functional deficits of the schizophrenic. Elucidation of the elemental cognitive and affective constituents of psychiatric diseases has been extremely difficult. It is possible that analysis of neurologic processes in which specific psychiatric symptoms and signs occur will be a preferable route to understanding psychiatric disease. Personality in temporal lobe epilepsy [Bear and Fedio, 1977] and depression in Parkinson's disease

[Mayeux et al., 1981] are two such routes. Obsessive-compulsive disorder in postencephalitic states and Gilles de la Tourette syndrome may be others.

The third aspect of CHI which seems appropriate for the goals of this paper is a consideration of the gaps in our understanding of brain-behavior issues in patients with CHI. This list could, of course, be very lengthy; it will, however, be limited to a few rather arbitrarily selected items.

The severity of DAI cannot be defined biologically in survivors. As outlined above, patients with CHI may suffer DAI as a consequence of rotatory inertial forces transmitted through the brain. Abrupt loss of consciousness is the hallmark clinical sign. CT may reveal one of several typical profiles. Severity is judged by an amalgamation of clinical observations, but there is no biologic measure of severity. Therefore, all neuropsychological investigations which purport to demonstrate the critical deficit after CHI are unsupportable because they have no objective measure of comparison. At the present time, MRI offers the best prospect of defining the extent of tissue damage. It is also possible that cognitive evoked potential [Karnaze et al., 1982] may reveal some defining decrement in functional activity which would serve as an objective measure of severity.

It is often suggested that DAI leaves a deficit in attention as a major residual – variously conceived of as sustained attention, vigilance or focused attention. The patients seem to have persistent deficits in concentrating for sustained periods, in shifting attention rapidly between competing sources, and in screening out insistent irrelevant stimuli, but what is this deficit [Brouwer and van Wolffelaar, 1985]? It has not been defined, measured or operationally demonstrated reliably. How does it contribute to the high level cognitive problems that even 'well-recovered' patients display?

Beyond troubles delineating severity and establishing the nature of a core deficit of DAI, there is the problem of establishing subsyndromes of DAI based on idiosyncratic differences in damage distribution. For instance, 15 years ago it was demonstrated that over 50% of patients dying of CHI had significant DAI lesions in the hypothalamus [Crompton, 1971], yet there is still no clinical, laboratory, or imaging technique to establish this injury in life, except in those rare cases with unequivocal diencephalic-posterior pituitary dysfunction. In a population in whom personality change, irritability, low motivation states, inappropriate behavior, sleep-wake disturbances and the like are common residuals, it seems unbelievable that no method to define hypothalamic injury has emerged.

In the section on FCC it was suggested that the depth of contusion extension might influence neurobehavioral sequelae, whatever the extent of cortical injury. In most other realms of behavioral neurology in which careful attention has been paid to lesion extent, this consideration (depth of damage) has been productive in understanding clinical disorders. Evaluation of the Kluver-Bucy syndrome (temporal neocortex versus temporal white matter versus amygdala) is an example [Akert et al., 1961]. Investigations of aphasia (big Broca's versus little Broca's) is another [Mohr et al., 1978]. Higher order visual disorders (temporal-occipital neocortex versus the occipitotemporal pathways) are others [Alexander and Albert, 1983]. In CHI with FCC there are probably very specific advances to be made in clinical-anatomical correlations simply by careful study of the white matter extent of orbitofrontal lesions.

The last gap in our understanding of CHI which will be considered here is the absence of scientific or clinical evidence about the interaction of lesions with age and sex. This problem may be particularly acute for CHI for two reasons. One, CHI occurs across the entire age span from infancy to senescence. Two, FCC after CHI has a predilection for limbic structures, which are critical for the modulation of basic drives and which mature across the early life. Damage to orbitofrontal regions in an adolescent male whose brain has only recently been exposed to increased testosterone, whose frontal cortical connections may still be incomplete, and whose motivated behaviors are dominated by one or two elemental biological drives, cannot be expected to have the same effect as the exact same CT injury in a late middle-aged man with mature frontal connections and weaker elemental drives but stronger abstract drives (making money, security for old age, etc.). Particularly in cases with hypothalamic DAI, age and sex might have powerful influences on residual deficit states.

In conclusion, I would like to reemphasize a few points. First, the neurobehavioral deficits of severe CHI are not 'dirty'. They are explicable residuals of at least three discrete neuropathologic processes. Each possesses distinct rules of clinical-anatomical correlation although many rules await definition. Second, because CHI may result in unique distributions of lesions in the limbic system, it may be a source of rare cases with combinations of lesions which offer particularly illuminating views of specific neurobehavioral deficits, such as delusions. Third, there are several areas ripe for clinical investigation in CHI which may even further clarify some basic brain-behavior principles.

References

Adams, J.H.: The neuropathology of head injuries; in Vinken, Bruyn, Handbook of clinical neurology, pp. 35–65 (North-Holland, Amsterdam 1975).

Adams, J.H.: Graham, D.I.; Murray, L.S.; Scott, G.: Diffuse axonal injury due to nonmissile head injury in humans: an analysis of 45 cases. Ann. Neurol. *12;* 564–574 (1982).

Adams, J.H.; Mitchell, D.E.; Graham, D.I.; Doyle, D.: Diffuse brain damage of immediate impact type. Brain *100:* 489–502 (1977).

Akert, K.; Gruesen, R.A.; Woolsley, R.N., et al.: Kluver-Bucy syndrome in monkey with neocortical ablations of temporal lobe. Brain *84:* 480–498 (1961).

Alexander, M.P.; Albert, M.L.: Visual agnosia; in Kertesz, Localization in Neuropsychology, pp. 393–415 (Academic Press, New York 1983).

Alexander, M.P.; Freedman, M.: Amnesia after anterior communicating artery aneurysm rupture. Neurology, Minneap. *34:* 752–757 (1984).

Alexander, M.P.; Stuss, D.T.; Benson, D.F.: Capgras' syndrome: a reduplicative phenomenon. Neurology, Minneap. *29:* 334–339 (1978).

Barth, J.T.; Macciocchi, S.N.; Giordani, B., et al.: Neuropsychological sequelae of minor head injury. Neurosurgery *13:* 529–533 (1983).

Bear, D.M.; Fedio, P.: Quantitative analysis of interictal behavior in temporal lobe epilepsy. Archs Neurol., Chicago *34:* 454–467 (1977).

Benson, D.F.; Gardner, H.; Meadows, J.C.: Reduplicative paramnesia. Neurology, Minneap. *26:* 147–151 (1976).

Botez, M.I.; Barbeau, A.: Role of subcortical structures and particularly the thalamus in the mechanisms of speech and language. Int. J. Neurol. *8:* 300–320 (1971).

Brooks, D.N.; Aughton, M.E.; Bond, M.R., et al.: Cognitive sequelae in relationship to indices of severity of brain damage after severe blunt head injury. J. Neurol. Neurosurg. Psychiat. *43:* 529–534 (1980).

Brouwer, W.H.; van Wolffelaar, P.C.: Sustained attention and sustained effort after closed head injury: detection and 0.10 Hz heart rate variability in a low event rate vigilance task. Cortex *21:* 111–119 (1985).

Capgras, J.; Reboul-Lachaux, J.: Illusions des sosies dans un délire systématisé chronique. Bull. Soc. clin. méd. ment. *2:* 6–16 (1923).

Clifton, G.L.; Grossman, R.G.; Makela, M.E., et al.: Neurological course and correlated computerized tomography findings after severe closed head injury. J. Neurosurg. *52:* 611–614 (1980).

Colohan, A.R.T.; Dacey, R.G.; Alves, W.M., et al.: Neurological and neurosurgical implications of mild head injury. J. Head Trauma Rehabil. *1:* 13–21 (1986).

Crompton, M.R.: Hypothalamic lesions following closed head injury. Brain *94:* 165–172 (1971).

Gennarelli, T.A.; Thibault, L.E., Adams, J.H., et al.: Diffuse axonal injury and traumatic coma in the primate. Ann. Neurol. *12:* 564–574 (1982).

Graham, D.I.; Adams, J.H.; Doyle, D.: Ischaemic brain damage in fatal nonmissile head injuries. J. Neurosci. *39:* 213–234 (1979).

Greenblatt, S.H.: Localization of lesions in alexia; in Kertesz, Localization in neuropsychology, pp. 323–356 (Academic Press, New York 1983).

Gronwall, D.: Advances in the assessment of attention and information processing after head injury; in Levin, Grofman, Eisenberg, Neurobehavioral recovery from head injury, pp. 355–371 (Oxford University Press, New York 1987).

Gronwall, D.; Wrightson, P.: Delayed recovery of intellectual function after minor head injury. Lancet *ii:* 605–609 (1974).
Jane, J.; Stewart, O.; Gennarelli, T.A.: Axonal degeneration induced by experimental non-invasive minor head injury. J. Neurosurg. *62:* 96–100 (1985).
Karnaze, D.S.; Marshall, L.F.; McCarthy, S., et al.: Localizing and prognostic value of auditory evoked responses in coma after closed head injury. Neurology, Minneap. *32:* 299–302 (1982).
Kurtze, J.F.: The current neurologic burden of illness and injury in the United States. Neurology, Minnap. *32:* 1207–1214 (1982).
Levin, H.S.; Handel, S.F.; Goldman, A.M., et al.: Magnetic resonance imaging after 'diffuse' nonmissile head injury: a neurobehavioral study. Archs Neurol., Chicago *42:* 963–968 (1985).
Lobato, R.D.; Cordobes, F.; Rivas, J.J., et al.: Outcome of severe head injury related to the type of intracranial lesion. J. Neurosurg. *59:* 762–774 (1983).
Mayeux, R.; Stern. Y.; Rosen, J.; Leventhal, J.: Depression, intellectual impairment, and Parkinson's disease. Neurology, Minneap. *31:* 645–650 (1981).
Meyers, C.A.; Levin, H.S.; Eisenberg, H.M.: Early versus late ventricular enlargement following closed head injury. J. Neurol. Neurosurg. Psychiat. *46:* 1092–1097 (1983).
Milner, B.: Visual recognition and recall after right temporal lobe excision in man. Neuropsychologia *6:* 191–209 (1968).
Mohr, J.P.; Pessin, M.S.; Finkelstein, S., et al.: Broca's aphasia: pathologic and clinical. Neurology, Minneap. *28:* 311–324 (1978).
Nauta, W.J.H.; Feirtag, M.: Fundamental neuroanatomy, pp. 120–131 (Freeman, New York 1986).
Ommaya, A.K.; Grubb, R.L., Jr.; Naumann, R.A.: Coup and contre-coup injury: observations on the mechanics of visible brain injuries in the Rhesus monkey. J. Neurosurg. *35:* 503–503 (1971).
Oppenheimer, D.R.: Microscopic lesions in the brain following head injury. J. Neurol. Neurosurg. Psychiat. *31:* 299–306 (1968).
Rimel, R.W.; Giordani, B.; Barth, J.T., et al.: Disability caused by minor head injury. Neurosurgery *9:* 221–223 (1981).
Ross, E.D.; Stewart, R.M.: Akinetic mutism from hypothalamic damage: successful treatment with dopamine agonists. Neurology, Minneap. *31:* 1435–1439 (1981).
Rowe, M.J.; Carlson, C.: Brainstem auditory evoked potentials in postconcussion dizziness. Archs Neurol., Chicago *37:* 679–683 (1980).
Stuss, D.T.; Alexander, M.P.; Lieberman, A.; Levine, H.: An extraordinary form of confabulation. Neurology, Minneap. *28:* 1166–1172 (1978).
Teasdale, G.; Jennett, B.: Assessment of coma and impaired consciousness; a practical scale. Lancet *ii:* 81–84 (1974).
Victor, M.; Angevine, J.B.; Mancall, E.L.; Fisher, C.M.: Memory loss with lesions of the hippocampal formation. Archs Neurol., Chicago *5:* 244–263 (1961).
Weinstein, E.A.; Kahn, R.L.: Denial of illness: symbolic and physiological aspects (Thomas, Springfield 1955).

Michael P. Alexander, MD, Behavioral Neurology, Braintree Hospital,
250 Pond Street, Braintree, MA 02184 (USA)

Mueller (ed.): Neurology and Psychiatry: A Meeting of Minds,
pp. 192–209 (Karger, Basel 1989)

Post-Stroke Mood Disorders[1]

Sergio E. Starkstein[a, c], *Robert G. Robinson*[a, b]

Departments of [a] Psychiatry and Behavioral Sciences and [b] Neuroscience,
The Johns Hopkins University School of Medicine, Baltimore, Md., USA;
[c] University of Buenos Aires, Buenos Aires, Argentina

Stroke has an annual incidence of approximately 400,000 and is the third leading cause of death in the USA [Wolf et al., 1977]. Adams and Victor [1985] defined stroke as a sudden nonconvulsive focal neurological deficit produced by insufficiency of blood circulation to the brain. In spite of the major impact that stroke has had on our health care system, little attention has been paid to the recognition and treatment of emotional disorders which occur following stroke. Feibel and Springer [1982], for instance, reported that the great majority of stroke victims who developed depression in the first 6 months after stroke received no medical care for this problem. The failure to treat post-stroke emotional disorders is one of the great unmet needs of stroke victims.

Despite clinical neglect, the frequent appearance of emotional disorders following stroke has been recognized for many years. Kraepelin [1921] recognized that cerebrovascular infarction may 'engender states of depression'. Goldstein [1948] found that patients with left hemisphere injury developed depression, irritability and explosive outbursts, which he termed the 'catastrophic reaction'. In 1922, Babinski noted that indifference or euphoria can follow right hemisphere damage. Hecaen et al. [1951] and Denny-Brown et al. [1952] identified a similar emotional disorder associated with right hemisphere lesions, which they labeled the 'indifference reaction'.

Depressive disorders generally have been assumed to be an understandable reaction to impairment of function [Fisher, 1961]. Goldstein

[1] This work was supported in part by the following NIH grants: Research Scientist Development Award MH-00163 (RGR), NS-15178, MH-40355, NS-15080, and a grant from the University of Buenos Aires to Dr. Starkstein.

[1948] attributed depression to the, '... desparate reaction of the organisms confronted with severe physical disability. The severity of the catastrophic reaction correlated with severity of the disability.' Fisher [1961] described the depression due to brain damage as reactive and understandable because, '... the brain is the most cherished organ of humanity.' This emphasis on psychological causation of post-brain injury mood disorders, however, contrasts sharply with early clinical observations on the relationship between lesion location and type of emotional disorder [Meyer, 1904]. Preoccupation with psychological causes also overlooks the emerging data from systematic studies of depression following brain injury.

Post [1962], in a study of 100 elderly patients with affective disorder, noted the high frequency of ischemic brain events in patients with first episodes of endogenous depressive disorder. He suggested that the causes of atherosclerotic disease and depression may be linked. Folstein et al. [1977] reported that patients with orthopedic impairments were not as depressed as stroke patients, when matched for severity of physical impairment. Gainotti [1972] demonstrated lateralized emotional syndromes associated with unilateral brain injury. Left hemisphere brain injury produced a depressive catastrophic reaction, while right hemisphere brain injury was associated with indifference and a tendency to joke. Gasparrini et al. [1978], using the Minnesota Multiphasic Personality Inventory (MMPI), found that subjects with left hemisphere dysfunction showed an elevation of the depression subscale when compared with right hemisphere damaged patients. The authors suggested that since no differences were found between the two groups in language, manual dexterity, logical memory, and verbal or performance IQ, the depression occurring with left hemisphere damage could not be ascribed to motor or cognitive disturbances. Ross and Rush [1981] described a right hemisphere neural network subserving emotion and analogized this to the language circuitry of the left hemisphere. In a retrospective study Sackheim et al. [1982] reported that patients with left hemisphere damage had a high incidence of disinhibited or 'pathologic' crying and negative mood changes, while patients with right hemisphere lesions showed 'pathologic' laughter. A high incidence of depression following left hemisphere damage was also reported recently by de Bonis et al. [1985]. Finkelstein et al. [1982] found that depression and failure to suppress serum cortisol after dexamethasone administration were significantly more common in stroke patients than in a control group of patients with equally disabling medical illnesses.

Some investigators, however, have been unable to show a specific relationship between ischemic brain injury and depression. Robins [1976] compared stroke patients with patients disabled from either spinal cord injury or orthopedic disorders. All groups had had their disorders for more than 5 years. Although all three groups reported high levels of depression, he found no differences in severity of depression between stroke patients and the two control groups. Two limitations of this study, however, were that the location of the stroke was not evaluated and the amount of time elapsed since injury was not taken into account. Other investigators have failed to show a significant relationship between hemispheric lesion location (left versus right hemisphere) and frequency or severity of depression [Folstein et al., 1977; Sinyor et al., 1986].

In an effort to determine which factors influence the expression of post-stroke emotional disorders, we have conducted two longitudinal studies of mood disorders following stroke. We have systematically studied the symptoms, course, and associated variables in the development of post-stroke depression (PSD). In this chapter we discuss findings on PSD with particular emphasis on its clinical manifestations, diagnosis, prevalence, course, mechanisms, and results of a treatment study.

Three Types of Post-Stroke Mood Disorders: Clinical Manifestations

We have separated depressed stroke patients into those with major and minor (dysthymic) depressive disorders using symptom criteria for major or dysthymic affective disorder. We did this because the DSM-III category of organic affective disorder makes no distinction of subtypes of affective disorder in terms of symptom severity. We were interested to see if mild to moderate depression would have different associated variables and etiologies than severe depression.

(a) Patients with severe PSD meet DSM-III symptom criteria for major affective disorder [American Psychiatric Association, 1980]. Clinical symptoms found in more than half of these patients with major affective disorder include: sadness, anxiety, tension, loss of energy, worrying, loss of interest, early morning awakening, weight loss, poor concentration, and preoccupation with death or suicide.

(b) Patients with minor depression (from RDC terminology) meet the DSM-III criteria for dysthymic disorder. Minor (dysthymic) depression is characterized by sadness, sleep disturbance, loss of energy, poor concentration, social withdrawal, loss of interest, brooding, pessimistic attitude toward the future, irritability, and tearfulness.

(c) A third mood disorder associated with stroke is an apathetic indifference associated with a cheerfulness which, although not true euphoria, is clearly inappropriate in patients who have suffered a recent stroke. Although it will not be the major focus of this chapter, this disorder is important to distinguish from the two depressive disorders we plan to describe in some detail. The full syndrome consists of anxiety, slowness, loss of interest, and worrying, accompanied by inappropriately cheerful mood. In a previous study [Robinson et al., 1983a] this disorder was found in 6 of 20 patients (30%) who sustained a single right hemisphere lesion, but in none of 28 patients with a single left hemisphere stroke.

Ross and Rush [1981] proposed that disorders of affective language, termed 'aprosodias', may prevent patients with right hemisphere lesions from recognizing, or cause them to actually deny symptoms of depression. Prosodic disturbances may partially explain our failure to find depression among patients with acute right anterior lesions. These patients, however, may also deny symptoms such as sleep or appetite disturbance and loss of libido. This makes the diagnosis of depression in these patients quite difficult.

Prevalence and Duration of Depressive Disorders

In an effort to address the prevalence and duration of PSD we have conducted two studies. The first was a follow-up study involving 103 unselected outpatients who regularly attended a stroke clinic [Robinson and Price, 1982]. The second study was a longitudinal evaluation of acute stroke patients in which we followed 103 patients (a totally different group from the first study) for 2 years after their stroke [Robinson et al., 1983b].

Prevalence

The prevalence of clinically important depression appears to depend on two important variables. The first is the location of the brain injury [Robinson et al., 1984a] and the second is the time elapsed since the stroke [Robinson and Price, 1982]. Although patients with any lesion location can have severe depression, we have demonstrated that patients with left frontal injury are more likely to develop severe depression than patients with any other lesion location [Robinson et al., 1984a]. In a study of 36

1 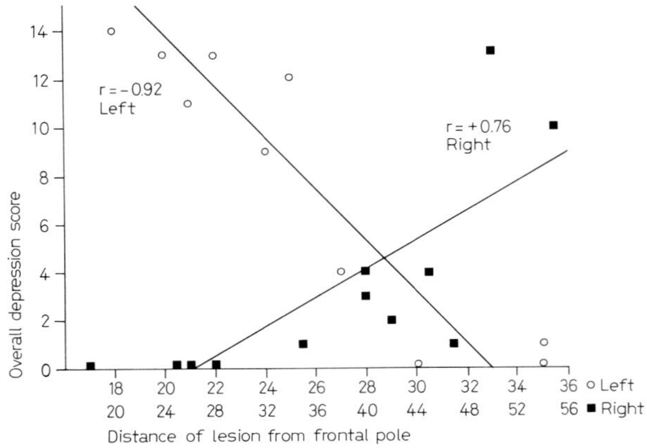

2 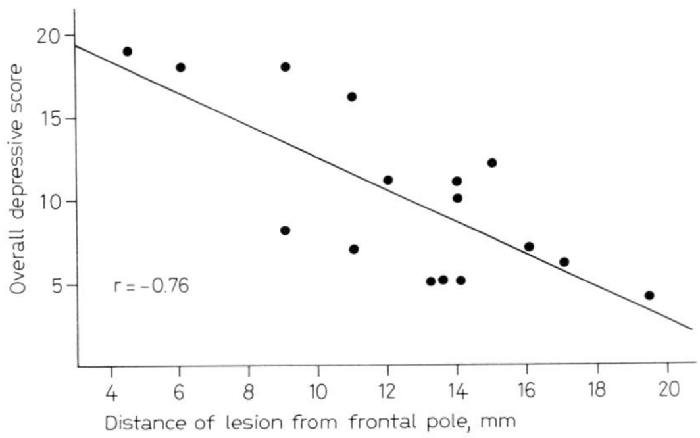

Fig. 1. Relationship between overall depression score and distance of the anterior border of the lesion from the frontal pole for patients with either left anterior hemisphere infarcts or right hemisphere infarcts. The distance from the frontal pole is expressed as a percentage of the total anteroposterior distance. The correlation coefficients are indicated in the figure. r left, $p < 0.001$; r right, $p < 0.01$. From Robinson et al. [1984a]. Reprinted by permission.

Fig. 2. Relationship between severity of depression as measured by overall depression score and mean distance of the lesion from the frontal pole for patients with either stroke or traumatic lesions that extended into the frontal lobe. The closer the lesion was to the frontal pole, the greater was the depression ($r = 0.76$, $p < 0.001$). From Robinson and Szetela [1981]. Reprinted by permission.

patients with computed tomography (CT) verified single lesions of the right or left hemisphere, 6 of 10 patients with left anterior brain injury had the symptoms of major depression and one had minor depression [Robinson et al., 1984a]. Among the patients with left anterior brain injury, CT showed that the closer the anterior border of the lesion was to the frontal pole, the

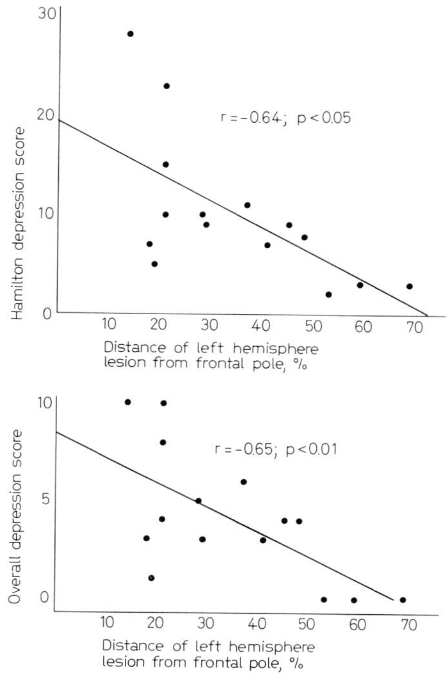

Fig. 3. Relationship between severity of depression as measured by Hamilton Depression Score and overall depression score and mean distance of left hemisphere lesion from the frontal pole. The closer the lesion was to the frontal pole, the greater the depression. Distance from frontal pole is expressed as percent of A-P distance. From Lipsey et al. [1983]. Reprinted by permission.

more severe the depression [Robinson et al., 1984a] (fig. 1). We have also recently confirmed these findings in patients with lesions restricted to either cortical or subcortical structures [Starkstein et al., 1987]. Patients with either cortical or subcortical lesions of the left anterior hemisphere were significantly more depressed than those with any other lesion location and the severity of depression was significantly correlated with the proximity of the lesion to the frontal pole in both cortical and subcortical groups.

We have also demonstrated a strong association between traumatic injury to the left frontal region and severity of depression in patients with both unilateral [Robinson and Szetela, 1981] (fig. 2) and bilateral brain trauma [Lipsey et al., 1983] (fig. 3). Among the patients with bilateral brain injury, the severity of depression depends on the location of the left hemisphere lesion (the more anterior the lesion, the greater the depression) and is independent of the location of the right hemisphere lesion and the temporal sequence of the lesions [Lipsey et al., 1983].

In contrast to patients with left hemisphere injury, only about 15% of patients with single lesions of the right hemisphere have depression during the acute post-stroke period [Robinson et al., 1983a]. In addition, those with right posterior brain injury have more depressive symptoms than those with right anterior brain injury [Robinson et al., 1984a] (fig. 1). Patients with right anterior lesions tend to be apathetic and unduly cheerful, while those with posterior lesions tend to have mild to moderate depressive symptoms. Thus, we have found that both anterior-posterior and left-right aspects of lesion location are important in determining the prevalence of PSD.

The other variable affecting the prevalence of PSD is time elapsed since stroke. When we divided the 103 patients in the first study (outpatient follow-up) into groups based on time since stroke, we found that patients who were between 6 months and 2 years post-stroke had more depressive symptoms than did other groups of patients who were up to 10 years post-stroke. Patients more than 10 years post-stroke, however, tended to have more depressive symptoms than those between 2 and 10 years post-stroke [Robinson and Price, 1982].

Duration

We found in our outpatient follow-up study that almost one third of the patients were depressed at the time of the initial interview, as determined by scores on the General Health Questionnaire [Robinson and Price, 1982]. Two thirds of these initially depressed patients remained depressed for 8–9 months. By one year after the initial evaluation, however, none of the patients continued to remain depressed (fig. 4).

Since depression may have been present for several months before the patients were identified in the clinic, this could have led us to underestimate the apparent duration of depression. This study suggested that depression following stroke is not simply a transient depression that mirrors the clinical course of the stroke. Rather, it appears to have a course of its own that persists at least 8–9 months.

Depression in our prospective 2-year study was determined according to DSM-III criteria for major or minor affective disorders. Patients were seen for initial evaluation at the time of their in-hospital care for acute stroke. This occurred at a mean of 10 days post-stroke with a standard

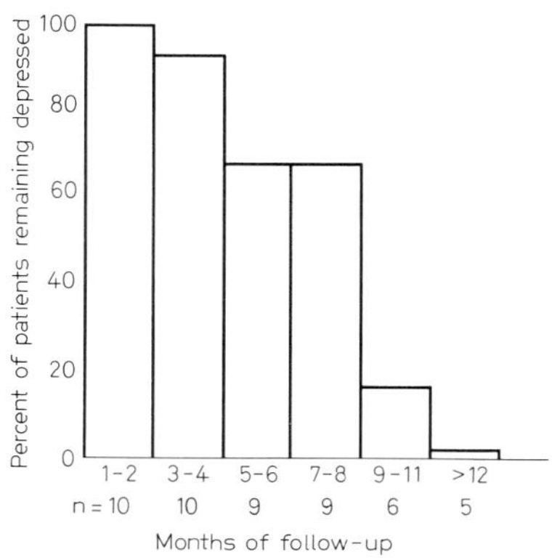

Fig. 4. The percent of patients who were found to be depressed at the initial interview and who continued to be depressed at various time intervals following the initial interview. The number of patients evaluated at each time period is indicated in the figure. From Robinson and Price [1982]. Reprinted by permission.

deviation of 11 days. Twenty-six percent of these 103 acute stroke patients had the symptom cluster of major depression, while 20% had the symptom cluster of minor depression (dysthymic disorder) [Robinson et al., 1983b]. We were able to do follow-up interviews on 86 of the initial 103 patients, performing four follow-up evaluations on subgroups of this population (i.e. 3 months, 6 months, 1 year and 2 years) (table I).

After 6 months about one third had symptoms of major depression, one quarter had minor depression, and 40% remained nondepressed [Robinson et al., 1984b].

We looked at the depressed patients individually and found that 21 of 22 patients with initial in-hospital depression (either major or minor) remained depressed at 6 months. Another 9 patients, who initially had not been depressed, had developed depression [Robinson et al., 1984c]. At one year follow-up, 7 of 12 patients who were depressed at the time of their in-hospital evaluation remained depressed, while 5 of 25 patients who had not been depressed during their acute stroke care developed depression [Robinson et al., 1987]. After 2 years all patients with major depression at the time of their in-hospital evaluation had improved (i.e. significantly lower mean depression scores and no diagnosis of major depression), while 7 of 10 patients with minor depression were still depressed (i.e. they had either major or minor depression and showed no improvement in mean depression scores) [Robinson et al., 1987].

Table I. Prevalence of depression at various time intervals following stroke[1]

	Time of clinical evaluation			
	initial in-hospital evaluation[2] (%)	6 months (%)	1 year (%)	2 years (%)
Number of patients	103	50	37	48
Major depression	28 (27)	17 (34)	5 (14)	6 (13)
Minor depression	21 (20)	13 (26)	7 (19)	19 (21)
No depression	53 (53)	20 (40)	24 (67)	32 (66)

[1] Eight patients died and 9 were lost to follow-up over the course of the study. Figures at 6 months, 1 year and 2 years reflect the prevalence of depression among the patients we were able to interview at those times.

[2] Initial evaluation was performed at a mean of 10 days post-stroke with a standard deviation of 11 days.

These two studies confirmed our earlier finding that major depressive disorders following stroke last for about one year. This study also demonstrated that the prognosis at 2 years for patients with untreated minor depression is less favorable than it is for patients with major depression. The reason for this relatively poor prognosis for minor depression is not known. One possibility is that minor depression after stroke reflects a characterologic vulnerability which leads to chronic depression.

Mechanisms of Mood Disorders

Just as functional depression may arise from several possible mechanisms, the causation of PSD is likely to represent a mixture of etiologic factors.

Physical, Intellectual and Social Functioning

In our stroke studies we also examined: (1) global intellectual impairment as measured by the Mini-Mental State Examination (MMSE) [Folstein et al., 1975], (2) functional physical impairment (i.e. activities of daily living) as measured by the Johns Hopkins Functioning Inventory (JHFI), and (3) social functioning as measured by the Social Functioning Examination (SFE) [Robinson et al., 1985a]. In the longitudinal 2-year study of 103 stroke patients, we found a weak association between severity of depression and severity of impairment or disturbance in social functioning. The mean correlation coefficients between depression score and intellectual impairment (MMSE) score [Robinson et al., 1983a] was r = –0.29; between severity of depression and impairment in activities of daily living as measured by the JHFI score was r = 0.36; between severity of depression and social functioning (SFE) score was r = –0.24; and between severity of depression and age was r = –0.28 [Robinson et al., 1983a]. Thus, it appears that at the time of detection of depression only 15% of the variance in depression could be explained by severity of intellectual impairment, severity of physical impairment, quality of available social supports, or age.

At six months follow-up, however, correlation between severity of depression and functional physical impairment, cognitive impairment or social functioning had increased [Robinson et al., 1984b]. Patients who were most severely impaired in the hospital were the most likely to have severe depression 6 months later. This suggests a reciprocal relationship between depression and impairment. In other words, depressed, patients may be less likely to recover from physical impairments, and these physical impairments may exacerbate the depression. Depression may also produce or exacerbate intellectual impairment [Robinson et al., 1986]. Both biologic and reactive elements therefore may contribute to the long-term outcome of depression and rehabilitation from stroke.

Aphasia

Language disorders are important symptoms in stroke patients since they serve to disconnect these patients from family, friends and the environment. Patients with comprehension deficits so severe that they could not participate in a verbal interview have been excluded from our studies. We have, however, examined aphasic patients who were capable of responding reliably to simple questions [Robinson and Benson, 1981]. In the longitudinal study of 103 acute stroke patients [Robinson et al., 1983a], the diagnosis of aphasia was made by a neurologist (TRP) who was unaware of the psychopathologic findings. Among 15 patients with left hemisphere lesions who had aphasia, only 7 had major or minor depression (table II). This percentage did not differ significantly from our findings in patients without aphasia. In the latter group, 16 of 33 left hemisphere lesion patients had diagnosable depression. Thus, depression may exist without aphasia, and aphasia may occur without depression. Interestingly, among patients with left frontal lesions, depression increases with proximity to the frontal

Table II. Aphasia and depression in patients with left hemisphere lesions (n = 48)

	Broca's aphasia	Wernicke's aphasia	Other aphasia	No aphasia	Total
Major depression	2	0	2	9	13
Minor depression	1	1	1	7	10
No depression	4	1	3	17	25
Total	7	2	6	33	48

pole, even though the motor speech area (Broca's area) lies in the posterior inferior region of the frontal lobe.

The greater frequency of depression in patients with Broca's aphasia as contrasted with other aphasias most likely represents the association between left frontal injury and *both* depression and Broca's aphasia. Two factors suggest that aphasia and depression are independent outcomes of stroke that may coexist, depending upon the lesion location: (1) the covariance of depression and aphasia is low; (2) depression continues to be associated with left frontal lesions in left-handed patients, regardless of hemispheric specialization for language [Robinson et al., 1985b].

It might be argued that our exclusion of patients with severe comprehension deficits (lesions generally involving the posterior superior temporal gyrus) skews our anatomic distribution to more anterior lesion locations and thus falsely associates left anterior lesions and depression. This explanation would assume very high prevalence of depression among patients with comprehension deficits. This conclusion is not supported by our available data. Among our 8 patients with mild comprehension deficits (these patients had either mild Wernicke-type or mixed receptive and expressive, that is, mild 'global' aphasia), only 4 were depressed, compared with 16 depressed persons among 33 nonaphasic patients. Furthermore, clinical reports suggest that post-stroke patients with comprehension deficits tend to be euphoric or paranoid, rather than depressed [Benson, 1976].

Biological Factors

Lesion Location and Neurochemistry. The correlation between lesion site and severity of depression was described previously in the prevalence section. The fact that patients with left anterior brain injury have a greater likelihood of developing a major depressive disorder than patients with any other lesions location suggests that the left anterior brain region is involved in mood regulation.

We have hypothesized that the development of PSD reflects pathologic changes in the catecholamine-containing neurons. Axons originating in cell bodies located in the brainstem nucleus locus ceruleus project anteriorly through the median forebrain bundle into the frontal cortex. They then pass in an anterior to posterior direction through the deep layers of the cortex with arborizations throughout all cortical layers [Morrison et al., 1979]. Focal cortical damage caused by stroke or other insult may cause partial injury to these norepinephrine containing neurons. Due to the anterior to posterior orientation of the catecholaminergic axons, anterior damage would be expected to cause greater disruption of these neurons than posterior damage, since the former would interrupt them closer to their origin. In fact, using a rat stroke model, we have reported significant decreases in norepinephrine (NE) and dopamine concentrations in widespread brain regions after a right middle cerebral artery ligation [Robinson et al., 1975]. We have also shown that lesions closer to the frontal pole produce greater depletion of NE than identical lesions which are more posterior [Pearlson et al., 1984].

Reis and Ross [1973] proposed that partially injured neurons may switch from the production of neurotransmitters to the synthesis of proteins required for regeneration and sprouting. Such a mechanism could diminish available neurotransmitters throughout both injured and uninjured branches of the system.

Study of experimental stroke in rats has also suggested that the biochemical response to focal cortical lesions may be lateralized [Robinson and Coyle, 1980]. That is, the degree of noradrenergic depletion depends on which hemisphere is injured. Somewhat surprisingly, right hemisphere lesions appear to produce greater depletion of NE concentrations throughout the brain than do identical lesions of the left hemisphere. Depression associated with left anterior injury, and undue cheerfulness or apathy related to right anterior lesions, may be the outcome of differential neurochemical responses to injury.

Dexamethasone Suppression Test. The dexamethasone suppression test (DST) has been investigated as a possible biologic marker for functional melancholic depression [Carroll et al., 1981]. We examined 65 patients with recent or remote stroke using the DST [Lipsey et al., 1985]. Sixty-seven percent of the patients with symptoms of major depression who were less than one year post-stroke failed to suppress serum cortisol following dexamethasone administration. Twenty-five percent of the patients with minor depression and 32% of the nondepressed patients failed to suppress cortisol. The sensitivity of the DST to major depression was 67% but specificity was only 70%. Abnormal DST tests seemed to be related to large lesion volumes. The DST thus did not appear to be useful diagnostically in PSD, but may provide a means of establishing more homogenous groups of post-brain injury depressed patients for future research studies.

Treatment of PSD

We have recently published the results of a double-blind, randomized treatment study of PSD using the tricyclic antidepressant, nortriptyline [Lipsey et al., 1984]. Patients were excluded from the study if they had: (1) heart block or other severe cardiac conduction abnormalities, (2) significant prostatism, (3) narrow angle glaucoma, or (4) been prescribed medications such as monoamine oxidase inhibitors or guanethidine that might interact adversely with nortriptyline. Fourteen patients were treated with nortriptyline, and 20 with placebo. Half of the patients had major depressive symptoms while the other half had minor depression. No differences were noted between the nortriptyline and placebo treated groups in demographic characteristics, impairment severity, time elapsed since stroke, size or location of the stroke lesion. During the first week of treatment, patients received nortriptyline 20 mg/day. This was subsequently increased by week two to 50 mg, by week four to 70 mg, and by week five to 100 mg, with identical placebo being given throughout to the comparison group. The 11 nortriptyline patients who completed the study showed significantly ($p = 0.006$) greater improvement in their Hamilton Depression score when compared to the 15 placebo-treated patients.

Successfully treated patients had serum nortriptyline levels between 50 and 150 ng/ml, which is the range required for treatment of depression in nonbrain-injured individuals [Ziegler et al., 1977]. These data suggest that patients treated for PSD require similar doses, have a similar therapeutic window (50 to 150 ng/ml), and should be treated as long as other depressed patients (i.e. at least 4–6 weeks) before deciding whether lack of response to a particular medication represents a treatment failure. Patients receiving nortriptyline had no greater frequency of adverse effects, including episodes of dizziness or another stroke, than the placebo-treated groups. However, three of the nortriptyline patients developed delirium characterized by confusion, drowsiness, and intermittent agitation. Although symptoms abated when the drug was discontinued, these complications underline the need for cautious treatment with antidepressant medication in elderly stroke patients, who often have numerous medical problems.

Summary

Conclusions

PSD is a frequent consequence of brain injury. Between a third and a half of stroke patients develop a clinically significant depression during the acute post-stroke period. These are equally divided between major and minor depressive disorders, which can be diagnosed using DSM-III criteria. In addition to these two conditions, a third disorder characterized by apathy, indifference, and inappropriate cheerfulness can be seen in about one fourth of patients with right hemisphere stroke.

The prevalence of PSD is influenced by two major factors: lesion location and time elapsed since injury. Patients with left frontal brain injury are more frequently and more severely depressed than patients with any other lesion location. Among patients with left frontal brain injury, the severity of depression is significantly correlated with proximity of the lesion to the frontal pole; i.e. lesions closer to the frontal pole are associated with more severe depression than more posterior lesions. This correlation between depression and left frontal lesion location appears to be independent of the presence of lesions in the other hemisphere, etiology of the focal injury (i.e. trauma versus stroke), or cerebral dominance (handedness). Since prevalence of depression is highest during the first 2 years post-stroke, this suggests that the risk period for developing PSD lasts for at least 2 years. The duration of untreated post-stroke major depression is approximately one year. Minor depression, however, will last for more than 2 years after stroke in about 70% of cases if no intervention is made.

The impairments associated with stroke do not appear to be a cause of depression. They interact with depression in such a fashion that by 6 months after stroke the most depressed patients also have the most severe impairments. The mechanisms of depression are uncertain, but we have hypothesized that alteration of biogenic amine neurons by stroke may lead to the development of depression or apathy. The depressive disorders can be treated successfully with the tricyclic antidepressant, nortriptyline. This represents a significant therapeutic modality for stroke patients and may play an important role in speeding recovery and rehabilitation.

Issues for Future Study

We have found it helpful to use DSM-III criteria to subtype patients with PSD. Consideration should be given, however, to whether these diagnostic subtypes, derived from a nomenclature designed to characterize nonstroke-induced depression, may be useful among the brain-injured either as indicators of etiology or as predictors of outcome and response to treatment. Since denial and inability to express emotions may play a significant role in the clinical presentation of mood disorders after right hemisphere stroke, methods need to be established whereby reliable and valid diagnoses can be made in these patients. The relationship of the post-stroke symptoms of apathy, indifference and undue cheerfulness to the physiological determinants of depression must be explored, particularly with regard to possible response to medications. Study of personal and/or family histories of depression may help to elucidate why some but not all individuals with left anterior lesions develop depression, and why some patients develop PSD with other lesions. Finally, the role of neuropeptides, neuromodulators and neurotransmitters other than NE deserves to be studied as potential factors in what may turn out to be a cascade of mechanistic events underlying the genesis of PSD.

References

Adams, R.A.; Victor, M.: Principles of neurology; 3rd ed., pp. 569–640 (MaGraw-Hill, New York 1985).

American Psychiatric Association: Diagnostic and statistical manual of mental disorders (DSM-III), 3rd ed. (APA, Washington 1980).

Babinski, J.: Reflexes de défence. Brain *45:* 149–184 (1922).

Benson, D.F.: Psychiatric aspects of aphasia. Br. J. Psychiat. *123:* 555–566 (1976).

Bonis, M. de; Dellatolas, G.; Rondot, P.: Mood disorders in left and right brain damaged patients: comparison between ratings and self-ratings on the same adjective mood scale: some methodological problems. Psychopathology *18:* 286–292 (1985).

Carroll, B.J.; Feinberg, M.; Gredent, J.F.; Tarika, J.; Albala, A.A.; Haskett, R.F.; James, N.N.; Kronfol, Z.; Lohr, N.; Steiner, M.; de Vigne, J.P.; Young, E.: A specific laboratory test for the diagnosis of melancholia: standardization, validation and clinical utility. Archs gen. Psychiat. *38:* 15–22 (1981).

Denny-Brown, D.; Meyer, J.S.; Horenstein, S.: The significance of perceptual rivalry resulting from parietal lesions. Brain *75:* 434–471 (1952).

Feibel, J.H.; Springer, C.J.: Depression and failure to resume social activities after stroke. Archs phys. Med. Rehabil. *63:* 276 (1982).

Finkelstein, S.; Benowitz, L.J.; Baldessarini, R.G.; Arana, G.W.; Levine, D.; Woo, E.; Baer, D.; Moya, K.; Stoll, A.L.: Mood, vegetative disturbance and dexamethasone suppression test after stroke. Ann. Neurol. *12:* 463–468 (1982).

Fisher, S.: Psychiatric considerations of cerebral vascular disease. Am. J. Cardiol. *7:* 379 (1961).

Folstein, M.F.; Folstein, S.E.; McHugh, P.R.: Mini-mental state: a practical method for grading the cognitive state of patients for the clinician. J. psych. Res. *12:* 189–198 (1975).

Folstein, M.F.; Maiberger, R.; McHugh, P.R.: Mood disorder as a specific complication of stroke. J. Neurol. Neurosurg. Psychiat. *41:* 470–473 (1977).

Gainotti, G.: Emotional behavior and hemispheric side of the lesion. Cortex *8:* 41–55 (1972).

Gasparrini, W.G.; Satz, P.; Heilman, K.M.; Coolidge, F.L.: Hemispheric asymmetries of affective processing as determined by the Minnesota Multiphasic Personality Inventory. J. Neurol. Neurosurg. Psychiat. *41:* 470–473 (1978).

Goldstein, K.: Language and language disturbances (Grune & Stratton, New York 1948).

Hécaen, H.; Ajuriaguerra, J. de; Massonet, J.: Les troubles visuoconstructives par lésion pariétooccipitale droit. Encéphale *40:* 122–179 (1951).

Kraepelin, E.: Manic depressive insanity and paranoia (Livingstone, Edinburgh 1921).

Lipsey, J.R.; Robinson, R.G.; Pearlson, G.D.; Rao, K.; Price, T.R.: Mood change following bilateral hemisphere brain injury. Br. J. Psychiat. *143:* 266–273 (1983).

Lipsey, J.R.; Robinson, R.G.; Pearlson, G.D.; Rao, K.E.; Price, T.R.: Nortriptyline treatment for post-stroke depression: a double-blind study. Lancet *i:* 297–300 (1984).

Lipsey, J.R.; Robinson, R.G.; Pearlson, G.D.; Rao, K.; Price, T.R.: Dexamethasone suppression test and mood following stroke. Am. J. Psychiat. *142:* 318–323 (1985).

Meyer, A.: The anatomical facts and clinical varieties of traumatic insanity. Am. J. Insanity *60:* 373 (1904).

Morrison, J.M.; Molliver, M.E.; Grzanna, R.: Noradrenergic innervation of cerebral cortex: widespread effects of local cortical lesions. Science *205:* 313–316 (1979).

Pearlson, G.D.; Kubos, K.L.; Robinson, R.G.: Effect of anterior-posterior lesion location on the asymmetrical behavioral and biochemical response to cortical suction ablations in the rat. Brain Res. *293:* 241–250 (1984).

Post, F.: The significance of affective symptoms in old age. Maudsley Monogr., No. 10 (Oxford University Press, London 1962).

Reis, D.J.; Ross, R.A.: Dynamic changes in brain dopamine β-hydroxylase activity during anterograde and retrograde reactions to injury of central noradrenergic axons. Brain Res. *57:* 307–326 (1973).

Robins, D.M.; Are stroke patients more depressed than other disabled subjects? J. chron. Dis. *29:* 479–482.

Robinson, R.G.; Benson, D.F.: Depression in aphasic patients: frequency, severity and clinical-pathological correlations. Brain Lang. *14:* 282–291 (1981).

Robinson, R.G.; Bolduc, P.L.; Price, T.R.: A two-year longitudinal study of post-stroke mood disorders: diagnosis and outcome at one- and two-year follow-up. Stroke *18:* 837–843 (1987).

Robinson, R.G.; Bolduc, P.L.; Starr, L.B.; Kubos, K.L.; Price, T.R.: Social functioning assessment in stroke patients: responses of patients and other informant and relationship of initial evaluation to six months follow-up. Archs. phys. Med. Rehabil. *66:* 496–500 (1985a).

Robinson, R.G.; Bolla-Wilson, K.; Kaplan, E.; Lipsey, J.R.; Price, T.R.: Depression influences intellectual impairment in stroke patients. Br. J. Psychiat. *148:* 541–547 (1986).

Robinson, R.G.; Coyle, J.T.: The different effects of right versus left hemispheric infarction on catecholamines and behavior in the rat. Brain Res. *188:* 63–78 (1980).

Robinson, R.G.; Kubos, K.L.; Starr, L.B.; Rao, K.; Price, T.R.: Mood changes in stroke patients: relationship to lesion location. Compreh. Psychiat. *24:* 555–566 (1983a).

Robinson, R.G.; Kubos, K.L.; Starr, L.B.; Rao, K.; Price, T.R.: Mood disorders in stroke patients: importance of location of lesion. Brain *107:* 81–93 (1984a).

Robinson, R.G.; Lipsey, J.R.; Bolla-Wilson, K.; Bolduc, P.L.; Pearlson, G.D.; Rao, K.; Price, T.R.: Mood disorders in left-hand stroke patients. Am. J. Psychiat. *142:* 1424–1429 (1985b).

Robinson, R.G.; Price, T.R.: Post-stroke depressive disorders: a follow-up study of 103 stroke out-patients. Stroke *13:* 635–641 (1982).

Robinson, R.G.; Shoemaker, W.J.; Schlumpf, M.; Valk, T.; Bloom, F.E.: Effect of experimental cerebral infarction in rat brain on catecholamines and behavior. Nature *255:* 332–333 (1975).

Robinson, R.G.; Starr, L.B.; Kubos, K.L.; Price, T.R.: A two-year longitudinal study of post-stroke mood disorders: findings during the initial evaluation. Stroke *14:* 736–741 (1983b).

Robinson, R.G.; Starr, L.B.; Lipsey, J.R.; Rao, K.; Price, T.R.: A two-year longitudinal study of post-stroke mood disorders: dynamic changes in associated variables over the first six months of follow-up. Stroke *15:* 510–517 (1984b).

Robinson, R.G.; Starr, L.B.; Lipsey, J.R.; Rao, K.; Price, T.R.: A two-year longitudinal study of post-stroke mood disorders: in-hospital prognostic factors associated with six-month outcome. J. nerv. ment. Dis. *173:* 221–226 (1985c).

Robinson, R.G.; Starr, L.B.; Price, T.R.: A two-year longitudinal study of mood disorders following stroke: prevalence and duration at six months follow-up. Br. J. Psychiat. *144:* 256–262 (1984c).

Robinson, R.G.; Szetela, B.: Mood change following left hemisphere brain injury. Ann. Neurol. *9:* 447–453 (1981).

Ross, E.D.; Rush, A.J.: Diagnosis and neuroanatomical correlates of depression in brain patients. Archs gen. Psychiat. *38:* 1344–1354 (1981).

Sackheim, H.D.; Greenburg, M.S.; Weiman, A.L.; Gur, R.C.; Hungerbühler, J.P.; Geschwind, N.: Hemispheric asymmetry in the expression of positive and negative emotions: neurologic evidence. Archs Neurol. *39:* 210–218 (1982).

Sinyor, D.; Jacques, P.; Kaloupek, D.G.; Becker, R.; Goldenberg, M.; Coopersmith, H.M.: Poststroke depression and lesion location: an attempted replication. Brain *109:* 537–546 (1986).

Starkstein, S.E.; Robinson, R.G.; Price, T.R.: Comparison of cortical and subcortical lesions in the production of post-stroke mood disorders. Brain *110:* 1045–1059 (1987).
Wolf, P.A.; Dawber, T.R.; Thomas, H.E.; Colton, T.; Kannel, W.B.: Epidemiology of stroke; in Thompson, Green, Advances in neurology, vol. 16, pp. 5–19 (Raven Press, New York 1977).
Ziegler, V.E.; Clayton, P.J.; Biggs, J.T.: A comparison study of amitriptyline and nortriptyline with plasma levels. Arch gen. Psychiat. *34:* 607–612 (1977).

Robert G. Robinson, MD, Departments of Psychiatry and Behavioral Sciences and Neuroscience, The Johns Hopkins University School of Medicine,
Baltimore, MD 21205 (USA)

Mueller (ed.): Neurology and Psychiatry: A Meeting of Minds,
pp. 210–246 (Karger, Basel 1989)

AIDS and the Central Nervous System: A Challenge for the New Neuropsychiatry

Robert M. Levy[a], *Dale E. Bredesen*[b], *Mark L. Rosenblum*[c]

[a] Departments of Surgery (Neurosurgery) and Physiology, Northwestern University Medical School, Chicago, Ill.; [b] Department of Neurology and [c] Department of Neurological Surgery, University of California, San Francisco, Calif., USA

Although in restrospect the first cases of the acquired immunodeficiency syndrome (AIDS) were seen as early as 1978, the first reports of this new illness did not appear until late 1981 [Friedman-Kien et al., 1982; Gottlieb et al., 1981; Masur et al. 1981]. These reports described the unusual occurrence of Kaposi's sarcoma, *Pneumocystis carinii* pneumonia and other opportunistic infections in previously healthy homosexual males and intravenous drug abusers. Common to all of these patients was a defect in cellular immunity which was considered to be important in the pathogenesis of the disease. This led the disease to be designated the 'acquired immunodeficiency syndrome'. The Centers for Disease Control (CDC), for the purposes of epidemiological surveillance, first defined AIDS in 1982 as a 'reliably diagnosed disease that is at least moderately indicative of an underlying cellular immunodeficiency in a person who has no known underlying cause of cellular immunodeficiency nor any other cause of reduced resistance reported to be associated with that disease' [CDC, 1983]. This definition has recently undergone major revision based upon further experience with the disease.

Early reports focused upon the high incidence of malignant tumors, including Kaposi's sarcoma and non-Hodgkin's lymphoma, and opportunistic infections, including *Pneumocystis carinii* pneumonia and atypical mycobacteriosis, in these otherwise healthy patients. It soon became evident that the appearance of these opportunistic processes was related to suppression of the cellular immune system following infection with one of a group of retroviruses, now known as the human immunodeficiency virus (HIV) [Barré-Sinoussi et al., 1983; Gallo et al., 1984; Levy et al., 1984a]. In the attempt to develop preventive and therapeutic strategies for this fatal illness, much work has been done in the past few years to elucidate the mechanism of infection and subsequent immunosuppression by this virus.

Reports of neurologic dysfunction in patients with AIDS [Snider et al., 1983; Bredesen and Messing, 1983] have appeared from the beginning of the AIDS epidemic. Only recently have the frequency and breadth of the neurologic manifestations of the acquired immunodeficiency syndrome become apparent [Levy et al., 1985b; Levy and Bredesen, 1988]. The demonstration that these neurologic illnesses arise not only from opportunistic processes which affect the nervous system but also from primary HIV infection of the nervous system is of great import [Ho et al., 1985; Levy et al., 1985a; Resnick et al., 1985]. Thus, HIV has as a target both the immune and nervous system. Moreover, primary infection with HIV can produce a number of previously unrecognized neurologic illnesses. As the AIDS epidemic spreads and the number of patients increases dramatically, physicians must become familiar with the broad spectrum of the neurologic and neuropsychiatric manifestations of this disease.

Incidence of AIDS-Related CNS Illness

By the end of 1984, we had evaluated 318 patients at the University of California, San Francisco (UCSF). One hundred and twenty-four (39%) had neurologic symptoms [Levy et al., 1985b]. Updated through June 1986, the UCSF series included 1,286 patients treated with AIDS or the AIDS-related complex (ARC). Of these, 482 patients were identified with either significant neurologic complaints or neurologic illness (37%). In these 482 patients, 553 neurologic diseases were identified, of which 474 affected the CNS and 79 affected the peripheral nervous system. Sixty-five patients had multiple neurologic illnesses. We have thus seen three times as many neurologically symptomatic AIDS patients in the past 2 years as we had during the preceding 5 years. The annual incidence of AIDS-related neurologic illness at UCSF has more than doubled over each of the 6 years that we have evaluated patients with AIDS.

Of the 37% of AIDS patients with neurologic illness, one third presented with these neurologic complaints as their initial manifestation of AIDS. Thus, 10% of all AIDS patients first presented with symptoms of neurologic illness. A similar incidence of overall AIDS-related neurologic illness [Snider et al., 1983; Koppel et al., 1985] and neurologic illness at presentation with AIDS [Levy et al., 1988] has been reported in other groups of AIDS patients. The incidence of AIDS-related neuropathology is much higher in autopsy series, which suggest that 75% of AIDS patients have significant nervous system pathology on postmortem evaluation [Levy et al., 1986c; Urmacher and Nielsen, 1985; Moskowitz et al., 1984].

Epidemiology of AIDS-Related CNS Illness

Recent epidemiologic studies [Levy et al., 1988] have confirmed the empiric observation that patients from different risk groups and geographical locations are at different risks for contracting AIDS-related neurologic illnesses. These data suggest that toxoplasmosis occurs most frequently in Florida, in both Haitian and non-Haitian AIDS patients. In general, Haitian AIDS patients are more frequently reported to have central nervous system (CNS) complications than are patients in other risk groups. Cryptococcal meningitis is reported most frequently in New Jersey, possibly because of the higher percentage of AIDS patients in that state who are black or intravenous drug abusers. Progressive multifocal leukoencephalopathy (PML) and primary CNS lymphoma do not appear to preferentially affect any single risk group or geographical location.

Diagnosis of AIDS-Related CNS Illness

After obtaining a history, physical examination and cognitive assessment, radiologic and cerebrospinal fluid (CSF) examinations are the mainstays of the diagnosis of AIDS-related nervous system illness. Positive HIV antibody titers indicate only exposure to the AIDS virus and not active disease. Serologic tests are of little value in the differential diagnosis of AIDS-related CNS disease [Levy et al., 1984b].

CSF examination is critical for the evaluation and therapy of the AIDS patient with CNS disease. The CSF examination may provide the definitive diagnosis in several of these processes, including HIV or other viral infections and cryptococcal meningitis. We have evaluated the CSF profiles of our AIDS patients with neurologic illness to determine whether findings, apart from the direct identification of organisms (by titers, stains or culture), can be of value in differential diagnosis. Mean CSF protein ranged from 62 to 97 mg/dl, implying that all of these CNS diseases produce a mild elevation of CSF protein. The mean CSF glucose concentration ranged from 43 to 63 mg/dl, this being within normal limits. CSF cell count was normal in patients with HIV encephalopathy, PML and toxoplasmosis. A minimal pleocytosis was noted in patients with primary CNS lymphoma, while more marked CSF pleocytoses were noted in patients with cryptococcal meningitis and opportunistic viral infections. In all cases, these white blood cells were almost exclusively monocytes or lymphocytes. Thus, in those patients with nonfocal radiologic studies and no CSF pleocytosis, the diagnosis of HIV encephalopathy is suggested.

Computerized tomographic (CT) brain scans have, until recently, been the most widely used radiologic examination in neurologically symptomatic AIDS patients. In our review of 200 cases [Levy et al., 1986a], CT scans were normal in 39.5% of cases, revealed focal lesions in 25.5% of cases, and demonstrated diffuse cerebral atrophy only in 35% of cases. These findings were of some prognostic value: patients with diffuse cerebral atrophy were three times more likely than patients with normal CT scans to manifest neurologic progression and to subsequently demonstrate CNS pathology. Review of the literature reveals that patients with focal abnormalities on CT scans were subsequently shown to have toxoplasmosis (50–70%), primary CNS lymphoma (10–25%), PML (10–22%) or had either nondiagnostic biopsies (10%) or other disease (9%) [Levy et al., 1986a; DeLapaz and Enzmann, 1988].

In those patients with no focal CT abnormalities, cryptococcal meningitis was by far the most frequent diagnosis (28%). While these studies report an incidence of CMV and HIV encephalitis in 11 and 3% of these patients, respectively, this probably reflects a lack of rigor in pursuing these diagnoses. Our experience would suggest that more than one third of neurologically symptomatic AIDS patients with nonfocal CT scans actually have HIV encephalitis.

The CT findings in our 482 patients with AIDS-related neurologic illness were evaluated in an attempt to determine whether these findings could be of value in the specific differential diagnosis of these disease. This evaluation identified two major groups of patients: those with normal scans or with diffuse cerebral atrophy only and those with focal lesions on CT. Nonfocal examinations were obtained in patients with HIV encephalopathy (92%), opportunistic viral infection (82%) and cryptococcal meningitis (84%). Focal CT abnormalities were identified in patients with toxoplasmosis (88%), primary CNS lymphoma (86%) and PML (80%). Within this latter group, patients with low-density lesions that demonstrated little or no enhancement after the administration of iodinated contrast material tended to have PML or primary CNS lymphoma. Restriction of these lesions to the white matter suggested the diagnosis of PML, while the presence of mass effect tended to suggest lymphoma. The demonstration of ring-enhancing lesions, especially within the basal ganglia, suggested the diagnosis of toxoplasmosis. Unfortunately, there were many cases in which ring-enhancing lesions were proven to be primary CNS lymphomas and in which toxoplasma brain abscesses did not enhance. Thus, CT scans alone cannot provide a definitive diagnosis in AIDS-related CNS disease.

Our studies have demonstrated that magnetic resonance imaging (MRI) is more sensitive than CT to intracranial pathology in the patient with AIDS and neurologic symptoms [Levy et al., 1986b]. MRI also more accurately reflects the extent and distribution of histologically verified CNS disease. This increased sensitivity and accuracy has been demonstrated to have a significant impact on the evaluation and therapy of patients with AIDS-related CNS illness. Interestingly, in all but one of our cases of histologically proven toxoplasmosis, MRI has demonstrated multiple bilateral intracranial abnormalities [Levy et al., 1986b]. Thus, a single lesion on MRI probably reflects an illness other than toxoplasmosis. On the basis of these findings, we recommend that MRI be used as the initial radiologic screening procedure in these patients.

AIDS-Related CNS Syndromes

CNS syndromes associated with AIDS or ARC may arise from primary HIV infection or secondary opportunistic processes. Neurologic disease may occur as part of a diffuse systemic illness or as an isolated illness. These processes may manifest neurologic illness by virtue of nonfocal, diffuse CNS involvement, focal involvement by a space-occupying lesion, or by the production of obstructive hydrocephalus. CNS syndromes include focal or diffuse encephalopathy, myelopathy, meningitis, cranial neuropathy and retinopathy. The specific symptoms related to AIDS-related CNS illness includes virtually all those related to nervous system dysfunction (table I).

Disorders of consciousness or cognition, including dementia, are most common, being evident in 68% of neurologically symptomatic patients. Headaches are only slightly less frequent, being significant complaints in 55% of these patients. Also common are complaints of focal weakness (18%), incoordination (18%) and seizures (17%). Less frequently, patients

Table I. Symptoms related to central neurologic illness in AIDS

Headache	Pain
Altered mental status	Seizures
Weakness	Aphasia
Sensory loss	Dizziness
Paresthesias	Visual disturbances
	Disordered gait

present with aphasia (12%), incontinence (10%), cranial neuropathies (9%), sensory loss (8%) and visual disturbances (8%).

Although the neurologic symptoms associated with AIDS-related CNS illness are many and varied, patients' clinical profiles appear to overlap to such a degree that clinical findings are of little value in the differential diagnosis of these diseases. Of greatest utility, in our experience, is either the presence of focal weakness or sensory loss, suggestive of a focal process, such as toxoplasmosis or primary CNS lymphoma, or the presence of cranial neuropathies, suggesting lymphoma or opportunistic viral illness.

AIDS-Related CNS Diseases

The spectrum of diseases known to affect the CNS in AIDS is listed in table II.

Primary Viral Infection

HIV-Encephalopathy

The most common CNS illness associated with AIDS is also one that is unique to this syndrome. First reported by Snider et al. [1983] as 'subacute encephalitis', this fatal dementing illness has also been called 'AIDS-encephalopathy' and the 'AIDS-dementia complex'. The first step towards understanding the pathogenesis of this illness was made by Shaw et al. [1985], who demonstrated the presence of viral RNA in the brains of demented AIDS patients using in situ hybridization techniques. Ho et al. [1985] subsequently demonstrated that HTLV-III could be isolated from the CSF and neural tissues of patients with AIDS-related neurologic

Table II. Illnesses affecting the CNS in AIDS

Primary viral (HIV)
HIV encephalopathy
Atypical aseptic meningitis
Vacuolar myelopathy
Secondary viral (encephalitis, retinitis, vasculitis)
Cytomegalovirus
Herpes simplex virus, I and II
Herpes varicella zoster
Papovavirus (progressive multifocal leukoencephalopathy)
Nonviral infections (encephalitis, meningitis, abscess)
Toxoplasma gondii
Cryptococcus neoformans
Candida albicans
Coccidioides immitis
Aspergillus fumigatus
Histoplasma capsulatum
Mycobacterium avium intracellulare
Mycobacterium tuberculosis hominis
Listeria monocytogenes
Nocardia asteroides
Neoplasms
Primary CNS lymphoma
Metastatic systemic lymphoma
Metastatic Kaposi's sarcoma
Cerebrovascular
Infarction
Hemorrhage
Vasculitis
Complications of systemic AIDS therapy

syndromes. Levy et al. [1985a] also isolated HIV from the brains and CSF of neurologically symptomatic AIDS patients. At the same time, Resnick et al. [1985] demonstrated the synthesis of intra-blood-brain-barrier synthesis of HTLV-III-specific immunoglobulin G in 10 of 11 patients with AIDS-related mental status alterations. Sharer and co-workers [1985] reported the presence of multinucleated giant cells and HTLV-III in patients with

AIDS encephalopathy, and more recently, Koenig et al. [1986] detected HIV within macrophages in brain tissue from patients with HIV-encephalopathy. Thus, it appears that HIV-encephalopathy results from primary infection of the brain by HIV and the predominant cells containing this virus appear to be of macrophage origin. The precise mechanism whereby this infection results in dementia remains to be elucidated.

Price et al. [1987] have carefully studied the clinical profile of patients with AIDS-related dementia. He has coined the term 'AIDS dementia complex' or ADC. ADC may be the presenting or sole manifestation of HIV infection [Navia and Price, 1987] or may occur in the setting of other AIDS-related illnesses. All patients with ADC initially present with cognitive impairment. The syndrome is characterized by a progressive dementia often first appearing as a confusional state and frequently accompanied by fever or mild metabolic derangement. Less commonly, patients demonstrate weakness (34%), personality change (38%), transient dysarthrias or movement disorders (7%). Price reports that brain atrophy and white matter changes can be evident on CT or MRI [Navia et al., 1986a]. Neuropathologic studies reveal diffuse white matter changes, multinucleated cell and macrophage infiltrates. HIV can be isolated from blood, brain or CSF [Navia et al., 1986b]. The reported frequency of HIV-encephalopathy varies from series to series, but Price and co-workers indicate that as many as 90% of their patients with AIDS have some degree of dementia.

While the presence of neurologic and neuropsychiatric illness in patients with AIDS has been recognized from the beginning of the AIDS epidemic, the occurrence of cognitive dysfunction in patients with AIDS-related complex (ARC) and the possible occurrence and frequency of these disorders in asymptomatic HIV-1 infected individuals or those with persistant generalized lymphadenopathy has only been recently addressed [Jansen et al., 1988; Grant et al., 1987]. While there is some evidence to the contrary, the available data strongly support the hypothesis that cognitive deficits do not occur with any singnificantly increased frequency in HIV-1 seropositive, otherwise asymptomatic people as compared to seronegative controls. It is, however, premature to make absolute conclusions based upon the available data. In fact, the clinical experience of many physicians is that, although the frequency may be rare and the cause may not be HIV-1 infection per se but rather the associated stress and anxiety associated with the recent diagnosis of HIV-1 infection, there are some otherwise asymptomatic HIV-1 infected individuals who do exhibit and complain of cognitive dysfunction.

At UCSF, 100 patients with HIV-encephalopathy were seen from 1979 until mid-1986. The typical patient with AIDS-encephalopathy treated at UCSF is a 39-year-old homosexual male. He presents with complaints referable to diminished intellectual function and his neurologic examination is nonfocal. The only significant finding is his progressive dementia, which typically has been present for 6–7 weeks. His disease is rapidly progressive and invariably fatal, with mean survival being little over 3 months. As these figures reflect, there is no effective therapy for AIDS-encephalopathy at the present time. Trials of azidothymidine (AZT), an antiviral compound which crosses the blood-brain barrier, are currently underway.

Atypical Aseptic Meningitis

In 1983, we first reported 15 homosexual patients with an aseptic meningitis [Bredesen et al., 1983]. We have now documented 26 such cases at UCSF. These cases were atypical in that they were often chronic and tended to recur. They often included cranial neuropathies, especially of the fifth, seventh and eighth cranial nerves, or long tract findings. Several patients had evidence of elevated intracranial pressure and all, by definition, had CSF pleocytosis. CSF profiles were otherwise similar to those of patients with AIDS-related encephalopathy. Prior to the availability of culture techniques for HIV, the etiology of this syndrome was unclear. It now appears that the name atypical aseptic meningitis is something of a misnomer. Recent studies have demonstrated that HIV can be cultured from the CSF in the majority of these patients [Ho et al., 1985; Levy et al., 1985a]. Thus, this syndrome may be better named acute HIV meningitis.

Aseptic meningitis presents clinically in an entirely different manner from AIDS-related encephalopathy. Common features include headache, fever and meningeal signs. The clinical course is also different, being self-limited or recurrent rather than progressive. It has been suggested that the occurrence of AIDS-related encephalopathy or atypical meningitis as a manifestation of HIV infection may be a reflection of the patient's degree of immunosuppression [Snider et al., 1983; Levy et al., 1985b]. Both illnesses, however, have been seen in otherwise asymptomatic patients [Navia and Price, 1987] and autopsy findings indicate a remarkable similarity between these clinical entities.

Spinal Vacuolar Myelopathy

Vacuolar myelopathy, reported by Snider et al. [1983] and Goldstick et al. [1984] and characterized by Petito et al. [1985], appears to be a third unique AIDS-related CNS syndrome. Several further reports of AIDS-related spinal cord degeneration have appeared [Goldstick et al., 1985; Horoupian et al., 1984]. Petito et al. [1985] reported a vacuolar myelopathy, most severe in the lateral and posterior columns of the thoracic spinal cord, in 20 of 89 patients with AIDS undergoing autopsy (22%). Pathologically, this syndrome resembled closely the subacute combined degeneration of vitamin B_{12} deficiency with loss of myelin and spongy degeneration of the cord substance.

The most common symptoms associated with vacuolar myelopathy include leg weakness and incontinence [Berger and Resnick, 1987; Petito et al., 1985]. Neurologic examination often reveals paraparesis, spasticity and ataxia. Berger and Resnick [1987] note that hyperreflexia and extensor plantar responses may be detected in the absence of weakness. They observe that muscle stretch reflexes are occasionally absent, presumably due to concomitant peripheral neuropathy.

Petito et al. [1985] noted that neurologic findings were present more frequently in those patients with more severe pathologic changes and occurred in 12 of the 20 patients. Interestingly, 14 of these patients (70%) were also demented. Patients with vacuolar myelopathy frequently present with acute myelopathy and undergo either myelography or MRI prior to their diagnosis. Recent studies [Ho et al., 1985; Levy et al., 1985a] have demonstrated that HIV can be cultured from the spinal cords of many of these patients, which suggests that primary HIV infection is required for the development of this syndrome.

Opportunistic Viral Infections

The spectrum of opportunistic infections in AIDS can be predicted on the basis of the known immunodeficiency. The types of viral infection are not dissimilar to those seen in immunosuppressed transplant patients [Armstrong and Wong, 1982].

Progressive Multifocal Leukoencephalopathy

PML is an unusual infectious central demyelinating disease caused by the papovavirus JC [Narayan et al., 1973]. Prior to the AIDS epidemic, affected patients were reported to present with mental status alterations, blindness, aphasia, hemiparesis, ataxia and other focal deficits which slowly progress until death [Armstrong et al., 1958]. The characteristic CT finding was that of low-density lesions without contrast enhancement, mass effect or associated edema. Autopsy findings revealed focal myelin loss with sparing of axon cylinders and the presence of bizarre astrocytes and enlarged oligodendrocytes containing eosinophilic intranuclear inclusions surrounding these areas of demyelination [Zu Rhein, 1969].

The first report of PML occurring in association with AIDS was that of Miller et al. [1982]. They described a male homosexual with a T-cell-immune deficiency, progressive brainstem dysfunction, and a lucent cerebellar lesion demonstrated by CT was shown on biopsy to have PML. Bedri et al. [1983] reported the electron microscopic demonstration of papovavirus virions in an AIDS patient with PML. In the single published series of these patients, Krupp et al. [1985] detailed 7 cases of PML; 4 of these patients also had AIDS. Of note was the observation that CT abnormalities were disproportionately less striking than clinical findings. While lesions were noted to enlarge progressively on CT, these findings lagged behind the rate of clinical evolution.

As of August 1986, 172 cases of AIDS-related PML had been reported to the CDC. Eight of these patients with AIDS and PML have been treated at UCSF. Clinically, PML in the AIDS patient appears to behave in a fashion similar to PML in other immunocompromised patients. Survival after diagnosis of PML is extremely short. Several patients have died within one month of diagnosis; the longest reported survivor lived for 5 months after biopsy. No effective therapy exists for PML. The early suggestion by Snider et al. [1983] that cytarabine therapy may be effective in these patients has not been confirmed [Krupp et al., 1985].

Other Viral Infections

The ubiquity of the herpes viruses as well as the specific defect in cellular immunodeficiency associated with AIDS suggest that these viruses could represent a significant cause of opportunistic infection in the AIDS patient population. In fact, infection with cytomegalovirus (CMV), herpes simplex viruses type I and II (HSVI and HSVII) and varicella zoster virus (HVZ) is a major source of central neurologic disease in AIDS patients.

HSVI is the most frequent agent causing sporadic (nonepidemic) viral encephalitis. Most cases in immunocompetent patients are caused by HSVI [Baringer and Swoveland, 1973], which produces a hemorrhagic necrotizing encephalitis usually confined to the medial temporal and inferior frontal lobes. Reported clinical manifestations of this illness include headache, fever, seizures, aphasia and other less common focal findings. Diagnosis can be reliably established by temporal lobe biopsy. Treatment with adenine arabinoside (Ara-A) or acyclovir has been shown to decrease the morbidity and mortality rates associated with this infection [Whitley et al., 1977]. Episodes of encephalitic illness have been associated with CMV [Bale, 1984], HVZ [McKendall and Klawans, 1978] and HSVII [Dix et al., 1985], although infection with HSVII usually produces a benign self-limited meningitis (Baringer, 1978].

Several reports of AIDS-related CNS infection with HSV [Britton et al., 1985; Dix et al., 1985; Levy et al., 1985b] or HSV combined with CMV [Pepose et al., 1984; Tucker et al., 1985] have recently appeared. We initially reported 8 AIDS patients with HSV encephalitis. These patients fell into four groups, with the rapidity of disease progression and the severity of inflammation being roughly proportional to the degree of immune competence [Levy et al., 1985b].

CMV meningoencephalitis has also been reported in patients with AIDS [Hawley et al., 1983; Edwards et al., 1985; Moskowitz et al., 1984]. In a study of 10 patients with CMV encephalitis, Post et al. [1986] reported that CMV infection of the CNS was the cause of death in 6 patients, was superimposed on systemic infection in 2 patients and was not clinically evident in 2 patients. Diffuse cerebral atrophy was evident on CT scans in all cases although CT significantly underestimated the degree of CNS involvement and frequently failed to demonstrate focal abnormalities when they were apparent on autopsy.

HVZ virus is also a significant opportunistic CNS pathogen in AIDS patients [Levy et al., 1985b; Cole et al., 1984]. Interestingly, Ryder et al. [1986] have reported the case of a patient with AIDS who developed progressive, ultimately fatal neurological deficits 12 weeks after a course of cutaneous zoster. Autopsy revealed a diffuse herpes zoster encephalomyelitis.

While viruses other than papovaviruses or herpes viruses are potential opportunistic CNS pathogens in patients with AIDS, very few such cases have been reported. West and co-workers [1985] report the case of a bisexual man with a history of intravenous drug abuse who developed an encephalitis. Adenovirus type 2 was isolated from brain tissue obtained by biopsy while systemic infection with Epstein-Barr virus (EBV) was demonstrated. Infection with more than one opportunistic viral pathogen is now a well recognized entity [Levy et al., 1985b; Tucker et al., 1985; Pepose et al., 1984].

At UCSF, 28 patients have presented with AIDS-related opportunistic viral infections of the CNS. The presence of opportunistic CNS viral infection was associated with a poor prognosis. Despite the availability of acyclovir for the treatment of herpes viral infections and the development of anti-CMV agents, such as DHPG, therapy for opportunistic viral encephalidities has been largely ineffective.

Nonviral Infection

Toxoplasma gondii

Toxoplasmosis, an infection caused by the obligate intracellular protozoan *Toxoplasma gondii,* is one of the most common infections of animals and man [Anderson, 1979]. In immunocompetent patients, infection of the CNS with *T. gondii* produces acute focal or diffuse meningoencephalitis with cellular necrosis, microglial nodules and perivascular mononuclear inflammation associated with both intra- and extracellular trophozoites [Remington and Desmonts, 1976]. Thrombosis of blood vessels causing large areas of coagulation necrosis may produce mass lesions in the brain. In immunodeficient hosts, the lack of cell-mediated immunity may result in a persistent acute infection with severe necrotizing lesions. Pathological analysis of biopsy specimens from AIDS patients reveals necrotizing granulomas, usually within thin capsules and little inflammation [Sher, 1983]. Encysted *T. gondii* and tachyzoites are usually present.

The first report of cerebral toxoplasmosis in a patient with AIDS was that by Rutsaert et al. [1980]. Several series of such patients have since appeared [Chan et al., 1983; Handler et al., 1983; Post et al., 1983; Luft et al., 1983] which point to the increased risk of toxoplasmosis in the Haitian AIDS patients, the frequency of multiple deep ring-enhancing lesions on CT scans, and the common clinical findings of lethargy, seizures and weakness. In general, they reported the conclusion that early aggressive diagnosis and therapy with pyrimethamine and sulfadiazine resulted in a dramatic clinical and radiographic response, although most patients went on to die of other AIDS-related illnesses.

Several groups have recommended the routine biopsy of all patients with presumed cerebral toxoplasmosis [Levy et al., 1984; Rodan et al., 1984]. The remarkable sensitivity of biopsy techniques for the diagnosis of toxoplasmosis was addressed by Chan et al. [1983]. The morbidity of biopsy techniques, however small, and the sheer number of affected patients have led some groups to suggest that empiric therapy be initiated prior to biopsy [Wong et al., 1984]. We agree that in stable patients with strong clinical and radiologic evidence for cerebral toxoplasmosis, an empiric trial of pyrimethamine and sulfadiazine may establish the diagnosis without the need for cerebral biopsy.

By August 1986, 625 cases of cerebral toxoplasmosis had been reported to the CDC. The incidence of cerebral toxoplasmosis ranges between 2 and 13% depending upon patient risk group and geographic location. At UCSF, 53 patients with AIDS and proven cerebral toxoplasmosis have been treated. The typical patient with AIDS and cerebral toxoplasmosis in San Francisco is a 40-year-old homosexual male who presents with a 2- to 3-week history of headaches and altered mental status. CT scan reveals multiple bilateral enhancing intracerebral lesions while CSF analysis reveals a mildly elevated protein and few lymphocytes. Therapy with pyrimethamine and sulfadiazine at maximal doses is quite effective in controlling this illness. Meaningful survival of as long as one year after diagnosis has been reported.

Cryptococcus neoformans

Cryptococcus neoformans, a common soil fungus, causes the most common fungal infection of the CNS. Despite appropriate treatment with amphotericin B, the mortality rate of CNS cryptococcal infection in immunocompetent hosts is 40%. Pathologically, cryptococcal meningitis results in a granulomatous meningitis with additional granulomas and cysts which form within the cerebral cortex and deeper brain structures [Adams and Victor, 1977].

Seventy-nine cases of cryptococcal meningitis have been reported by various authors in patients with AIDS [Levy et al., 1985b; Snider et al., 1983; Kovacs et al., 1985]. Kovacs et al. [1985] have characterized the clinical, radiologic and therapeutic aspects of this most common nonviral opportunistic AIDS-related CNS infection. Of 27 patients with AIDS and cryptococcal meningitis, it was the initial manifestation of AIDS in 7 (26%). Meningitis was the most common clinical feature (67%). Studies of CSF frequently revealed normal leukocyte count, protein and glucose concentrations; CSF cryptococcal antigen and culture were diagnostic in all cases. Only 10 of 24 patients had no evidence of clinical activity of cryptococcal infection after the completion of therapy; 6 of these 10 had either clinical or autopsy-demonstrated relapses. The authors concluded, somewhat contrary to our experience, that standard therapy with amphotericin B with or without additional 5-flucytosine were ineffective.

1,252 cases of AIDS-related cryptococcal meningitis had been reported to the CDC by August 1986. These data, reflecting best the incidence of cryptococcosis at presentation with AIDS, represent an overall incidence of approximately 5% of all patients with AIDS. At particular risk are AIDS patients from New Jersey and those that are black or intravenous drug users; these risk factors may increase the risk of contracting cryptococcal meningitis to as high as 10% [Levy et al., 1988].

At UCSF, 68 reliably diagnosed cases of AIDS-related cryptococcal meningitis have been recorded as of June 1986. This represents an institutional incidence of 5.29%. The typical AIDS patient with cryptococcal meningitis in San Francisco is a 38-year-old homosexual male who already carries the diagnosis of AIDS. He has had 20 days of decreasing mental status, 10 days of headache and 5 days of meningismus. Cranial CT scan is normal; the diagnosis of cryptococcosis is made by CSF examination. He responds well initially to antibiotic therapy with amphotericin B, but his survival is still limited. Recurrent cryptococcal meningitis is a significant problem; mean survival is 2–3 months.

Other Fungal Infections

Candida albicans. Candidiasis, usually associated with diabetes, leukemia, lymphoma and intravenous drug abuse, is a relatively rare CNS pathogen [Thompson, 1974]. Nine cases of cerebral candidiasis have been reported in patients with AIDS. In light of the frequency of oral candidiasis in these patients, it is perhaps surprising that so few cases of intracerebral candidiasis have been observed. Three patients with AIDS and CNS candidiasis have been treated at UCSF; one of these has been reported previously [Levy et al., 1985b]. The combination of surgical abcess excision followed by amphotericin B appears to be the only effective therapy.

Aspergillus fumigatus. Infections with the mold *Aspergillus fumigatus* are uncommon, even in immunocompromised patients. Aspergillosis infecting the CNS may present as meningitis, encephalitis or abcess. Four cases of AIDS-related CNS aspergillosis have been reported.

Coccidioides immitis. Meningeal infection occurs in nearly one half of all cases of disseminated coccidioidomycosis. Although in immunocompetent patients the majority of cases have a subclinical or chronic, relapsing, long-lasting meningitis, coccidioidal meningitis can present as a rapid, fulminant illness in the immunocompromised patient. Treatment involves the long-term administration of intrathecal amphotericin B; frequently this requires the placement of an Ommaya reservoir. We have treated 2 cases of coccidioidomycosis in patients with AIDS at UCSF. One of these presented with coccidioidal meningitis while the other, with disseminated coccidioidal infection, was found to harbor multiple coccidioidal microabcesses throughout the cerebellum. A few other cases of AIDS-related CNS infection with *Coccidioides immitis* have been reported [Post et al., 1985].

Miscellaneous Fungal Infections. We have treated one child with AIDS and cerebral mucormycosis. Micozzi and Wetli [1985] have reported 5 cases of mucormycosis and intravenous drug users; these cases may well be AIDS-related. Two cases of cerebral infection with *Rhizopus species* and one case of cerebral infection with *Acremonium alabamensis* have been reported by Wetli et al. [1984]; these patients also probably had AIDS. There are also scattered case reports of intracranial infection with *Histoplasma capsulatum* [Post et al., 1985].

Mycobacterial Infections

Mycobacterium tuberculosis. The pathology and presentation of *Mycobacterium tuberculosis* meningitis have been well described [Adams and Victor, 1977]; mycobacterial infection can result in meningitis, encephalitis or brain abcess formation. Fifteen patients with AIDS and *M. tuberculosis* infections of the CNS have appeared in the literature [Bisburg et al., 1986]. These patients were uniformly either Haitians or intravenous drug abusers; these reports are consistent with the endemic nature of tuberculosis in the Caribbean basin and with epidemiologic data which indicate that Haitians are at higher risk of contracting any AIDS-related neurologic illness. The clinical profiles of these patients have not been fully reported; of note is that roughly two thirds presented with CNS mass lesions while one third presented with signs and symptoms of meningitis only. Of nearly 1,300 patients treated at UCSF, we have seen only one case of tubercular meningitis.

Mycobacterium avium intracellulare. While *Mycobacterium avium intracellulare* (MAI) infection is extremely common in the AIDS patient population, CNS infection with MAI is rare. Fourteen such cases have been reported [Zakowski et al., 1982). Four patients with AIDS and MAI infections of the nervous system have been treated at UCSF. In contrast to

CNS *M. tuberculosis* infection, there does not appear to be a Haitian prediliction for AIDS-related CNS MAI infection. Of patients reported in the literature, most had disseminated systemic MAI infection prior to their neurologic presentation with diffuse encephalitis. Meningitis, cranial neuropathy (facial nerve) and peripheral neuropathy have also been reported in association with MAI infection of the CNS. Survival after contracting CNS MAI infection is extremely limited; results with both standard tuberculosis chemotherapeutic agents and experimental regimens have been uniformly poor [Hawkins et al., 1986].

One patient with AIDS and CNS infection with *M. kansasii* has been reported [Armstrong et al., 1985].

Bacterial Infections

Reports of AIDS-related CNS complications from common bacterial pathogens have been conspicuously absent from the literature. None of the patients in the series presented by Snider et al. [1983] or that of Levy et al. [1985b] had bacterial infections of the CNS. Nervous system infections with opportunistic bacterial pathogens in patients with AIDS have rarely been reported. Thus, the immunologic defect initiated by HIV infection does not appear to place the AIDS patient at increased risk for contracting bacterial infections of the CNS.

Listeria monocytogenes. Lysteria, the most common cause of bacterial meningitis in immunocompromised patients, has only rarely been the cause of AIDS-related neurologic disease. We have treated 3 patients with AIDS and Listeria infections of the CNS at UCSF.

Nocardia asteroides. Nocardia infection of the CNS usually accompanies pulmonary infection in immunosuppressed patients; as with Listeria, Nocardia CNS infection in the AIDS patient population is extremely rare. Sharer and Kapila [1985] reported a single case of Nocardia brain abcess in a 34-year-old female intravenous drug abuser with AIDS.

Other Bacterial Infections. CNS infection with common bacterial pathogens is extremely rare in the AIDS patient population. One case each of AIDS-related *Escherichia coli* meningitis and meningoencephalitis have been reported [Berger et al. 1984; Post et al., 1985]; the clinical profiles of these patients are lacking. One case of syphilitic meningoencephalitis has been reported in a patient with AIDS [Berger et al., 1984].

Neoplasms

Primary CNS Lymphoma

Primary malignant lymphomas are rare tumors of the CNS, representing less than 1.5% of primary brain tumors [Henry et al., 1974]. While systemic lymphoma frequently invades the meninges [Griffin et al., 1971], primary CNS lymphomas more frequently involve the brain parenchyma [Bunn et al., 1976]. These neoplasms are more commonly seen in immunosuppressed patients; prior to the recognition of AIDS, primary CNS lymphomas were frequently seen in both renal and cardiac allograft recipients [Penn, 1975].

The risk of developing CNS lymphoma in the general population has been estimated at 0.0001% [Henry et al., 1974]. In immunosuppressed patients, this risk increases to 0.2% and in the population of patients with AIDS, the risk is roughly 1.5%. The annual incidence of primary CNS lymphoma in the USA prior to the AIDS epidemic was approximately 225 cases; in 1986, an estimated 240 cases were reported and, by 1988, projections suggest that 960 cases will occur. Thus, primary CNS lymphoma is becoming a disease predominantly affecting the AIDS patient population.

Three large series of patients with AIDS-related primary CNS lymphomas have appeared, summarizing the experience at UCSF [Levy et al., 1985b; So et al., 1986] and at the University of Southern California [Gill et al., 1985]. One hundred and seventy-two cases of AIDS-related primary CNS lymphoma were reported to the CDC by August 1986. This represents an incidence at presentation of 0.74%. At UCSF, 25 (1.9%) patients with AIDS-related primary CNS lymphomas have been treated. The average San Francisco AIDS patient with primary CNS lymphoma is a 37-year-old homosexual male. He presents with a subacute onset of altered mental status, headaches and hemiparesis. His CT scan reveals multiple enhancing intercranial lesions while CSF examination is remarkably only for a mild lymphocytic pleocytosis. Empiric therapy with pyrimethamine and sufadiazine for toxoplasmosis fails and the diagnosis of primary CNS lymphoma is made by biopsy. Until recently, such a patient has tended to survive for less than 2 months; his death has been related to his CNS neoplasm. Our recent experience with a protocol for the aggressive early treatment of these patients with radiation therapy [Rosenblum et al., 1988] suggests that these tumors are radiation-sensitive and that radiation therapy may have a significant effect on survival.

Systemic Lymphoma with CNS Involvement

Systemic lymphoma most frequently affects the CNS by invasion of the meninges [Griffin et al., 1971], resulting in meningitis or cranial neuropathies. Ziegler et al. [1982] first reported the outbreak of a Burkitt's-like lymphoma in homosexual men. Later reports firmly established the association of AIDS and systemic lymphomas. All of these first 4 patients had significant neurologic complications including epidural spinal block, meningitis and cranial neuropathies. Fernandez et al. [1983] reported a similar series of 6 patients with neurologic complications of systemic lymphomas, while the review by Snider et al. [1983] described 4 patients with meningeal lymphoma and one each with epidural thoracic lymphoma and epidural thoracic plasmacytoma. We have seen an additional 3 patients with metastatic systemic non-Hodgkin's lymphoma.

Neurologic manifestations of systemic lymphoma in these 19 patients included neoplastic meningitis in 9 patients, 5 of whom also had cranial neuropathies. Three other patients had isolated cranial neuropathies, 4 patients had epidural spinal cord compression by metastatic lymphoma, 2 patients had intracerebral hemorrhage from metastasis and one patient had brachial plexus invasion by tumor resulting in a brachial plexopathy. While transient improvement was noted in most cases following the institution of therapy, most patients were dead within one year after the onset of neurological symptoms.

Metastatic Kaposi's Sarcoma

Until the recent outbreak of AIDS, Kaposi's sarcoma was rarely documented in Europe or North America and had an annual incidence of 0.02–0.06 per 100.000 population [Rothman, 1962]. This neoplasm most often affected elderly Italian and Ashkenazic Jewish men. It responded well to therapy, with a mean survival ranging from 8 to 13 years. CNS involvement with Kaposi's sarcoma has been remarkably rare [Rwomushana et al., 1975].

The Kaposi's sarcoma associated with AIDS is characteristically much more aggressive than the classical form of the disease. It progresses rapidly and manifests widespread visceral involvement. Although Kaposi's sarcoma has been a primary feature of AIDS, CNS presentation of this neoplasm has been extremely rare. Four patients with AIDS and Kaposi's sarcoma metastatic to the brain have appeared in the literature [Gorin et al., 1985].

Cerebrovascular Complications

We have treated 20 patients with AIDS and documented cerbrovascular complications at UCSF (1.6% of all AIDS patients). Our recent neuropathologic study [Levy et al., 1986c] suggests this to be an extreme underestimate. In our series, 18 of 94 unselected patients with AIDS (19%) had cerebral infarctions. These infarcts varied from small multifocal infarctions to large infarcts, suggesting acute embolic phenomena. Of our 20 patients, 6 presented with transient ischemic attacks, 4 had hemorrhagic infarcts, 5 had ischemic cerebral infarcts and 4 had multifocal small infarcts. One patient presented with a subdural hematoma. Snider et al. [1983] reported 6 of 50 patients with AIDS who had cerebrovascular disease (12%). Three patients each had bland infarction or hemorrhagic infarction; 2 of the patients with intracerebral hemorrhage also had thrombocytopenia. Two patients had nonbacterial thrombotic endocarditis.

The majority of the hemorrhages have occurred in the setting of CNS neoplasia, with hemorrhages tending to occur within tumors. The ischemic infarcts have been more difficult to explain. Marantic endocarditis was not present in the vast majority of these patients. While there have been occasional cases of cerebral vasculitis in AIDS (DeLapaz and Enzmann, 1988], these appear to be uncommon and probably do not explain the large number of infarcts in the AIDS patient population. Circulating coagulating inhibitors have recently been isolated from some HIV-infected patients [Cohen et al., 1986]. The presence of such factors may explain the unusually high frequency of multifocal infarction in this young patient population.

CNS Complications as a Result of AIDS Therapy

Several groups have reported neurological symptoms arising as complications of AIDS therapy. Hollander et al. [1985] reported the development of extrapyramidal motor symptoms in AIDS patients treated with low-dose antiemetic therapy. Bates et al. [1985] have reported acute myelopathy following intrathecal chemotherapy for lymphoma in an AIDS patient. Antiviral therapy in AIDS patients has also been reported to produce startle myoclonus, dysphasia and delirium [Gold et al., 1984].

Multiple Intracranial Pathologic Processes

The evaluation and treatment of the AIDS patient with neurologic illness has been complicated by the observation that multiple intracranial pathologic processes may be present in patients with AIDS [Levy and Bredesen, 1988; Pitlik et al., 1984; Fischl et al., 1985]. Of 482 neurologically symptomatic AIDS patients treated at UCSF, 65 patients were identified with multiple intracranial pathologic processes (13.5%). In a more carefully studied group of patients, 29% of AIDS patients with nervous system illness had more than one CNS pathologic process identified at autopsy [Levy et al., 1986c]. Of note is that these processes were identified both within the same lesion and within spatially separated lesions as well as both sequentially and simultaneously. The care of the AIDS patient with neurologic illness is thus further complicated. Patients treated following biopsy or with a correct presumptive diagnosis may have other intracranial pathologic processes that remain untreated.

Psychosocial Manifestations of AIDS

While the virologic, epidemiologic and medical studies of AIDS have been pursued rigorously since 1981, the tremendous psychological impact of this devastating illness has been realized only recently. Walter Batchelor, Program Officer for Health Policy of the American Psychological Association, has recently labelled AIDS a psychological emergency [Batchelor, 1984]. In response to this tremendous need, many psychiatric and psychological researchers have begun to examine and address the problem of AIDS and mental health.

The neuropsychological complications of AIDS can either be primary or reactive. In the former case, psychopathology results directly from the effect of the disease process on the brain. In the latter case, illness can result from the unique psychological stresses arising from this chronic, debilitating fatal illness. Differentiation between these organic diseases and behavioral illnesses associated with AIDS can be quite difficult.

Price et al. [1988] have estimated that between 75 and 90% of patients with AIDS will manifest some degree of dementia during their illness. While HIV has been cultured from the brains of half of these patients and is assumed to be the cause of the dementia, efforts to culture virus from half of the demented patients have been unsuccessful. Thus, in as many as half of these patients, dementia may have another cause. In addition, careful neuropsychological testing of patients infected with this virus but without apparent clinical illness has demonstrated subtle behavioral and memory deficits in an alarming percentage of patients. While only very preliminary data are available, it has been estimated that from 10 to 30% of HIV-infected, non-AIDS patients have cognitive dysfunction on neuropsychological testing. Thus, infection with the AIDS virus alone can produce significant neuropsychological deficits very early in the patient's illness. These deficits may easily be ascribed to psychological illness rather than to an organic dementia.

In an attempt to characterize the psychological problems which appear in patients with AIDS, Dilley et al. [1985] summarized their experience performing psychiatric consultations in 13 of 40 patients hospitalized with AIDS. None of the patients had had previous psychiatric illness and none were judged suicidal. The most frequent reason for consultation request was depression, while the most common psychiatric diagnosis given these patients was an adjustment disorder with depressed mood in reaction to their illness. Severe clinical depression, dementia and delirium were also noted.

Several themes recurred during their interviews with these AIDS patients. Anxiety, frustration and anger over the uncertainty surrounding their illness and treatment were the most frequently expressed feelings. Doctors and fellow patients were unable to supply information as to the cause, treatment and outcome of their illness. The second most common theme was that of isolation and anticipated social abandonment. Patients had been fired from their jobs and had been deserted by their friends and lovers. Hospital isolation rooms along with isolation procedures requiring the doctors to gown and glove prior to contact with AIDS patients only served to heighten this feeling of isolation.

Another frequent psychological theme raised by these patients was that of illness as retribution for their 'immoral' acts. These fears were elevated by the knowledge that AIDS is sexually transmissible. Patients with multiple sexual partners experienced guilt and felt that their sexual appetites were responsible for their illness. Batchelor [1984] further addresses this issue of morality, noting that people with AIDS are often presumed to fit every negative stereotype of hypersexuality, drug use and bizarre behavior. While these factors appear to increase the risk of AIDS, clearly all AIDS patients are not from the 'dregs' of society. The generally low social esteem in which homosexuals, bisexuals or intravenous drug abusers are held contributes to the emotional distress of these patients.

An additional nuance to the sexual stresses associated with the diagnosis of AIDS is that many homosexuals have maintained secrecy with respect to their sexual orientation and are still 'in the closet'. The diagnosis of AIDS forces individuals out of the closet. At a time when they are least able to cope with such issues, it forces them to confront all of the negative reactions which initially led them to remain sexually covert.

Finally, the patients were observed to have those fears common to most patients facing a life-threatening illness. The patients 'struggled with fears related to their illness-fears of disability, loss of body control, pain and death' [Dilley et al., 1985]. They all had a great sense of loss and mourned their loss of health, money, friends and lovers.

Several of the typical reactions to death, dying and bereavement described by Kübler-Ross [1969] have been expressed by homosexual patients with AIDS [Morin et al., 1984]. These reactions include denial, depression, anger, bargaining and, finally, acceptance. The youth of AIDS patients makes coping with this diagnosis particularly difficult and painful. As the median age for AIDS patients is 35, this is often their first experience with serious illness. Contracting a fatal illness shatters the illusion of immortality that many young people have [Furstenberg and Olson, 1984]. Other authors have noted that since body image may be almost pathologically important to some homosexuals, fear of the loss of positive body image is particularly terrifying [Smith and Ryan, 1984]. Many AIDS patients respond with massive denial of the diagnosis or its implications. Others react with anger and depression.

A further issue that therapists need to confront is the fact that the homosexual life-style itself perpetuates the illness. Clearly, traumatic anal sex and possibly other homosexual practices involving the exchange of semen are involved with the transmission of AIDS. In the past, therapists have frequently recommended free sexual expression as a way to explore the patient's homosexuality. Therapists now have an ethical responsibility to promote behavior which limits the spread of this fatal illness. 'Currently, psychologists are trying to maintain a delicate balance: to remain sex-positive and gay-affirmative while at the same time working toward an educational model of safe sex (no exchange of semen or blood-related secretions)' [Morin et al., 1984].

Thus, the patient faced with the diagnosis of AIDS often reacts with guilt, the fear of exposure of his life-style, and the fear of death and dying. He must also face the fear of contagion, the loss of self-esteem and the fear of loss of physical attractiveness. The diagnosis of AIDS

Table III. AIDS cases and mortality: CDC predictions

	1986	1991
New cases	13,189	71,000
Alive from prior years	7,787	74,000
Total (for calendar year)	20,976	145,000
Cumulative total	29,137	270,000
Cumulative deaths	16,481	179,000

appropriately triggers the fear of decreased social support and increased dependency, isolation and stigmatization and the loss of financial and occupational status. Profound confusion concerning available options for medical treatment is compounded by uncertainty regarding long-term prognosis. Most critically, an overriding sense of gloom and helplessness are inevitable concomitants of progressive incurable illness for most patients.

Finally, since a multitude of AIDS-related neuropathologic processes can produce confusional states and dementia syndromes with secondary affective and anxiety features, the clinician must not allow the very real existential and humanistic aspects of AIDS to lessen his vigilance for treatable neuropathology. This necessity for balancing diagnostic vigilance with an informed and flexible approach to psychodynamic issues represents a critical challenge for neuropsychiatry.

Implications for Neurology, Neurosurgery and Psychiatry

As the number of AIDS cases in the USA continues to increase logarithmically, and in light of the frequency of AIDS-related neurologic and neuropsychiatric illness, the impact of this epidemic on the practice of the clinical neurosciences promises to be profound. To estimate the impact of AIDS upon the practice of neurology, neurosurgery and psychiatry, 5-year projections provided by the CDC [Curran and Morgan, 1986] and our own neuroepidemiologic data [Levy and Bredesen, 1988] were used.

The total number of AIDS cases, both patients alive from prior years and those presenting during 1986 in the USA, is presented in table III. For projections through 1991, the CDC has used a polynomial mathematical model. Only confirmed AIDS cases were used in these calculations and it was assumed that no changes in the epidemiology of the disease will occur

Table IV. Cases of AIDS-related neurologic illness compared to the annual incidence of other neurologic diseases

Neurologic disease	Yearly incidence[1]	
Migraine headache	562,000	
Stroke	337,500	
Epilepsy	112,500	
		← neurologic AIDS (1991)
Parkinson's disease	45,000	
Meningitis	33,750	
Cerebral palsy	20,250	
Tic douloureux	9,000	
		← neurologic AIDS (1986)
Multiple sclerosis	6,750	
Guillain-Barré syndrome	4,500	
Muscular dystrophy	1,575	
Huntington's disease	900	
Myasthenia gravis	900	

[1] Incidence data adapted from Kurtzke [1984].

and that no effective intervention if forthcoming. The annual number of new cases, number of AIDS patients treated and number of deaths, as well as the cumulative number of cases and deaths are presented in table III, both for 1986 and 1991.

From the beginning of the AIDS epidemic to the end of 1986, 29,137 patients with AIDS has been reported to the CDC; of these 16,481 patients had died. During the calendar year 1986, 20,976 patients with AIDS were alive in the USA. With significant neurologic symptoms reported during lifetime in 37% of AIDS patients, we estimate that in 1986 there were 7,761 neurologically symptomatic AIDS patients. During the calendar year 1991, when 145,000 patients with AIDS will be alive in the USA, with 270,000 cumulative cases, the number of neurologically symptomatic AIDS patients will have risen to 53,650. The number of deaths from AIDS was virtually equal to the number of deaths from brain tumors in 1986; by 1991, it will surpass head injury as a cause of death.

The number of neurologically symptomatic AIDS patients relative to the number of patients in the USA with other neurologic illness is striking (table IV). In 1986, there were more patients with AIDS than with cerebral palsy. During the year 1991, there will be more patients alive with AIDS than with epilepsy and almost half as many as those with stroke. In 1986, neurologically symptomatic AIDS patients were intermediate in frequency between those with trigeminal neuralgia and those with multiple sclerosis.

Table V. Predicted number of neurosurgical operations on patients with AIDS

	1986	1991
Alive from prior year	7,787	71,000
New cases	13,189	74,000
(CNS masses, 3.5%)	462	2,590
Total at risk	20,976	145,000
(nontoxoplasmosis CNS mass lesions, 2.9%)	608	4,205
Total projected operations	1,070	6,795

By 1991, the number of neurologically symptomatic AIDS patients will be nearly half the number of all patients with epilepsy and will far exceed those with Parkinson's disease.

These figures take into account only those patients with AIDS and neurologic dysfunction. This may, however, be an extreme underestimate of the impact of AIDS on the practice of neurology. The large number of patients infected with HIV but without signs of systemic illness creates a unique problem. CDC predictions suggest that 1.5 million people were infected with the virus in 1986. In 1991, 15 million Americans may be infected with the virus. Several recent studies have documented cognitive dysfunction in these HIV-infected patients [Navia and Price, 1987]. As a significant number of HIV-infected patients will develop dementia in the absence of other HIV-related illness, the potential number of HIV-related neurologically symptomatic patients may rise into the millions.

The impact of AIDS on the practice of neurosurgery can be predicted from the number of CNS mass lesions estimated from our experience at UCSF combined with the case predictions from the CDC. Our indications for brain biopsy include the presence intracranial mass lesions that do not respond to empiric treatment for toxoplasmosis in patients with AIDS and the presence of intracranial masses in patients who have not yet been diagnosed as having AIDS. In 1986 and 1991, the number of cases that would fulfill these relatively conservative indications for biopsy are 1,070 and 6,795, respectively (table V). The number of biopsies performed for AIDS-related CNS mass lesions will, therefore, approximate the yearly incidence of malignant astrocytomas in the USA (table VI). The number of biopsy procedures for AIDS-related primary CNS lymphomas alone will approximate the number of meningiomas by 1991.

The impact upon the practice of psychiatry is more difficult to ascertain. Most if not all patients with AIDS experience appropriate and

Table VI. Projected AIDS-associated brain biopsies compared to the annual incidence of primary brain tumors in the USA

Tumor	Yearly incidence	
Malignant astrocytoma	6,000	←——— AIDS brain Bx (1991)
Meningioma	2,250	
Astrocytoma	1,500	
Pituitary tumor	1,500	←——— AIDS brain Bx (1986)
Neurinoma/fibroma	750	
Medulloblastoma	600	
Congenital	600	
Ependymoma	300	
Lymphoma	225	

significant problems in coping with a fatal illness. Many of them will seek psychiatric assistance. In addition, more than 75% of AIDS patients will be demented [Price et al., 1987] and this dementia will frequently require psychiatric assessment. Finally, the potential impact of dementia in HIV-infected, non-AIDS patients is tremendous.

The distinction among and differential weighting of biologic, psychologic and social factors in this increasingly vast patient population will pose a major diagnostic task for neuropsychiatrists. Widely divergent therapeutic approaches exist for both organic and psychosocial HIV-related illness. Only through careful neurologic, psychiatric and cognitive assessment can the complex needs of patients with AIDS be best addressed.

Summary and Conclusions

AIDS is no longer a rare disease affecting only a small segment of our population. It has now been observed throughout the USA as well as most other countries in the world and already is recognized as a major public health menace in the USA, Western Europe and Africa. AIDS has spread across boundaries of sex, race and socioeconomic status. Millions of people are already infected with HIV, an unknown number of whom will go on to develop AIDS.

As the number of AIDS cases increases dramatically, it becomes imperative that health care workers involved with the treatment of these patients become aware of the myriad and protean manifestations of this illness. As the current data demonstrate, the effect of AIDS upon the nervous system is profound and widespread. About 10% of all AIDS patients will first present with a neurologic complaint. Evaluation of this complaint will then lead to the diagnosis of AIDS. Nearly 40% of all AIDS patients will develop significant neurologic symptoms during their lifetime. These symptoms may be related to primary HIV infection or secondarily to any of a number of opportunistic processes. At autopsy, 75% of AIDS patients will have neuropathologic abnormalities.

The AIDS-related CNS syndromes are as numerous and varied as are their associated signs and symptoms. As is the case with radiologic and serologic examination, the findings resulting from clinical examination of the AIDS patient with neurologic illness are nonspecific. While there are clinical findings that suggest one or another class of AIDS-related neurologic illness, there is such overlap in their presentations as to make specific CNS diagnosis on the basis of clinical examination virtually impossible.

The differential diagnosis of AIDS-related neurologic illness is made even more difficult by the frequent observation of multiple CNS pathologic processes in the same AIDS patient. Nearly one third of all histologically examined AIDS cases had multiple intracranial pathologies. Multiple treatable pathologic abnormalities have been identified both within the same intracranial lesion and within different lesions, both simultaneously and sequentially.

The impact of AIDS-related neurologic illness on the practice of the clinical neurosciences will be profound. By 1991, AIDS will surpass head injury as a cause of death. By this time, neurologic consultations for AIDS-related problems will be nearly half those for epilepsy. Neurosurgeons will be asked to perform more AIDS-associated brain biopsies than operations on malignant astrocytoma. The impact on psychiatry may be even greater in that millions of patients with cognitive dysfunction and dementia may require neuropsychiatric evaluation.

Thus, the evaluation and treatment of the AIDS patient with central neurologic illness is a difficult challenge. Algorithms for the evaluation of the neurologically symptomatic AIDS patient are included in figures 1 and 2. Close attention must be paid to subtle neurologic complaints and careful neurologic examination is warranted in all AIDS patients. Once the patient complains of neurologic dysfunction or a neurologic abnormality is identified on clinical examination, a careful workup is indicated. Our current recommendation for initial evaluation is MRI. If this is not available, then

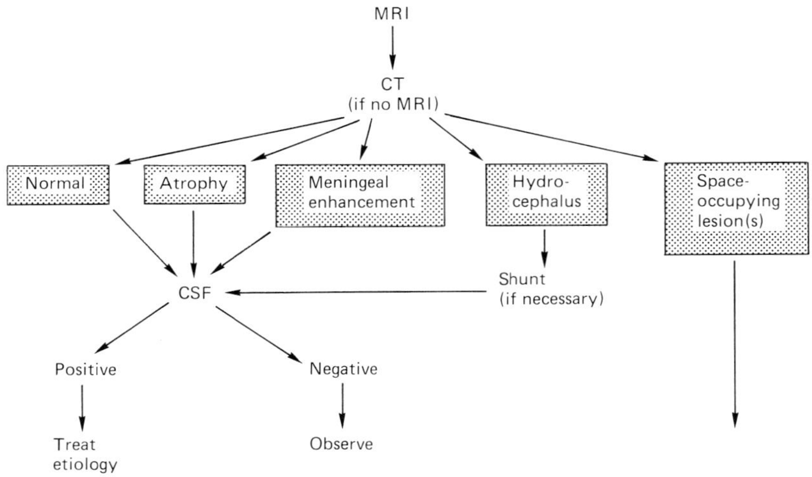

Fig. 1. Algorithm for the evaluation of the AIDS patient with CNS symptoms.

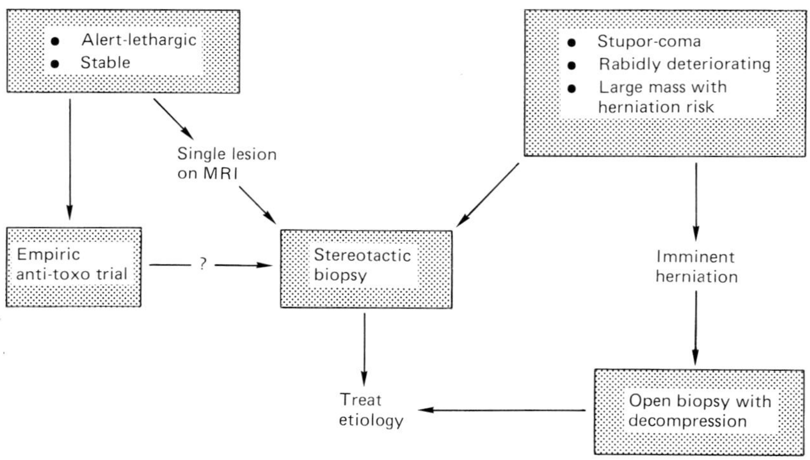

Fig. 2. Algorithm for the evaluation of the patient with space-occupying lesion(s).

CT brain scanning should be performed. If the neuroradiologic study is normal or reveals diffuse cerebral atrophy only, then CSF examination should be performed. In addition to routine chemistries, cytology and cultures, CSF examination should include studies for cryptococcus (antigen, culture and India ink) as well as full viral cultures. Treatment should be initiated based upon these findings. If not diagnosis is made, then careful, regular clinical and radiologic follow-up is indicated.

Those patients with focal lesions on MRI are divided into those who are stable (alert or lethargic) or those who are deteriorating. In stable patients a trial of empiric therapy for toxoplasmosis with pyrimethamine and sulfadiazine is initiated. If there is clear radiologic and clinical response after 3 weeks of therapy, maximal antibiotic therapy is continued for life. If the patient fails to respond, then stereotaxic biopsy is indicated. In patients who are neurologically unstable, we proceed directly to stereotaxic biopsy. Open craniotomy is reserved only for those patients with large mass lesions who are at risk of herniation and require emergent decompression.

Specific diagnosis is thus made on the basis of CSF findings, response to empiric therapy, or biopsy. These patients must then be followed with great diligence to evaluate the response to therapy. The very real possibility of multiple treatable intracranial pathologic processes may necessitate a repetition of the patient's diagnostic evaluation and the institution of additional therapies. While such a diagnostic and therapeutic program requires extreme care and diligence, such an approach is necessary to treat optimally the patient with AIDS-related neurologic illness. Only with such optimal therapy can we offer hope to patients with AIDS.

Acknowledgements

The author would like to thank his collaborators, Drs. Dale Bredesen and Mark Rosenblum, and Ravi Gupta, clinical research assistant, whose efforts have made this work possible. Portions of this chapter have appeared in *AIDS and the Nervous System,* Rosenblum, M.L.; Levy, R.M.; Bredesen, D.E. (editors), Raven Press, New York 1988), and Rosenblum, M.L.; Levy, R.M.; Bredesen, D.E.: Neurosurgical implications of the acquired immunodeficiency syndrome. Clinical neurosurgery, vol. 34 (Williams & Wilkins, Baltimore 1987).

References

Adams, R.A.; Victor, M.: Principles of neurology, p. 100 (McGraw-Hill, New York 1977).

Anderson, S.: *Toxoplasma gondii;* in Mandell, Douglas, Bennett, Principles and practice of infectious diseases, pp. 2127–2137 (Wiley & Sons, New York 1979).

Armstrong, D.; Gold, J.W.M.; Drjyanski, J.; Whimbey, E.; Polsky, B.; Hawkins, C.; Brown, A.E.; Bernard, E.; Kiehn, T.E.: Treatment of infections in patients with acquired immunodeficiency syndrome. Ann. intern. Med. *103:* 738–743 (1985).

Armstrong, D.; Wong, B.: Central nervous system infection in immunocompromised hosts. Annu. Rev. Med. *33:* 293–308 (1982).

Astrom, K.E.; Mancall, E.L.; Richardson, E.P., Jr.: Progressive multifocal leukoencephalopathy: a hitherto unrecognized complication of chronic lymphatic leukemia and Hodgkin's disease. Brain *81:* 93–111 (1958).

Bale, J.F., Jr.: Human cytomegalovirus infection and disorders of the nervous system. Archs Neurol. *41:* 310–320 (1984).

Baringer, J.R.: Herpes simplex infection of the nervous system; in Vinken, Bruyn, Handbook of clinical neurology, vol. 34, pp. 145–159 (North-Holland, Amsterdam 1978).

Baringer, J.R.; Swoveland, P.: Recovery of herpes-simplex virus from human trigeminal ganglions. New Engl. J. Med. *288:* 648–650 (1973).

Barré-Sinoussi, F.; Chermann, J.C.; Rey, F.; Nugeyre, M.T.; Chamaret, S.; Gruest, J.; Gauguet, C.; Axler-Blin, C.; Brun-Vezinet, F.; Rouzioux, C.; Rozenbaum, W.; Montagnier, L.: Isolation of a T-lymphotropic retrovirus from a patient at risk for acquired immune deficiency syndrome (AIDS). Science *220:* 868–871 (1983).

Bates, S.; Mc Keever, P.; Masur, H.; Levens, D.; Macher, A.; Armstrong, G.; Magrath, I.T.: Myelopathy following intrathecal chemotherapy in a patient with extensive Burkitt's lymphoma and altered immune status. Am. J. Med. *78:* 697–702 (1985).

Batchelor, W.F.: AIDS: a public health and psychological emergency. Am. Psychol. *39:* 1279–1284 (1984).

Bedri, J.; Weinstein, W.; DeGregorio, P.; Verity, M.A.: Progressive multifocal leukoencephalopathy in acquired immunodeficiency syndrome (letter). New Engl. J. Med. *309:* 492–493 (1983).

Berger, J.R.; Moskowitz, L.; Fischl, M.; Kelley, R.E.: The neurologic complications of AIDS; frequently the initial manifestation. Neurology *34:* suppl. 1, pp. 134–135 (1984).

Berger, J.R.; Resnick, L.: HTLV-III/LAV-related neurological disease; in Broder, AIDS: modern concepts and therapeutic challenges, pp. 263–283 (Dekker, New York 1987).

Bishburg, E.; Sunderam, G.; Reichman, L.B.; Kapila, R.: Central nervous system tuberculosis with the acquired immunodeficiency syndrome and its related complex. Ann. intern. Med. *105:* 210–213 (1986).

Bredesen, D.E.; Lipkin, W.I.; Messing, R.: Prolonged, recurrent aseptic meningitis with prominent cranial nerve abnormalities: a new epidemic in gay men? (Abstract). Neurology *33:* suppl. 2, p. 85 (1983).

Bredesen, D.E.; Messing, R.: Neurological syndromes heralding the acquired immune deficiency syndrome (Abstract). Ann. Neurol. *14:* 141 (1983).

Britton, C.B.; Mesa-Tejeda, R.; Fenoglio, C.M.; Hays, A.P.; Garvey, G.G.; Miller, J.R.: A new complication of AIDS: thoracic myelitis caused by herpes simplex. Neurology *35:* 1071–1074 (1985).

Bunn, P.A., Jr.; Schein, P.S.; Banks, P.M.; DeVita, V.T., Jr.: Central nervous system complications in patients with diffuse histiocytic and undifferentiated lymphoma: leukemia revised. Blood *47:* 3–10 (1976).

Centers for Disease Control: Prevention of acquired immune deficiency syndrome (AIDS): report of interagency recommendations. MMWR *32:* 101–103 (1983).

Chan, J.C.; Moskowitz, L.B.; Olivella, J.; Hensley, G.T.; Greeman, R.L.; Hoffman, T.A.: Toxoplasma encephalitis in recent Haitian entrants. Sth. med. J. *76:* 1211–1215 (1983).

Cohen, A.J.; Phillips, T.; Keffler, C.: Circulating coagulation inhibitors in the acquired immune deficiency syndrome. Ann. intern. Med. *104:* 175–180 (1986).

Cole, E.L.; Meisler, D.M.; Calabrese, L.H.; Holland, G.N.; Mondino, B.J.; Conant, M.A.: Herpes zoster ophthalmicus and acquired immune deficiency syndrome. Archs. Ophthal. *102:* 1027–1029 (1984).

Curran, J.: The epidemiology of AIDS: current status and future prospects. Proc. 2nd Int. Conf. on AIDS, Paris 1986, p. 7.

DeLapaz, R.; Enzmann, D.: Neuroradiology of acquired immunodeficiency syndrome; in AIDS and the nervous system, pp. 121–153 (Raven Press, New York 1988).

Dilley, J.W.; Ochitill, H.W.; Perl, M.; Volberding, P.: Findings in psychiatric consultations with patients with acquired immune deficiency syndrome. Am. J. Psychiat. *142:* 82–86 (1985).

Dix, R.D.; Waitzman, D.M.; Follansbee, S.; Pearson, B.S.; Mendelson, T.; Smith, P.; Davis, R.L.; Mills, J.: HSV type 2 encephalitis in two homosexual men with persistent lymphadenopathy. Ann. Neurol. *17:* 203–206 (1985).

Edwards, R.H.; Messing, R.; McKendall, R.R.: Cytomegalovirus meningoencephalitis in a homosexual man with Kaposi's sarcoma: isolation of CMV from CSF cells. Neurology *35:* 560–561 (1985).

Fernandez, R.; Mouradian, J.; Moore, A.; Asch, A.: Malignant lymphoma with central nervous system involvement in six homosexual men with acquired immunodeficiency syndrome (Abstract). Lab. Invest. *48:* 25A (1983).

Fischl, M.A.; Pitchenik, A.E.; Spira, T.J.: Tuberculous brain abscess and Toxoplasma encephalitis in a patient with the acquired immunodeficiency syndrome. J. Am. med. Ass. *253:* 3428–3430 (1985).

Friedman-Klien, A.E.; Laubenstein, L.J.; Rubinstein, P.; Buimovic-Klein, E.; Marmor, M.; Stahl, R.; Spigland, I.; Kim, K.S.; Zolla-Pazner, S.: Disseminated Kaposi's sarcoma in homosexual men. Ann. intern. Med. *96:* 693–700 (1982).

Furstenberg, A.L.; Olson, M.M.: Social work and AIDS. Soc. Work Hlth Care *9:* 45–63 (1984).

Gallo, R.C.; Salahuddin, S.Z.; Popovic, M.; Shearer, G.M.; Kaplan, M.; Haynes, B.F.; Palker, T.J.; Redfield, R.; Oleske, J.; Safai, B.; White, G.; Foster, P.; Markham, P.D.: Frequent detection and isolation of cytopathic retroviruses (HTLV-III) from patients with AIDS and at risk for AIDS. Science *224:* 500–503 (1984).

Gill, P.S.; Levine, A.M.; Meyer, P.R.; Boswell, W.D.; Burkes, R.L.; Parker, J.W.; Hofman, F.M.; Dworsky, R.L.; Lukes, R.J.: Primary central nervous system lymphoma in homosexual men. Clinical, immunologic, and pathologic features. Am. J. Med. *78:* 742–747 (1985).

Gold, J.W.M.; Leyland-Jones, B.; Urmacher, C.; Armstrong, D.: Pulmonary and neurologic complications of treatment with FIAC (2'fluoro-5-iodo-aracytosine) in patients with acquired immune deficiency syndrome (AIDS). AIDS Res. *1:* 243–252 (1984).

Goldstick, L.; Mandybur, I.T.; Bode, R.: Spinal cord degeneration in AIDS. Neurology *35:* 103–106 (1985).

Goldstick, L.; Mandybur, T.I.; Means, E.: Spinal cord long tract degeneration in AIDS (Abstract). J. Neuropath. exp. Neurol. *43:* 294 (1984).

Gorin, F.A.; Bale, J.F., Jr.: Hawks-Miller, M.; Schwartz, R.A.: Kaposi's sarcoma metastatic to the CNS. Archs Neurol. *42:* 162–165 (1985).

Gottlieb, M.S.; Schroff, R.; Schanker, H.M.; Weisman, J.D.; Fan, P.T.; Wolf, R.A.; Saxon, A.: *Pneumocystis carinii* pneumonia and mucosal candidiasis in previously healthy homosexual men. Evidence of a new acquired cellular immunodeficiency. New Engl. J. Med. *305:* 1425–1431 (1981).

Grant, I.; Atkinson, J.H.; Hesselink, J.R; Kennedy, C.J.; Richman, D.D.; Spector, S.A.; McCutchan, J.A.: Evidence for early central nervous system involvement in the acquired immunodeficiency syndrome (AIDS) and other human immunodeficiency virus (HIV) infections. Ann. int. Med. *107:* 828–836 (1987).

Griffin, J.W.; Thompson, R.W.; Mitchinson, M.J.; Kiewiet, J. de; Welland, F.H.: Lymphomatous leptomeningitis. Am. J. Med. *51:* 200–208 (1971).

Handler, M.; Ho, V.; Whelan, M.; Budzilovich, G.: Intracerebral toxoplasmosis in patients with acquired immune deficiency syndrome. J. Neurosurg. *59:* 994–1001 (1983).

Hawkins, C.; Gold, J.M.; Whimbey, E.; Kiehn, T.E.; Brannon, P.; Cammarata, R.; Brown, A.E.; Armstrong, D.: *Mycobacterium avium* complex infections in patients with acquired immunodeficiency syndrome. Ann. intern. Med. *105:* 184–188 (1986).

Hawley, D.A.; Schaefer, J.F.; Schulz, D.M.; Muller, J.; Cytomegalovirus encephalitis in acquired immunodeficiency syndrome. Am. J. clin. Path. *80:* 874–877 (1983).

Henry, J.M.; Heffner, R.R., Jr.; Dillar, S.H.; Earle, K.M.; Davis, R.L.: Primary malignant lymphomas of the central nervous system. Cancer *34:* 1293–1302 (1974).

Ho, D.D.; Rota, T.R.; Schooley, R.T.; Kaplan, J.C.; Allan, J.D.; Groopman, J.E.; Resnick, L.; Felsenstein, D.; Andrews, C.A.; Hirsch, M.S.: Isolation of HTLV-III from cerebrospinal fluid and neural tissues of patients with neurologic syndromes related to the acquired immunodeficiency syndrome. New Engl. J. Med. *313:* 1493–1497 (1985).

Hollander, H.; Golden, J.; Mendelson, T.; Cortland, D.: Extrapyramidal symptoms in AIDS patients given low-dose metoclopramide or chlorpromazine (Letter). Lancet *ii:* 1186 (1985).

Horoupian, D.S.; Pick, P.; Spigland, I.; Smith, P.; Portenoy, R.; Katzman, R.; Cho, S.: Acquired immune deficiency syndrome and multiple tract degeneration in a homosexual man. Ann. Neurol. *15:* 502–505 (1984).

Janssen, R.S.; Saykin, A.J.; Kaplan, J.E.; Spira, T.J.; Pinsky, P.F.; Sprehn, G.C.; Hoffman, J.C.; Mayer, W.B.; Schonberger, L.B.: Neurological complications of human immunodeficiency virus infection in patients with lymphadenopathy syndrome. Ann. Neurol. *23(1):* 49–55 (1988).

Keonig, S.; Gendelman, H.E.; Orenstein, J.M.; Dal Canto, M.C.; Pezeshkpour, G.H.; Yungbluth, M.; Janotta, F.; Aksamit, A.; Martin, M.A.; Fauchi, A.S.: Detection of AIDS virus in macrophages in brain tissue from AIDS patients with encephalopathy. Science *233:* 1089–1093 (1986).

Koppel, B.S.; Wormser, G.P.; Tuchma, A.J.; Maayan, S.; Hewlett, D., Jr.; Daras, M.: Central nervous system involvement in patients with acquired immune deficiency syndrome (AIDS). Acta neur. scand. *71:* 337–351 (1985).

Kovacs, J.A.; Kovacs, A.A.; Polis, M.; Wright, W.C.; Gill, V.J.; Tuazon, C.U.; Gelmann, E.P.; Lane, H.C.; Longfield, R.; Overturf, G.; Macher, A.M.; Fauci, A.S.; Parrillo, J.E.; Bennett, J.E.; Masur, H.: Cryptococcosis in the acquired immunodeficiency syndrome. Ann. intern. Med. *103:* 533–538 (1985).

Krupp, L.B.; Lipton, R.B.; Swerdlow, M.L.; Leeds, N.E.; Llena, J.: Progressive multifocal leukoencephalopathy: clinical and radiographic features. Ann. Neurol. *17:* 344–348 (1985).

Kübler-Ross, E.: On death and dying. (Macmillan, London 1969).

Kurtzke, J.F.: Neuroepidemiology. Ann. Neurol. *16:* 265–277 (1984).

Levy, J.A.; Shimabukuro, J.; Hollander, H.; Mills, J.; Kaminsky, L.: Isolation of AIDS associated retroviruses from cerebrospinal fluid and brain of patients with neurological symptoms. Lancet *ii:* 586–588 (1985a).

Levy, R.M.; Bredesen, D.E.: Central nervous system dysfunction in acquired immunodeficiency syndrome. AIDS and the nervous system, pp. 29–63 (Raven Press, New York 1988).

Levy, R.M.; Bredesen, D.E.; Rosenblum, M.L.: Neurological manifestations to the acquired immunodeficiency syndrome (AIDS): experience at UCSF and review of the literature. J. Neurosurg. *62:* 475–495 (1985b).

Levy, R.M.; Bredesen, D.E.; Rosenblum, M.L.; Davis, R.L.: Postmortem neuropathology in the acquired immunodeficiency syndrome (AIDS): 106 consecutive AIDS autopsies. Congress of Neurological Surgeons Annual Meeting, New Orleans, September 1986 (Abstract) (1986c).

Levy, J.A.; Hoffman, A.D.; Kramer, S.M.; Landis, J.A.; Shimabukuro, J.M.; Oshiro, L.S.: Isolation of lymphocytopathic retroviruses from San Francisco patients with AIDS. Science *225:* 840–842 (1984a).

Levy, R.M.; Janssen, R.S.; Bush, T.J.; Rosenblum, M.L.: Neuroepidemiology of the acquired immunodeficiency syndrome; in Rosenblum, Levy, Bredesen, AIDS and the nervous system, pp. 13–28 (Raven Press, New York 1988).

Levy, R.M.; Mills, C.; Posin, J.; Moore, S.; Rosenblum, M.; Bredesen, D.E.: The superiority of MR to CT in the detection of intracranial pathology in the acquired immunodeficiency syndrome (AIDS). Proc. Int. Conf. on Acquired Immunodeficiency Syndrome (AIDS), Paris 1986b, p. 37, abstr.

Levy, R.M.; Pons, V.G.; Rosenblum, M.L.: Central nervous system mass lesions in the acquired immunodeficiency syndrome (AIDS). J. Neurosurg. *61:* 9–16 (1984b).

Levy, R.M.; Rosenbloom, S.; Perrett, L.V.: Neuroradiological findings in the acquired immunodeficiency syndrome (AIDS): A review of 200 cases. AJNR *7:* 833–839 (1986a).

Luft, B.J.; Conley, F.; Remington, J.S.: Outbreak of central-nervous-system toxoplasmosis in Western Europe and North America. Lancet *i:* 781–783 (1983).

Masur, H.; Michelis, M.A.; Greene, J.B.; Onorato, I.; Vande Stouwe, R.A.; Holzman, R.S.; Wormser, G.; Brettman, L.; Lange, M.; Murray, H.W.; Cunningham-Rundles, S.: An outbreak of community-acquired *Pneumocystis carinii* pneumonia. Initial manifestion of cellular immune dysfunction. New Engl. J. Med. *305:* 1431–1438 (1981).

McKendall, R.R.; Klawans, H.L.: Nervous system complications of varicella-zoster virus; in Vinken, Bruyn, Handbook of clinical neurology, vol. 34, pp. 161–183 (North-Holland, Amsterdam 1978).

Micozzi, M.S.; Wetli, C.V.: Intravenous amphetamine abuse, primary cerebral mucormycosis and acquired immunodeficiency. J. forens. Sci. *30:* 504–510 (1985).

Miller, J.R.; Barrett, R.E.; Britton, C.B.; Tapper, M.L.; Bahr, G.S.; Bruno, P.J.; Marquardt, M.D.; Hays, S.P.; McMurtry, J.G.; Weissman, J.B.; Bruno, M.S.: Progressive multifocal leukoencephalopathy in a male homosexual with T-cell immune deficiency. New Engl. J. Med. *307:* 1436–1438 (1982).

Morin, S.F.; Charles, K.A.; Malyon, A.K.: The psychological impact of AIDS on gay men. Am. Psychol. *39:* 1288–1293 (1984).

Moskowitz, L.B.; Hensley, G.T.; Chan, J.C.; Gregorios, J.; Conley, F.K.: The neuropathology of acquired immune deficiency syndrome. Archs Pathol. Lab. Med. *108:* 867–872 (1984).

Nafayan, O.; Penny, J.B., Jr.; Johnson, R.T.; Herndon, R.M.; Wiener, L.P.: Etiology of progressive multifocal leukoencephalopathy. Identification of papovavirus. New Engl. J. Med. *289:* 1278–1282 (1973).

Navia, B.A.; Cho, E.S.; Petito, C.K.; Price, R.W.: The AIDS dementia complex. II. Neuropathology. Ann. Neurol. *19:* 525–535 (1986a).

Navia, B.A.; Jordan, B.D.; Price, R.W.: The AIDS dementia complex. I. Clinical features. Ann. Neurol. *19:* 517–524 (1986b).

Navia, B.A.; Price, R.W.: The acquired immunodeficiency dementia complex as the presenting or sole manifestation of human immunodeficiency virus infection. Archs Neurol. *44:* 65–69 (1987).

Penn, I.: The incidence of malignancies in transplant recipients. Transplant. Proc. *7:* 323–326 (1975).

Pepose, J.S.; Hilborne, L.H.; Cancilla, P.A.; Foos, R.Y.: Concurrent herpes simplex and cytomegalovirus retinitis and encephalitis in the acquired immune deficiency syndrome (AIDS). Ophthalmology *91:* 1669–1677 (1984).

Petito, C.K.; Navia, B.A.; Cho, E.S.; Jordan, B.D.; George, D.C.; Price, R.W.: Vacuolar myelopathy pathologically resembling subacute combined degeneration in patients with the acquired immunodeficiency syndrome. New Engl. J. Med. *312:* 874–879 (1985).

Pitlik, S.D.; Rios, L.; Hersh, E.M.; Bolivar, R.; Mansell, P.A.: Polymicrobial brain abscess in a homosexual man with Kaposi's sarcoma. Sth. med. J. *77:* 271–272 (1984).

Post, M.J.D.; Kursunoglu, S.J.; Hensley, G.T.; Chan, J.C.; Moskowitz, L.B.; Hoffman, T.A.: Cranial CT in acquired immunodeficiency syndrome: spectrum of diseases and optimal contrast enhancement technique. AJNR *145:* 929–940 (1985).

Post, M.J.D.; Chan, J.C.; Hensley, G.T.; Hoffman, T.A.; Moskowitz, L.B.; Lippman, S.: Toxoplasma encephalitis in Haitian adults with acquired immunodeficiency syndrome: a clinical-pathologic-CT correlation. Am. J. Roentg. *140:* 861–868 (1983).

Post, M.J.D.; Hensley, G.T.; Moskowitz, L.B.; Fischl, M.: Cytomegalic inclusion virus encephalitis in patients with AIDS: CT, clinical and pathologic correlation. AJNR *7:* 275–280 (1986); Am. J. Roentg. *146:* 1229–1234 (1986).

Price, R.W.; Sidtis, J.J.; Navia, B.A.; Pumarola-Sune, T.; Ornitz, D.B.: The AIDS dementia complex. AIDS and the nervous system, pp. 203–219 (Raven Press, New York 1988).

Remington, J.S.; Desmonts, G.: Toxoplasmosis; in Remington, Klein, Infectious diseases of the fetus and newborn infant, pp. 191–332 (Saunders, Philadelphia 1976).

Resnick, L.; DiMarzo-Veronese, F.; Schupbach, J.; Tourtellotte, W.W.; Ho, D.D.; Muller, F.; Shapshak, P.; Vogt, M.; Groopman, J.E.; Markham, P.D.; Gallo, R.C.: Intra-blood-brain-barrier synthesis of HRLC-III-specific IgG in patients with neurologic symptoms associated with AIDS or AIDS-related complex. New Engl. J. Med. *313:* 1498–1504 (1985).

Rodan, B.A.; Cohen, F.L.; Bean, W.J.: CT biopsy of cerebral toxoplasmosis in AIDS. J. Fla. med. Ass. *71:* 158–160 (1984).

Rosenblum, M.L.; Levy, R.M.; Bredesen, D.E.; So, Y.T.; Wara, W.; Ziegler, J.L.: Primary central nervous system lymphomas in patients with the acquired immunodeficiency syndrome (AIDS). Ann. Neurol. *23:* suppl., S13–S26 (1988).

Rothman, S.: Remarks on sex, age and racial distribution of Kaposi's sarcoma and on possible pathogenetic factors. Acta Un. int. Cancr. *18:* 326–329 (1962).

Rutsaert, J.; Melot, C.; Ectors, M.; Cornil, A.; De Prez, C.; Flament-Durant, J.: Complications infectieuses pulmonaires et neurologiques d'un sarcome de Kaposi. Annls Anat. path. *25:* 125–138 (1980).

Rwomushana, R.J.W.; Bailey, I.C.; Kyalwazi, S.K.: Kaposi's sarcoma of the brain. Cancer *35:* 1127–1131 (1975).

Ryder, J.W.; Croen, K.; Kleinschmidt-DeMasters, B.K.; Ostrove, J.M.; Straus, S.E.; Cohn, D.L.: Progressive encephalitis three months after resolution of cutaneous zoster in a patient with AIDS. Ann. Neurol.*19:* 182–188 (1986).

Sharer, L.R.; Cho, E.S.; Epstein, L.G.: Multinucleated giant cells and HTLV-III in AIDS encephalotpathy. Human Pathol. *16:* 760 (1985).

Sharer, L.R.; Kapila, R.: Neuropathologic observations in acquired immunodeficiency syndrome (AIDS). Acta neuropath. *66:* 188–198 (1985).

Shaw, G.; Harper, M.E.; Hahn, B.H.; Epstein, L.G.; Gajdusek, D.C.; Price, R.W.; Navia, B.A.; Petito, C.K.; O'Hara, C.J.; Groopman, J.E.; Cho, E.-S.; Oleske, J.M.; Wong-Staal, F.; Gallo, R.C.: HTLV-III infection in brains of children and adults with AIDS – encephalopathy. Science *227:* 177–182 (1985).

Sher, J.H.: Cerebral toxoplasmosis (Letter). Lancet *i:* 1225.

Smith, R.W.; Ryan, C.C.: Psychosocial issues for people with AIDS. J Med Assn GA *73:* 535–536 (1984).

Snider, W.D.; Simpson, D.M.; Nielsen, S.; Gold, J.W.M.; Metroka, C.E.; Posner, J.B.: Neurological complications of acquired immune deficiency syndrome: analysis of 50 patients. Ann. Neurol. *14:* 403–418 (1983).

So, Y.T.; Beckstead, J.H.; Davis, R.L.: Primary central nervous system lymphoma in acquired immune deficiency syndrome: a clinical and pathologic study. Ann. Neurol. *20:* 566–572 (1986).

Thompson, R.A.: Clinical features of central nervous system fungus infection. Infectious diseases of the central nervous system. Adv. Neurol., vol. 6, pp. 93–100 (Raven Press, New York 1974).

Tucker, T.; Dix, R.D.; Katzen, C.; Davis, R.J.; Schmidley, J.W.: Cytomegalovirus and herpes simplex virus ascending myelitis in a patient with acquired immune deficiency syndrome. Ann. Neurol. *18:* 74–79 (1985).

Urmacher, C.; Nielsen, S.: The histopathology of the acquired immune deficiency syndrome. Pathol. A. *20:* 197–220 (1985).

Wetli, C.V.; Weiss, S.D.; Cleary, T.J.; Gyori, E.: Fungal cerebritis from intravenous drug abuse. J. forens. Sci. *29:* 260–268 (1984).

West, T.E.; Papsian, C.J.; Park, B.H.; Parker, S.W.: Adenovirus type-2 encephalitis and concurrent Epstein-Barr virus infection in an adult man. Archs. Neurol. *42:* 815–817 (1985).

Whitley, R.J.; Soong, S.F.; Dolin, R.; Galasso, G.J.; Ch'ien, L.T.; Alford, C.A.; and the Collaborative Study Group: Adenine arabinoside therapy of biopsy-proved herpes simplex encephalitis. National Institute of Allergy and Infectious Diseases Collaborative Antiviral Study. New Engl. J. Med. *297:* 289–294 (1977).

Wong, B.: Gold, J.W.M.; Brown, A.E.; Lange, M.; Fried, R.; Grieco, M.; Mildvan, D.; Giron, J.; Tapper, M.L.; Lerner, C.W.; Armstrong, D.: Central-nervous-system toxoplasmosis in homosexual men and parental drug abusers. Ann. intern. Med. *100:* 36–42 (1984).

Zakowski, P.; Fligiel, S.; Berlino, G.W.; Johnson, B.L.: Disseminated *Mycobacterium avium* centracellulare in homosexual men dying of acquired immunodeficiency syndrome. J. Am. med. Ass. *248:* 2980–2982 (1982).

Ziegler, J.L.; Drew, W.L.; Miner, R.C.; Rosenbaum, E.; Lennette, E.T.; Shilltoe, E.; Casavant, C.; Mintz, L.; Gershow, J.; Greenspan, J.; Beckstead, J.; Yamamoto, K.: Outbreak of Burkitt's-like lymphoma in homosexual men. Lancet *ii:* 631–633 (1982).

Zu Rhein, G.M.: Association of papova-virions with a human demyelinating disease (progressive multifocal leukoencephalopathy). Prog. med. Virol., vol. 11, pp. 185–247 (Karger, Basel 1969).

Robert M. Levy, MD, PhD, Division of Neurosurgery, Northwestern University Medical Center, Suite 811, Chicago, IL 60611 (USA)

Neuropsychologic Approaches

Mueller (ed.): Neurology and Psychiatry: A Meeting of Minds,
pp. 248–265 (Karger, Basel 1989)

Cognitive Status Testing: History, Present Status and Future Directions

Ralph J. Kiernan
San Francisco Veterans Administration Medical Center, San Francisco, Calif., USA

Psychiatry, neurology and neuropsychology are clinical specialties that share an interest in the cognitive functioning of their patients. These fields, however, have evolved relatively independently (table I). Each has developed a different approach to assessing cognition, and, as a result, they are presently unable to communicate easily with each other regarding this area of shared concern.

Neurology

Neurology traditionally has been oriented toward an anatomically based conception of cerebral functioning. In its most extreme form this approach has resulted in a mosaic mapping of cerebral centers [Kleist, 1934] reminiscent of phrenological diagrams. Even as careful a thinker as Liepmann [1905] proposed a 'center' for intellectual functions. As our understanding of the functional or cognitive side of the brain-behavior correlation becomes increasingly refined, anatomical approaches continue to enhance our understanding of brain-behavior relationships. Geschwind's [1965] synthesis of the localizationist approach to the study of higher cortical dysfunction exemplifies the contributions that can be made from such a perspective. This approach, however, is largely independent of the main thrust of this chapter, and its history will not be reviewed further.

Present-day neurologists continue to utilize an anatomical framework in their conceptual approach to cognitive functions. Localized brain lesions must be identified as quickly and accurately as possible. Such lesions can be life-threatening and their early detection must have the highest priority. As a result, the neurologist's examination of cognitive functions is often little more than a collection of techniques aimed at discovering pathognomonic signs of focal damage. In this way, neurologists screen for specific aphasic, agnostic, apraxic, and amnestic syndromes. A collection of such screening techniques, however, does not constitute a coherent cognitive evaluation. Thus, neurologists employ cognitive screening procedures that meet the pressing need for pathoanatomic diagnosis within their specialty but fail to provide a more general framework for understanding cognition. Present understanding of anatomically based functional systems is very limited and many of the most important cognitive functions (e. g. reasoning) are so complex that an adequate anatomical understanding may never be reached.

Psychiatry

Psychiatry also has a long tradition of interest in cognitive function. Prior to the turn of the century a number of clinical researchers developed cognitive assessment procedures with the hope that they would prove useful in clinical diagnosis. Kraepelin and his associate Oehrn [1896], for instance, reported a variety of 'mental capacity' tests which evaluated sensory functions, fatiguability, calculations, time sense and memory. Reiger [1889] reported the extensive evaluation of a brain-injured patient with an enormous battery of tests. These included measures of simple perceptual skills, musical ability, memory, repetition, word finding, writing, gestural expression, logical analysis, and a number of additional skills. His monograph clearly showed the utility of investigating complex skills in order to understand the deficits associated with brain dysfunction. In his 1894 text, *Psychiatrie,* Ziehen attempted to organize the testing procedures developed by Kraepelin, Reiger and Ebbinghaus into a coherent examination that could be used more routinely with patients.

All of these early attempts at cognitive testing in psychiatry predated the testing revolution that took place within psychology. In the early 1900s the question of how to assess individual differences in human abilities was redefined by Binet and Henri [1895]. Binet believed strongly that the tasks traditionally used in assessment to evaluate the most basic or elemental sensory and motor functions failed to capture the major variations in skills among individuals. Binet insisted that only complex tasks, such as problem solving, could distinguish individual differences

Table I. The history of cognitive status testing

	Psychiatry	Psychology	Neurology
			The localizationists
			(the identification of
			specific behavior)
1875		*Experimental psychology*	Broca
		(the measurement of indi-	Wernicke
	The alienists	vidual differences)	Jackson (?)
	(special studies of	Wundt	
	pathologic states)	Galton	
	Kraepelin and Oehrn	Titchener	
	Rieger	Cattell	
	Rauschberg	Ebbinghaus	
			Specific function tests
			(quantitative procedures)
			Grashey
	The development of	*The Cattell-Binet debate*	Proust
	modern psychiatry	*and the testing movement*	Liepmann
	(the first formal cognitive	Binet	
1900	exams)	Ferrari	
	Ziehen	Stern	
	White and Franz		
	Hoch	*Statistical methods*	*Early test batteries*
	Meyer	(the standardized test)	(qualitative test batteries)
	Kirby	Spearman	Heilbronner
		Pearson	Rossolimo
	Stagnation and neglect of	Thrustone	Poppelreuter
	mental status		Gelb and Goldstein
	Bleuler		
	Henderson and Gillespie		*Aphasia test batteries*
1925	Noyes		Marie
	Strecker and Ebaugh		Head
	Starr		Weisenburg and McBride
		Neuropsychology	
		(the application of stan-	
		dardized tests to brain	
		dysfunction)	
		Halstead	
		Luria (?)	
		Hécaen	
		Teuber	
		Zangwil	

Table I (cont.)

	Psychiatry	Psychology	Neurology
1950	*The development of consultation psychiatry*		*Behavioral neurology* (the study of specific behavioral signs and symptoms) Critchley Geschwind Benson
1975	*A renewal of interest in cognitive status* Jacobs and Strain Folstein and McHugh		

meaningfully. His first test of intelligence [Binet and Simon, 1905] demonstrated that complex tasks could differentiate school children in a way that had direct relevance to their potential for academic success. This result led to a new era within psychology which can be best labeled the 'testing movement'.

Psychologists quickly immersed themselves in test development, measurement, and statistics. They established themselves by employing a unique set of skills that had very wide potential application. This eventually led the whole field of psychology in a direction that was far removed from the modest sensory-motor experimental laboratories of the 19th century. It is from the testing movement that the subspeciality of neuropsychology derives.

The testing movement had hardly begun in 1907 when William Alanson White hired S. I. Franz to head an experimental psychology laboratory at St. Elizabeth's Hospital in Washington, D. C. White had a vision of experimental psychology as a laboratory that could function as an adjunct to clinical specialities within the hospital setting. Franz's first assignment [Franz, 1933] was to construct a standard method of cognitive assessment procedures. These procedures were published as chapter 7 in White's book, *Outline of Psychiatry* [White, 1907].

The examination that resulted from Franz's work was much more than a simple attempt to use procedures devised by others within a broader framework. Franz developed many original procedures and organized them into a complete and modern looking cognitive screening examination. His thorough language examination assessed speech articulation, spontaneous speech production, word finding ability, word and phrase repetition, comprehension, reading and writing. He included an attention task and an assessment of memory. Sections requiring mental calculations, logical reasoning, and ethical judgment completed the evaluation. His examination predates the testing movement in that it includes no scoring or standardization. It is, however, a surprisingly thorough screening examination that has no comparable antecedent.

Psychiatrists, in general, responded to Franz's examination enthusiastically. In fact, he was besieged with requests to elaborate on his chapter, and in 1912 he published his *Handbook of Mental Examination Methods* [Franz, 1912]. The chapters of this book were organized according to each of the important areas of functioning that Franz had incorporated in his examination. This examination was the first abilities-based conceptualization of cognitive status, and it could have served as the basis for a sophisticated development of cognitive evaluation procedures. There was, however, no such continuing development.

The rise of dynamic psychiatry in the first half of this century led to a focus on the individual and on dynamic formulations. Formalized testing was discouraged and there was little inclination to refine assessment techniques. The popular psychiatry textbooks of the 1920s and 1930s [Strecker and Ebaugh, 1925; Henderson and Gillespie, 1927; Noyes, 1935] made no attempt to build on Franz's beginnings. Some authors restated procedures such as Franz's in abbreviated form while others simply described the basic functions which must be tested.

Only recently has a renewal of interest in cognitive testing appeared within psychiatry. Both the Mini-Mental State Examination (MMSE) [Folstein et al., 1975] and the Cognitive Capacity Screening Examination (CCSE) [Jacobs et al., 1977] were developed in response to this renewed interest. They are typical of the new cognitive screening examinations in that they produce a single, total score which reflects the overall status of brain function. They have an advantage over Franz's examination in that they are briefer and provide a rough quantification. They are, however, far more cursory than Franz's examination and cannot characterize many important details of cognitive functioning.

It made sense in the section above to discuss the psychological testing movement within the context of psychiatry's budding interest in clinical assessment. It was only with the rise of neuropsychology that the testing movement began to address the clinical problem of assessing cognitive skills.

Neuropsychology

Neuropsychology grew out of the psychological testing movement and developed following World War II in response to the need to understand the acquired deficits of brain-injured soldiers. Two quite different approaches to assessment evolved during this period. The first emphasized loosely connected assemblages of complex tasks, performance on which was evaluated qualitatively [Goldstein and Sheerer, 1941]. The second utilized groups of tasks with concrete rules for highly quantified scoring and interpretation [Halstead, 1947]. Neither approach provides a sound conceptual basis for understanding brain functions. In the years since then a wide variety of testing procedures have been developed that have not been grouped into organized testing systems. The majority of these are lengthy, cumbersome, and inappropriate as bedside screening instruments. Indeed, neuropsychologists have not been overly concerned with the issue of brief cognitive screening.

A conceptual scheme for cognitive assessment, however, has gradually emerged from within neuropsychology. Lezak [1983] organizes the plethora of neuropsychological tests into major ability areas that represent a common focus in any cognitive evaluation. These include: intellectual ability in general, verbal functions, perceptual functions, constructional functions, memory functions, conceptual functions, executive functions, and attention. Albert [1984] recently described the task of neuropsychology as the evaluation of specific ability areas: attention, language, memory, visuospatial ability, and conceptualization. Cummings et al. [1986] have defined 'dementia syndrome' as decreased functioning in three or more of the basic spheres of mental activity: language, memory, visuospatial skills, personality/behavior, and cognition.

Over the past 8 years my colleagues and I have developed a cognitive screening examination based on an abilities model of brain function. The Neurobehavioral Cognitive Status Examination (NCSE) [Kiernan et al., 1983, submitted; Mueller et al., 1984; Kiernan et al., 1987, and Appendix, this volume, pp. 262–265] independently evaluates functioning in five major ability areas: language, constructions, memory, calculations and reasoning. In addition, it assesses level of consciousness, orientation and attention. The NCSE utilizes a screen and metric approach which minimizes testing in intact areas while providing a more detailed, graded assessment in areas of possible disability. Despite its comprehensiveness, the NCSE is relatively brief. It requires less than 5 min to administer to intact individuals and 10–20 min to administer to moderately or severely impaired patients. The NCSE may be given easily at the bedside or in the office.

The NCSE differs from most previous cognitive screening examinations in that it provides a differentiated assessment of abilites and disabilities. NCSE subtest scores are plotted on a profile which appears on the front of the examination booklet. Since isolated dysfunction is not buried in an overall summed score, this screening examination is sensitive to even quite subtle patterns of brain dysfunction. A recent study [Schwamm et al., 1987] compared the sensitivity of the NCSE to that of two widely utilized cognitive screening examinations, the CCSE and the MMSE, in a group of neurosurgical patients who had well-documented brain lesions. The CCSE and MMSE both had a roughly 50% detection rate, while the NCSE detected dysfunction in 28 (87%) of the 30 patients evaluated.

The NCSE brings cognitive screening examination into the modern age by defining specific abilities and disabilities. The overall pattern of abilities and disabilities provides a sound basis for diagnostic hypotheses. It also provides direct information about the nature of a patient's functional limitations. This information can be used to: (1) counsel patients and family members; (2) assist hospital staff who work with the patient; (3) highlight specific areas that may benefit from cognitive rehabilitation, and (4) formulate appropriate discharge or transfer plans.

The remainder of this chapter will describe the NCSE in some detail. Three general factors – level of consciousness, orientation, and attention – are important to assess in any examination of cognitive functions. Level of consciousness is graded according to standard neurological criteria. Patients who are less than fully alert may have difficulty with many of the NCSE subtests because of fluctuating arousal rather than as a reflection of specific disabilities. A brief measure of orientation is included in deference to traditional cognitive examinations and as an additional test of memory. A 12-point scale of orientation allows the examiner to detect changes in orientation over the course of time. Attention span is assessed with a digit repetition task. Attention is a basic factor that is required in varying degrees by all of the other subtests.

Within the five major ability areas, all but memory are given in a screen and metric format. The patient is first presented with the screen, a single test item which demands a high level of skill within the area involved. Screen items were selected so that approximately 20% of the normal population would fail them. If the patient succeeds on the screen item, skill within the particular ability area is assumed normal and no further testing is done in that area. If the patient fails the screen, however, this raises the question of possible dysfunction within that area and the metric is then administered. The metric consists of a series of test items that are graded in difficulty from relatively simple to quite difficult. Performance on the metric yields a score which reflects the level of functioning within the particular ability area.

The five major ability areas of the NCSE were chosen on the basis of a careful review of the literature in psychiatry, neurology and neuropsychology. Indeed, professionals from each of these specialities were intimately involved in the early stages of test development. It was decided, for example, that the prevailing model of aphasia in the behavioral neurology literature [Benson, 1979] was the optimal one to follow in brief language assessment. Accordingly, the language examination was divided into four sections: spontaneous speech, comprehension, repetition, and naming. These allow for differential diagnosis within the major divisions of the aphasias.

In the spontaneous speech section the patient is asked to describe a complex picture of a fishing scene. The response is recorded verbatim and any speech errors such as paraphasias or circumlocutions are noted. No score is computed for this section. The comprehension screen item is a three-step command. The comprehension metric consists of a series of one-, two-, and three-step commands. The screen for repetition is a complex sentence that is quite difficult to repeat. The repetition metric consists of a series of sentences and phrases which are read aloud to the patient and must be repeated exactly. The screen for naming requires the patient to name a pen and three of its parts: cap, clip, and point. The metric consists of eight pictured objects to be named. It was decided that spelling and reading could not be adequately assessed in a brief screening examination, and we elected to omit tests for these language skills.

Although construction tasks are often minimized or omitted altogether in cognitive status testing, the neuropsychology literature clearly documents their sensitivity to brain dysfunction [Benson, 1979]. Often such constructional tasks are the only sign of right hemisphere dysfunction, and their omission from brief cognitive assessment increases the likelihood of missing such disorders. Indeed, a recent review of cognitive screening examinations concluded that they were insensitive to focal brain disorders in general and focal right hemisphere dysfunction in particular [Nelson et al., 1986]. The screen item employed by the NCSE for the construction section consists of two line drawings that must be reproduced from memory following a 10-second study period. Both designs must be reproduced with all of the major features drawn correctly in order to pass the screen. The metric for this section consists of a series of mosaic design constructions. This task is similar to the block design subtest of the revised Wechsler Adult Intelligence Scale [Wechsler, 1981] but uses tiles instead of cubes. The block design test is known to be one of the tests most sensitive to brain dysfunction [Spreen and Benton, 1965].

Calculations have been included in almost every cognitive screening examination since Franz, and dyscalculia can be of important localizing significance [Hécaen, 1962]. The NCSE uses the single question, 'How much is 5 times 13?' as the screen item for the calculation section. The metric consists of four verbally presented arithmetic problems that include addition, subtraction and division, and are of graded difficulty.

Memory has always proven difficult to evaluate, even in extensive neuropsychological evaluations. Cognitive screening examinations are often particularly weak in assessing this important area. Examinations such as the MMSE and the CCSE fail to discriminate between inadequate registration due to poor concentration or attention and truly defective recall. The NCSE utilizes a standard four-word memory task, but it incorporates administration procedures designed to accentuate the distinction between registration and recall.

Patients are first given four words to learn and then are asked immediately to repeat them. The vast majority of patients are able to do this, but simple repetition ability does not itself guarantee that proper registration has taken place. In order to ensure adequate registration we require that the patient be able to repeat the four words again after a brief interference interval. The examiner creates this interference by briefly describing the memory task and stressing the importance of remembering the list of four words. If the patient fails to produce all four words on the second trial, the complete registration procedure is repeated. This process continues until the patient either shows adequate registration of the four words or clearly demonstrates that he/she will be unable to do this. In most cases the patient is able to register the four words, and the examiner can meaningfully interpret the results of the recall procedure in terms of memory. If the patient is unable to register the four words, the examiner gains important information about attention and concentration.

Recall of the four words follows the construction subtest. The memory score is based on the amount of cueing necessary. The patient is first simply requested to recall as many of the four words as possible. If the patient cannot recall one or more of the words, a category cue is presented (e. g. if the patient fails to recall the word 'piano', he or she is told that one of the words was a musical instrument). If the category cue does not enable the patient to recall the correct word, he/she is next asked to select the correct word from a three-word multiple choice list which contains the correct choice. Three points are awarded for each word recalled correctly without need of a cue or list; two points are given for each word recalled in response to a category cue; and one point is scored for each word correctly selected from a list. This scoring system creates a twelve-point scale which allows the examiner to quantify the degree of memory dysfunction.

A variety of reasoning tasks that differ widely in terms of their neuropsychological demands are available. We chose two types of verbal reasoning tasks since they are easy to administer at the bedside. The first is a similarities task in which the patient is asked to state how two objects, such as a rose and a tulip, are alike. The screen item for this subtest is rather abstract: it asks how painting and music are alike. The metric for this section is a series of word pairs of increasing complexity. This type of task has been shown to be sensitive to brain dysfunction in general [Spreen and Benton, 1965] and to left temporal lobe dysfunction in particular [McFie, 1975].

The second reasoning task consists of situational or 'practical' judgment questions presented in the form. 'What would you do if...?'. The screen item for this section is, 'What would you do if you were stranded in the Denver Airport with only $1 in your pocket?'. This is followed by the metric which consists of three additional problem situations. Such questions are frequently useful in detecting abnormal thought processes that may occur in psychiatric patients. On the other hand, these questions are relatively insensitive to both focal and generalized brain dysfunction. When we compared a normal geriatric group to a neurosurgical patient group with proven brain pathology, this subtest alone failed to significantly differentiate the two groups [Kiernan et al., 1987; Schwamm et al., 1987].

The figures that follow illustrate how NCSE profiles that display the pattern of a patient's abilities and disabilities may aid in the diagnostic process.

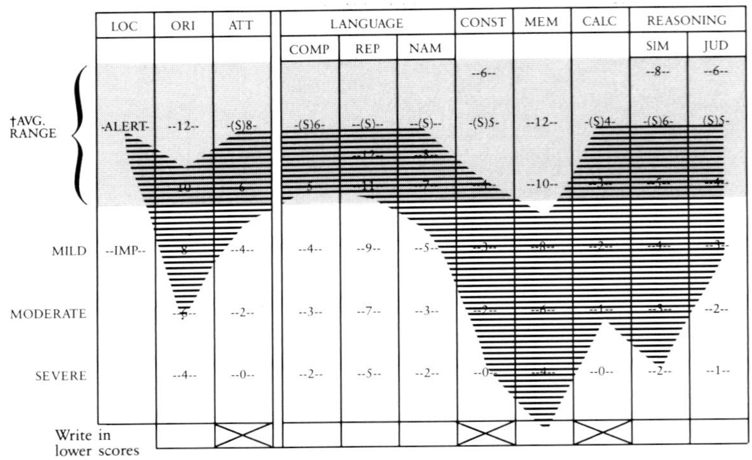

Fig. 1. Range of typical cognitive status profiles in mild to moderate dementia of the Alzheimer type. S = Screen; LOC = level of consciousness; ORI = orientation; ATT = attention; COMP = comprehension; REP = repetition; NAM = naming; MEM = memory; CONST = constructions; CALC = calculations; SIM = similarities; JUD = judgment; IMP = impaired.

Figure 1 illustrates the range of NCSE scores typical of mild to moderate dementia of the Alzheimer type. Such individuals are usually alert and attentive and demonstrate relatively preserved language functions. They frequently show evidence of mild disorientation and have difficulty with constructional and memory tasks. Their performance on calculation and verbal reasoning tasks is highly variable and often remains largely unimpaired in early stages of the disease.

Figure 2 illustrates the highly articulated and dramatically different profiles that can be obtained in individual cases. Figure 2a is a Korsakoff's amnestic syndrome in a 75-year-old chronic alcoholic man. This patient was alert, attentive, and had essentially normal language, constructions, calculations and reasoning. His disorientation was secondary to his dramatic memory dysfunction. Figure 2b shows the profile of a 65-year-old woman who had sustained a major infarction in the territory of the left middle cerebral artery 8 years prior to the date of testing. The NCSE profile demonstrates her alertness and fairly well-preserved intellectual abilities, as contrasted to her continuing language impairment.

a

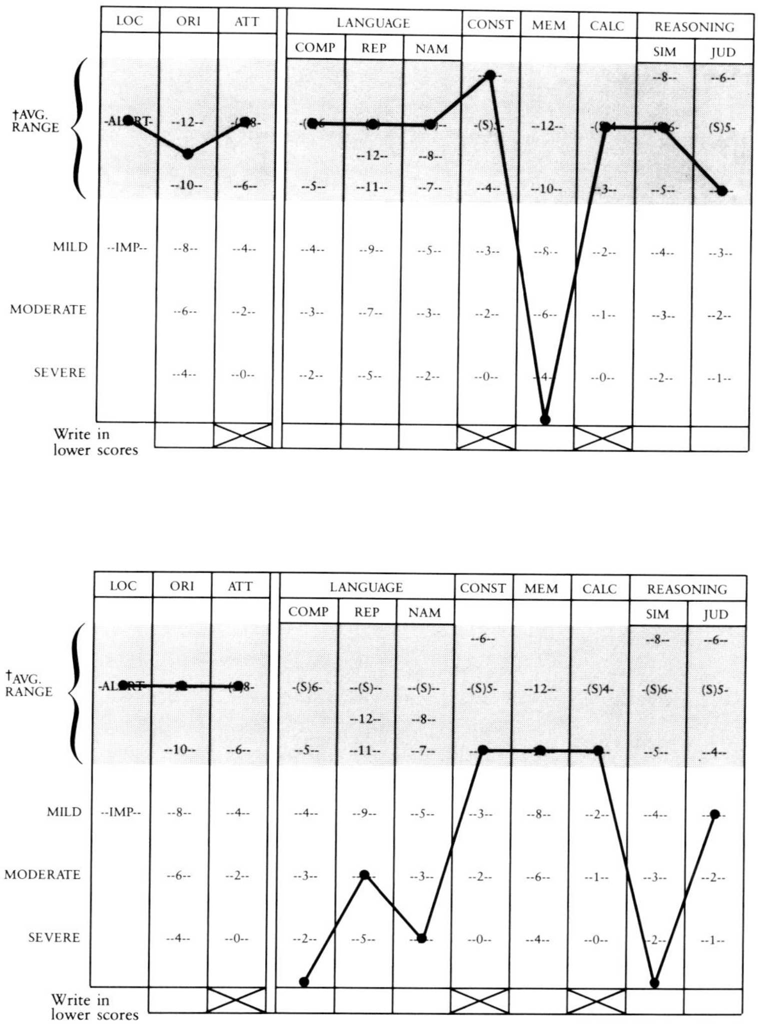

Fig. 2. a 75-year-old man with longstanding memory disturbance associated with chronic alcohol abuse. *b* 65-year-old woman with residual aphasia 8 years after left middle cerebral artery infarction.

These cases illustrate the utility of the NCSE in clinical assessment. They also show the power of a differentiated approach to cognitive assessment that accentuates rather than obscures areas of specific disability.

References

Albert, M.: Cognitive function assessment in the elderly. Psychosom. *25:* 310–317 (1984).

Benson, D.F.: Aphasia, alexia, and agraphia (Churchill-Livingstone, New York 1979).

Binet, A.; Henri, V.: La psychologie individuelle. Ann. Psychol. *2:* 411–463 (1895).

Binet, A.; Simon, T.: Méthodes nouvelles pour le diagnostic du niveau intellectuel des anormaux. Ann. Psychol. *11:* 191–244 (1905).

Cummings, J.L.; Benson, D.F.: Dementia of the Alzheimer type. J. Am. Geriat. Soc. *34:* 12–19 (1986).

Ebbinghaus, H.: Über eine neue Methode zur Prüfung geistiger Fähigkeiten und ihre Anwendung bei Schulkindern. Z. Psychol. *13:* 401–459 (1897).

Folstein, M.F.; Folstein, S.E.; McHugh, P.R.: Mini-mental state. J. psychiat. Res. *12:* 189–198 (1975).

Franz, S.I.: Handbook of mental examination methods. Nervous and Mental Disease Publishing, Washington (1912).

Franz, S.I.: in Murchison, The history of psychology in autobiography, pp. 89–113 (Russell & Russell, New York 1961).

Geschwind, N.: Disconnexion syndromes in animals and man. Brain *88:* 237–294 (1965).

Goldstein, K.; Scheerer, M.: Abstract and concrete behavior: an experimental study with special tests. Psychol. Monogr. *53:* (2, whole No. 239) (1941).

Halstead, W.C.: Brain and intelligence (University of Chicago Press, Chicago 1947).

Hécaen, H.: Clinical symptomatology in right and left hemisphere lesions; in Mountcastle, Interhemispheric relations and cerebral dominance in man (Johns Hopkins University, Baltimore 1962).

Henderson, D.K.; Gillespie, R.D.: A test-book of psychiatry (Oxford University Press, London 1927).

Jacobs, J.W.; Bernhard, M.R.; Delgado, A.; Strain, J.J.: Screening for organic mental syndromes in the medically ill. Ann. intern. Med. *86:* 40–47 (1977).

Kiernan, R.J.; Langston, J.W.; Mueller, J.: A brief, yet specific and quantitative mental status examination. Proc. 91st Annu. Meet. Am. Psychological Association, 1983.

Kiernan, R.J.; Mueller, J.; Langston, J.W.; Van Dyke, C.: The neurobehavioral cognitive status examination. I. A brief but quantitative approach to cognitive status Testing. Ann. Neurol. *105:* 481–486 (1987).

Kleist, K.: Gehirnpathologie (Barth, Leipzig 1934).

Lezak, M.D.: Neuropsychological assessment; 2nd ed. (Oxford University Press, New York 1983).

Liepmann, H.: Über Störungen des Handelns bei Gehirnkranken (Berlin 1905).

McFie, J.: Assessment of organic intellectual impairment (Academic Press, London 1975).

Mueller, J.; Kiernan, R.J.; Langston, J.W.: Mental status examination; in Goldman, Review of general psychiatry, pp. 206–220 (Lange, Los Altos 1984).

Nelson, A.; Fogel, B.S.; Faust, D.: Bedside cognitive screening instrumentation. J. nerv. ment. Dis. *174:* 73–83 (1986).
Noyes, A.P.: Modern clinical psychiatry (Saunders, Philadelphia 1935).
Oehrn, A.: Experimentelle Studien zur Individualpsychologie. Psychol. Arbeiten *1:* 92–151 (1896).
Reiger, K.: Beschreibung der Intelligenzstörungen in Folge einer Hirnverletzung. Verh. Phys. Med. Ges. Würzburg *22:* 65–134; *23:* 95–150 (1889).
Schwamm, L.H.; Van Dyke, C.; Kiernan, R.J.; Merrin, E.L.; Mueller, J.: The neurobehavioral cognitive status examination. II. Comparison with the CCSE and MMSE in a neurosurgical population. Ann. Neurol. *105:* 486–491 (1987).
Spreen, O.; Benton, A.L.: Comparative studies of some psychological tests for cerebral damage. J. nerv. ment. Dis. *110:* 323–333 (1865).
Strecker, E.A.; Ebaugh, F.G.: Practical clinical psychiatry for students and practitioners (Blakiston, Philadelphia 1925).
Wechsler, D.: WAIS-R manual (Psychological Corporation, New York 1981).
White, W.A.: Outlines of psychiatry (Nervous and Mental Disease Publishing, Washington 1907).
Ziehen, T.: Psychiatrie (Berlin 1894).

Ralph J. Kiernan, PhD, San Francisco Veterans Administration Medical Center, 4150 Clement Street, San Francisco, CA 94121 (USA)

Appendix

TEST BOOKLET
for
THE NEUROBEHAVIORAL COGNITIVE STATUS EXAMINATION (NCSE)

______________________ Addressograph

NAME: ______________________
AGE AND DATE OF BIRTH: ______________________
NATIVE LANGUAGE: ______________________
HANDEDNESS (circle): L R
LEVEL OF EDUCATION: ______________________

OCCUPATIONAL STATUS: ______________________
DATE: ______________________
TIME: ______________________
EXAMINER: ______________________
EXAMINATION LOCATION: ______________________

COGNITIVE STATUS PROFILE*

	LOC	ORI	ATT	LANGUAGE			CONST	MEM	CALC	REASONING	
				COMP	REP	NAM				SIM	JUD
† AVG. RANGE							--6--			--8--	--6--
	-ALERT-	--12--	-(S)8-	-(S)6-	--(S)--	--(S)--	-(S)5-	--12--	-(S)4-	-(S)6-	(S)5-
					--12--	--8--					
		--10--	--6--	--5--	--11--	--7--	--4--	--10--	--3--	--5--	--4--
MILD	--IMP--	--8--	--4--	--4--	--9--	--5--	--3--	--8--	--2--	--4--	--3--
MODERATE		--6--	--2--	--3--	--7--	--3--	--2--	--6--	--1--	--3--	--2--
SEVERE		--4--	--0--	--2--	--5--	--2--	--0--	--4--	--0--	--2--	--1--
Write in lower scores			X				X		X		

ABBREVIATIONS

ATT	Attention	JUD	Judgment	ORI	Orientation
CALC	Calculations	LOC	Level of Consciousness	REP	Repetition
COMP	Comprehension	MEM	Memory	S	Screen
CONST	Constructions	NAM	Naming	SIM	Similarities
IMP	Impaired				

*The validity of this examination depends on administration in strict accordance with the NCSE Manual.

†For patients over age 65 the average range extends to the "mild impairment level" for Constructions, Memory and Similarities.

Note: Not all brain lesions produce cognitive deficits that will be detected by the NCSE. Normal scores, therefore, cannot be taken as evidence that brain pathology does *not* exist. Similarly, scores falling in the mild, moderate, or severe range of impairment do not *necessarily* reflect brain dysfunction (see the section of the NCSE Manual entitled "Cautions in Interpretation").

The Northern California Neurobehavioral Group, Inc.
P.O. Box 460
Fairfax, CA 94930
Telephone: (415) 457-6400

THE NEUROBEHAVIORAL COGNITIVE STATUS EXAMINATION (NCSE)
Record patient's responses verbatim.

I. LEVEL OF CONSCIOUSNESS: Alert_______ Lethargic_______ Fluctuating_______
Describe patient's condition: ____

II. ORIENTATION (Score 2, 1, or 0.)

		Response	*Score*
A. Person	1. Name (0 pts.)	____________	___
	2. Age (2 pts.)	____________	___
B. Place	1. Current location (2 pts.)	____________	___
	2. City (2 pts.)	____________	___
C. Time	1. Date: mo. (1 pt.)____ day (1 pt.)____ yr. (2 pts.)____		___
	2. Day of week (1 pt.)	____________	___
	3. Time of day within one hour (1 pt.)	____________	___

Total Score _____

III. ATTENTION

A. Digit Repetition

1. Screen: 8-3-5-2-9-1 Pass____ Fail____
2. Metric: Graded digit repetition (Score 1 or 0; discontinue after 2 misses at one level.)

Score	*Score*	*Score*	*Score*
3-7-2____	5-1-4-9____	8-3-5-2-9____	2-8-5-1-6-4____
4-9-5____	9-2-7-4____	6-1-7-3-8____	9-1-7-5-8-2____

Total Score _____

B. Four Word Memory Task
Give the four unrelated words from Section VI: robin, carrot, piano, green.
(Alternate list: table, lion, orange, glove.) Have patient repeat the four words twice correctly (see Manual) and record the number of trials required to do this:_______

IV. LANGUAGE

A. Speech Sample

1. Fishing Picture (Record patient's response verbatim.)

____
____
____
____

B. Comprehension (Be sure to have at least 3 other objects in front of the patient for this test.) If a, b, and c are successfully completed, praxis for these tasks is assumed normal.

1. Screen: 3-step command: "Turn over the paper, hand me the pen, and point to your nose." Pass____ Fail ____
2. Metric: (Score 1 or 0.) If incorrect, describe behavior.

	Response	*Score*
a. Pick up the pen.	____________	___
b. Point to the floor.	____________	___
c. Hand me the keys.	____________	___
d. Point to the pen and pick up the keys.	____________	___
e. Hand me the paper and point to the coin.	____________	___
f. Point to the keys, hand me the pen, and pick up the coin.	____________	___

Total Score ____

C. Repetition

1. Screen: The beginning movement revealed the composer's intention.
____
Pass____ Fail____
2. Metric: (Score 2 if first try correct; 1 if second try correct; 0 if incorrect.)

	Response	*Score*
a. Out the window.	____________	___
b. He swam across the lake.	____________	___
c. The winding road led to the village.	____________	___
d. He left the latch open.	____________	___
e. The honeycomb drew a swarm of bees.	____________	___
f. No ifs, ands, or buts.	____________	___

Total Score ____

D. Naming

1. Screen: a) Pen____ b) Cap or Top____ c) Clip____ d) Point, Tip, or Nib____

Pass____ Fail____

2. Metric: (Score 1 or 0.)

	Response	*Score*		*Response*	*Score*
a. Shoe	________	____	e. Horseshoe	________	____
b. Bus	________	____	f. Anchor	________	____
c. Ladder	________	____	g. Octopus	________	____
d. Kite	________	____	h. Xylophone	________	____

Total Score ____

V. CONSTRUCTIONAL ABILITY

A. Screen: Visual Memory Task (Present stimulus sheet for 10 seconds, then have patient draw the two figures from memory. Must be perfect to pass. The examiner may wish to have patients who fail the screen copy the two figures.)

Pass____ Fail ____

B. Metric: Design Constructions (Score 2 if correct in 0-30 seconds; 1 if correct in 31-60 seconds; 0 if correct in greater than 60 seconds or incorrect.)

Place squares in front of patient as shown here:

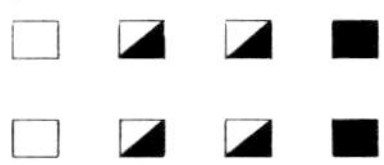

		Record incorrect attempts below	*Time*	*Score*
1. Design 1:		⊞ ⊞	____	____
2. Design 2:		⊞ ⊞	____	____
3. Design 3:		⊞ ⊞	____	____

Total Score ____

VI. MEMORY (Score 3 if recalled without prompting; 2 if recalled with category prompt; 1 if recognized from list; 0 if not recognized.) Check if correct.

Words	*Check*	*Category Prompt*	*Check of Response*	*List (circle)*	*Score*
Robin	____	Bird	____________	Sparrow, robin, bluejay	____
Carrot	____	Vegetable	____________	Carrot, potato, onion	____
Piano	____	Musical instrument	____________	Violin, guitar, piano	____
Green	____	Color	____________	Red, green, yellow	____

Incorrect initial response: ________________________ Total Score ____

VII. CALCULATIONS

A. Screen: 5 × 13 Response:____ Time:____ (Must be correct within 20 seconds.)

Pass____ Fail ____

B. Metric: (Score 1 point if correct within 20 seconds.) Problems may be repeated, but time runs continuously from first presentation.

	Response	*Time*	*Score*
1. How much is 5 + 3?	________	____	____
2. How much is 15 + 7?	________	____	____
3. How much is 39 ÷ 3?	________	____	____
4. How much is 31 − 8?	________	____	____

Total Score ____

VIII. REASONING

A. Similarities (Explain: "A hat and a coat are alike because they are both articles of clothing." If patient does not respond, encourage; if patient gives differences, score 0.)

1. Screen: Painting-Music (Must be abstract—only "art," "artistic," or "forms of art" are acceptable.)

________________________ Pass____ Fail ____

2. Metric: (Score 2 if abstract; 1 if imprecisely abstract or concrete; 0 if incorrect.) See manual for examples. Check if abstract.

	Check	*Abstract Concept*	*Other Responses*	*Score*
a. Rose-Tulip	____	Flowers	____________	____
b. Bicycle-Train	____	Transportation	____________	____
c. Watch-Ruler	____	Measurement	____________	____
d. Corkscrew-Hammer	____	Tools	____________	____

Total Score ____

B. Judgment

1. Screen: What would you do if you were stranded in the Denver Airport with only $1.00 in your pocket?

____

____

Pass____ Fail____

2. Metric: (Score 2 if correct; 1 if partially correct; 0 if incorrect.)

a. What would you do if you woke up one minute before 8:00 a.m. and remembered an important appointment downtown at 8:00?

____

____

Score____

b. What would you do if you were walking beside a lake and you saw a two-year-old child playing alone at the end of a pier?

____

____

Score____

c. What would you do if you came home and found that a broken pipe was flooding the kitchen?

____

____

Score____

Total Score ____

IX. MEDICATIONS

List *all* current medications and dosages:

1. __________ 2. __________ 3. __________ 4. __________

5. __________ 6. __________ 7. __________ 8. __________

X. GENERAL COMMENTS

Note any known or observed motor, sensory or perceptual deficits that may affect test performance (e.g., impaired visual or auditory acuity, tremor, apraxia, dysarthria):

____

____

____

Note "process features" such as distractability, frustration, exhaustion, and nature of cooperation. The patient's impression of his or her performance should also be noted here.

____

____

____

Space for Visual Memory Task

Mueller (ed.): Neurology and Psychiatry: A Meeting of Minds,
pp. 266–283 (Karger, Basel 1989)

Theories of Frontal Lobe Function

D. Frank Benson[a], *Donald T. Stuss*[b]

[a] Department of Neurology, UCLA School of Medicine, Los Angeles, Calif., USA;
[b] The Schools of Medicine (Neurology Division) and Psychology, University of Ottawa, and Ottawa General Hospital, Ottawa, Ont., Canada

Problem

In the human the frontal lobe represents a significant portion of the brain (estimates vary from 25 to 33% of total cerebral tissue). Despite the great size, the function of the frontal lobe has remained somewhat of a mystery. Because the frontal lobes represent so much of the total brain tissue and are proportionately so much greater in extent (particularly that portion known as the prefrontal cortex) than in any other animal species, it has been widely assumed that the highest human functions were the properties of the frontal lobes. Innumerable investigations, however, have failed to substantiate this reasonable assumption and the frontal lobes have been described as mysterious, illusive and enigmatic. In some well-studied cases, the psychometric measures of intelligence were as good or even better after significant frontal lobe damage than before. What, then, are the functions of this massive amount of brain tissue? This is the problem that will be addressed in this chapter.

Background

All investigators of frontal lobe functions agree that the area has proved difficult to study. Reasons behind this difficulty deserve note. For one, animal ablation studies, so successful in the investigation of functions of other portions of the brain, have only limited applicability to frontal disturbances. Two reasons are obvious; first, the frontal lobe is so vastly greater in size and complexity in the human that animal studies cannot be expected to be fully applicable. Second, the limited avenue of expression of animals, particularly their lack of language, hampers the use of animal experimentation for human frontal behavioral studies.

Additional problems are also present. For instance, few vascular infarcts involve the frontal lobes alone. Occlusion of the anterior cerebral artery (ACA) may fit this picture but since this disturbance is both unusual and variable in result, even patients with ACA territory infarction have provided only limited information concerning frontal lobe functions. The far more common infarctions of the middle cerebral artery (MCA) almost invariably involve brain tissue that is both deeper and more posterior than frontal lobe alone; MCA infarctions rarely make good study material for frontal abnormality. A third problem deserves attention. Most of the psychological test materials currently used to evaluate brain damage fail to probe selectively for frontal malfunction. In the face of these difficulties, clinical evaluation of frontally damaged patients has been the major investigational tool. Three major types of frontal pathology – trauma, tumor, and psychosurgery – have been studied extensively. Each has advantages and disadvantages.

Trauma, particularly the trauma from penetrating head injury from the major wars, has provided a great deal of the currently available information concerning frontal lobe function. The classic case of Phineas Gage [Harlow, 1868] provided elegant evidence of serious frontal lobe dysfunction in an individual whose pathology was primarily, if not entirely, localized to the frontal lobes. Many additional cases of trauma to the frontal lobes have been recorded and over the years a sizeable body of knowledge concerning the behavioral disturbances with frontal trauma has arisen [Feuchtwanger, 1923; Kleist, 1934; Marie and Foix, 1917; Salazar et al., 1985]. This body of work has proved somewhat difficult to interpret. No two lesions are exactly alike and almost all major trauma to the brain, no matter where the skull is struck, produces distant effects of pertinence. Most often useful premorbid information is unavailable for comparison with the post-injury behavior. Despite these limitations, frontal trauma does produce sufficiently consistent behavioral residua that a number of attributes of frontal function have been outlined and are rather reliably reproduced in additional trauma cases [Lishman, 1966; Russell, 1951].

The second major source for frontal behavioral observations comes from brain tumor cases. The frontal lobes remain relatively silent to intracranial neoplasm and the defect may grow to rather tremendous size before diagnostic clinical manifestations are noted. Many cases of frontal tumor have been reported and two investigators, Luria [1965] and Hécaen [1964] have reported extensively on the behavioral disturbances seen in patients with massive frontal brain tumors. Unfortunately, like the trauma cases, the large frontal brain tumors produce distant effects through pressure, infiltration or infarction, making the correlation of the behavioral change with an individual frontal tumor somewhat questionable. Once again, however, sufficient consistency in the reports of carefully investigated patients with frontal tumors provides an overview of frontal symptomatology.

Finally, frontal lobotomy (leukotomy) procedures performed as a means of treating psychiatric abnormality in the mid-20th century produced a sizeable number of individuals with relatively clean, well-localized frontal lobe lesions. These cases were never extensively studied, however, for psychological deficits. Inasmuch as all had psychiatric abnormality, the focus of follow-up studies concerned psychiatric disability; only a few reported results beyond one year following surgery. Few studies of psychological residua have been made. The most extensive, the Columbia-Greystone Associates study [Mettler, 1949], used standard psychological tests and other pertinent procedures and demonstrated deficient function in only a limited number of tests and these were apparently location-specific. Few studies of patients over a longer term have been performed and these have proved difficult to interpret because of the underlying psychiatric disturbance, the lack of premorbid performance data and the lack of control standards. All told, despite the fact that over 100,000 individuals were subjected to frontal destructive surgery during the 1940s and 1950s, limited useful evidence of frontal dysfunction has come from this literature.

Based on this background, most concepts of the functions of the frontal lobes have been limited by methodological problems. Nonetheless, theories concerning frontal lobe function have advanced considerably in the past several decades and deserve review. Before doing this, however, we will present a short description of one recent long-term follow-up study, utilizing extensive neuropsychological investigation, of patients who had undergone prefrontal leukotomy in the 1940s.

Northampton VAMC Experience

In 1976 and 1977 a group of individuals who had undergone prefrontal leukotomy as a treatment for intractable schizophrenia in the 1940s and early 1950s was studied. Of 180 patients who had undergone prefrontal leukotomy as a treatment for psychiatric disease at the Northampton (Mass.) Veterans Administration Medical Center, 56 were still registered with the hospital. From this group, 16 patients were selected for intensive study. They were divided into three groups: Group I – those who had made a good recovery, had been free of psychiatric hospitalization a minimum of 15 years, had been employed and were basically self-caring. Group II – those with a relatively good recovery, were out of hospital most of the time but had an occasional psychotic episode demanding reevaluation in the hospital. Hospitalizations had occurred at least once in the 6 years prior to study. These individuals were not employed and could not be considered self-caring but were able to exist successfully outside the hospital. Group III – these individuals had undergone leukotomy but had never been judged sufficiently improved to be allowed out of hospital. In addition to the three schizophrenic patient groups, two control groups were tested. The first consisted of individuals who also carried the diagnosis of schizophrenia and had been in the same hospital for approximately 25–30 years. They were essentially identical to group III except that they had not undergone prefrontal leukotomy. The final group were age- and education-matched control subjects. They had no psychiatric history, had worked all of their adult life and been both self-supporting and self-caring.

An extensive battery of tests was administered including neurologic and psychiatric evaluations, two electroencephalograms, a CT scan and neuropsychological testing (39 tests taking from 8 to 12 h for administration). Psychological tests were presented in segments over 5 days to avoid excessive fatigue or belligerence on the part of the psychotic patients.

Results of these tests have been extensively reviewed [Benson et al., 1981; Naeser et al., 1981; Stuss and Benson, 1984; Stuss et al., 1981] but can be summarized briefly. The neurological examinations showed no abnormality. Of a large series of 'frontal release signs' described in the literature, only one patient showed a positive sign, a snout reflex. Psychiatric examination revealed that most of the patients still showed psychiatric symptomatology, including delusions, hallucinations, paranoia and loose associations. In fact, all of the leukotomized subjects showed some difficulties, the only difference being that group III, the poorest result group, showed far more severe problems than did group I, the best recovery group. The electroencephalographic results did not correlate with recovery: patients in each of the leukotomized subgroups had abnormal EEGs while others within each subgroup had normal EEGs. There was a trend for more group III patients to show EEG abnormality but the difference was minimal. The CT scan, however, did demonstrate striking differences. Although all lesions were located in exactly the same spot (the anterior, inferior, medial frontal lobe), the sizes of the lesions varied considerably, and size of lesion appeared to be a pertinent factor in recovery [Benson et al., 1981]. The patients in group I – the best recovery group – had the largest lesions while those in group III had the smallest lesions. In fact, there was an almost linear correlation between the size of the lesion and the degree of recovery. In reviewing the neuropsychological data, it must be recognized that the patients with the largest bifrontal lesions were those in the best recovery group.

The neuropsychological tests were most striking for their normality. Many of the tests showed no statistically significant difference between the performance of the leukotomized patients and the normal control group. Even more striking, group I, those with the largest bifrontal lesions performed very nearly at the level of the normal controls in almost all tests. In some instances they performed better than the normals. The poorest neuropsychological test results came from group III, those with the smallest frontal lesions. In most instances, the poor scores in the neuropsychological tests could be correlated with the degree of mental illness, not the degree of frontal abnormality. In fact, it was difficult to demonstrate specific frontal malfunction based on the leukotomy procedures. Several examples demonstrate these negative results.

It was anticipated that disordered attention would be a major problem in these subjects inasmuch as attention disturbance has been reported in both frontal damage [Goldstein, 1936; Hécaen and Albert, 1978] and schizophrenia [McGhie and Chapman, 1961; Venables, 1963]. A sizeable series of attention tasks were presented, ranging from simple digit span to complex and difficult attention problems [Stuss et al., 1981]. Except for the nonleukotomized schizophrenic group (and a few examples in group III patients), all attention tests in leukotomized patients gave results that were not statistically different from those of the normal control group. Clinical observations, however, showed that these patients were distractible, were stimulus-bound and had obvious problems in maintaining attention in ordinary ward activities. It was concluded that the neuropsychological tests for attention failed to demonstrate abnormality in these patients, not because there was no abnormality but because the artificial means in which the test was presented interfered with the results. In simple terms, the examiner acted as the frontal lobes for the patient during the test procedure.

A series of cognitive tests was presented and careful review provides some insights into disturbances caused by the frontal abnormality. Only two of the series of cognitive tests will be reviewed [see Stuss et al., 1982, 1983, for additional details]. In the first, the Wechsler Adult Intelligence Scale (WAIS) [Wechsler, 1955], the results were inconclusive. Group I – the well-recovered leukotomy patients – and the normal control group had scores that were not statistically different. The other leukotomy groups scored somewhat more poorly, and the nonleukotomized schizophrenics were the poorest of all. The only thing clearly demonstrated by the WAIS was a schizophrenia effect. In a more complicated test, the Wisconsin Card Sorting Test [Grant and Berg, 1948; Milner, 1963], different results were obtained. For the administration the test was divided into two halves with the first 64 cards being presented without any instructions. The test was then stopped, the patient asked what strategy was being used and then told that there were three categories – color, number and form – and the second 64 cards were presented. In the first half of the test no statistically significant difference was demonstrated between the performance of the normal controls and the leukotomized subjects (in contrast, none of the nonleukotomized schizophrenics completed the test). The normal subjects performed slightly better than group I who were slightly better than group II, etc., but the differences were slight and there was an overlap with the best performer of one group doing better than the poorest of the other groups, including the normal controls. In the second half, after the categories has been outlined, a striking difference became apparent. The normal control group immediately scored far better but all three of the leukotomized groups performed considerably poorer than they had in the first half. This was most striking for group I subjects who performed the poorest of all of the groups. The total number of correct responses was the same in the first and the second half for all of the leukotomized patients but the number of times 3–5 correct responses were given, followed by an incorrect response, was far greater in the second half for the leukotomized groups. It appeared that the additional information had interfered with the leukotomized patients' ability to carry on the tasks, an apparent frontal lobe disturbance. The poorest results in the second half of the Wisconsin Card Sorting Test were those of group I, the patients with the largest frontal defect.

In summary, an extensive evaluation of the neuropsychological residuals of prefrontal leukotomy confirmed earlier observations that most standard psychological tests did not reflect frontal abnormality. Nonetheless, these patients were distinctly abnormal and on some tests (e.g. the Wisconsin Card Sorting Test) a frontal effect could be demonstrated.

Theories of Frontal Lobe Function

Despite many declarations that frontal lobe functions represent the highest aspect of human brain function [Goldstein, 1944; Tilney, 1928; Worster-Drought, 1931], demonstration of these functions has proved remarkably illusive. Neuroscientists have not refrained from postulating (or fantasizing) on frontal lobe functions, however. Over the years both clinical observations and scientific research have been able to support or confirm some aspects of these postulates, producing a limited body of respectable theories concerning what the frontal lobes actually do. Relative to other portions of the brain, demonstrations of the frontal functions remain sketchy and hypotheses prevail. This presentation will now review selected theories.

Basic Theories of Brain Function

While many theories have been developed over the years, most fit into one of two groups, related to the era in which they were produced. The first group emanated from the great clinical/anatomical correlation studies of the 19th century and continued into the first part of the 20th century. The second is more recent, encompassing the past 20 or 25 years, the golden age of neuroscience. Despite this schism, development has been a slow and steady, not a sudden 'aha' occurrence. The separation of the two periods represents a hiatus during which more holistic (psychodynamic) explanations were preferred to explain mental operations [Chapman and Wolff, 1959; Lashley, 1929; Monakow, 1905].

The earliest suggestion of a specific frontal function came from the demonstration of the difference in anterior and posterior cerebral hemisphere functions. Meynert [1884] stressed the sensory/receptive/perceptual functions of the posterior portions of the cerebral hemisphere and the motor/executive function of the anterior or frontal brain. The frontal aspects were confirmed and studied by many anatomists and physiologists who concluded that external stimuli were received and processed in the posterior brain and then transmitted to the frontal lobes where a final common pathway for a motor response was established [Bianchi, 1895; Flechsig, 1896; Franz, 1907; Wernicke, 1874]. It was posited that the frontal lobes did more than merely respond to the information gathered and processed in the posterior lobes but the additional functions of the frontal lobe remained unknown. While considerable work on frontal function was subsequently performed [Denny-Brown, 1951; Fulton, 1951], most probed the complex motor responses of the precentral and premotor areas, not the functions of the much larger prefrontal cortex. The importance of the prefrontal lobes was accepted but little evidence of their function was demonstrated in this early era of frontal lobe investigation. Indeed, it was questioned whether experimental procedures could access the true functions of the frontal lobes [Hebb and Penfield, 1940].

Interest in the function of the prefrontal cortex was strongly whetted with publication of a symposium on the prefrontal granular cortex [Warren and Akert, 1964] that gathered experimental results and clinical observations of recent origin. Most were animal experiments, limited in behavioral complexity. At about this same time, collected observations of patients who survived frontal brain injury in World War II and of individuals who had been treated with prefrontal psychosurgical procedures became available. From this material, new, more complex theories of prefrontal function were formulated. Many theories have been offered in the past two decades, only a few of which have been selected for this presentation.

Pribram [1960], *Pribram and Melges* [1969], *Miller et al.* [1960]. Karl Pribram accepted the major anatomical subdivision of the brain – a posterior system involved with the search to delineate a basic problem and an anterior (frontal) system that subserved intentional behavior – but he emphasized that behavior could not be explained as a simple reflex arc. He posited a more complex system featuring a feedback loop for monitoring brain activity. A Test-Operate-Test-Exit (TOTE) system (see fig. 1) was suggested. This feedback loop could become quite complex with multiple functioning feedback loops providing a good deal of prefrontal control for brain activity before effecting a single response mechanism. The feedback loop was suggested as a fundamental functional unit for brain activity. In later writings, Pribram [1973] further emphasized the importance of the prefrontal regions for producing mental responses while maintaining appropriate awareness of the environmental context.

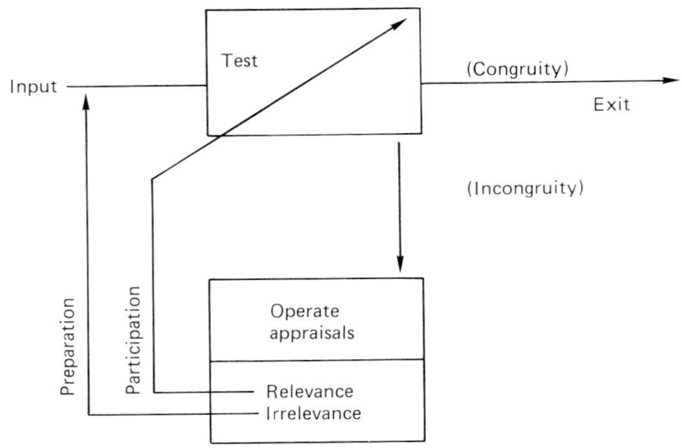

Fig. 1. Schematic illustration of brain effort hypothesized in the TOTE hypothesis suggested by Pribram and colleagues. Modified from Miller et al. [1960].

Teuber [1964, 1966, 1972]. Teuber presented a new and radically different theory of frontal lobe function. While previous investigators had universally considered brain functions to be initiated posteriorly and move forward to the motor system for the final common pathway, Teuber hypothesized that an anterior, anticipatory process both precedes and influences much posterior sensory processing. In his view, these 'corollary discharges' travelled from the anterior to the posterior brain areas to prepare the sensory structures for anticipated changes from voluntary movement. His classic example concerned volitional versus passive eye movement. When the eye is moved normally, the environment never appears to move. It is suggested that the corollary discharge from the frontal motor region to the posterior sensory regions presets the latter for the sensory consequences of a motor input. In contrast, when the eye is pushed (moved passively) the environment appears to relocate. To effect the corollary discharge the frontal lobes must monitor the external stimuli, first by feedback and then, by a feed-forward step, predict and prepare for the consequences of an upcoming motor act. Voluntary movements require two sets of feed-forward signals. The first is a direct signal to effector areas (prefrontal to motor); the second is a simultaneous signal (prefrontal to posterior) to preset the sensory system for the anticipated effect (fig. 2). Teuber's corollary discharge theory considerably complicated the postulated func-

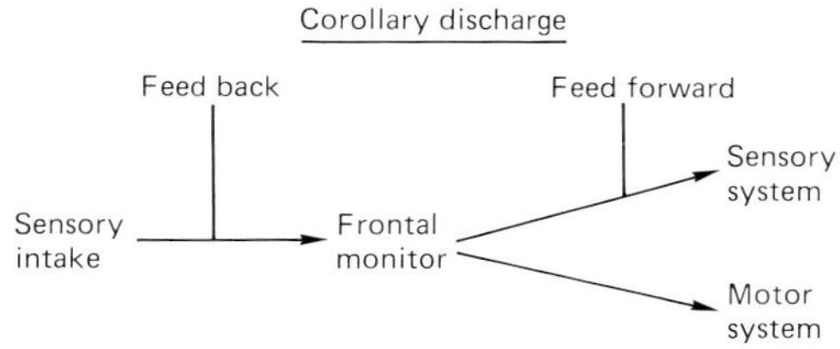

Fig. 2. Schematic illustration of corollary discharge mechanism proposed by Teuber.

tions of the prefrontal area and also suggested explanations for a number of complex brain activities.

Nauta [1971, 1972]. Nauta added a neuroanatomical basis for the theories posited by Pribram and Teuber. In particular, he emphasized the rich association of the limbic and somatosensory systems in the frontal lobe. In a series of papers describing frontal anatomical connections, he demonstrated that the prefrontal cortex was the only area in which the limbic system had strong reciprocal connections with association cortex and was also the only area in which the limbic and all somatosensory systems had strong associations. He not only provided a neuroanatomical basis for the feedback and corollary discharge theories proposed earlier but went on to suggest two major corollary discharge systems – one exteroceptive in which the influence was on the posterior cortical sensory system, and the second interoceptive in which the major influence concerned visceral activities. Nauta's anatomical demonstrations provided a structure for the internal testing of a proposed behavior, an important aspect of prefrontal function.

Damasio [1979]. In his discussion of frontal lobe function, Damasio emphasized that a guiding principle of behavior is the preservation of equilibrium and suggested that the frontal lobes are crucial for this task. The frontal lobes appear to fulfill three major functions: (1) they act as a judge of external stimuli; (2) they plan appropriate responses; (3) they regulate behavior. Each of these tasks can be demonstrated and an anatomical basis can be presented for their activity. Damasio went on to posit two significant gating systems for the control of human brain activity. The first is a hypothalamic gating system, primarily responsive to pleasure/pain, that actively monitors most automatic and autonomic functions. While this gating system is almost constantly active, most of this activity is performed unconsciously. The second is a frontal gating system in which complex environmental contingencies are monitored and responses prepared. This system handles novel and more complicated gating problems, at least some of which reach partial consciousness.

Fuster [1980]. In a relatively recent monograph based primarily on contemporary animal physiologic and anatomical investigations, Fuster emphasized that the temporal structuring of behavior was a key frontal lobe function. He further suggested that the frontal lobe functions in anticipation, provisional memory and control of interference. Provisional memory was described as the ability to maintain small bits of information for later response. Laboratory (animal) studies suggest that both anticipation and provisional memory can be localized to the dorsal lateral aspects of the frontal lobe. In addition to these basic activities, Fuster also postulated that the frontal lobes initiate, give intent, motivate and provide vigor to complex behaviors. Thus, he suggests that the prefrontal cortex exerts a strong executive control function.

Shallice [1978, 1982]. The British psychologist, Tim Shallice, using a combination of information theory and cognitive psychological approaches, constructed an information processing model of brain function. His model goes well beyond the functions of the prefrontal lobes but emphasizes the importance of these structures. Shallice posits four major component stages in mental activity: (1) Cognitive units, those brain functions associated with recognized anatomical/functional systems (e.g. memory, language, etc.), the mental activities that have been well studied in both recent and older behavioral and psychological studies. (2) Schemas, information from combinations of the cognitive units that is used in routine behavior. Thus, driving a car from work to home on a regular basis would demand the integrative activity of a number of cognitive units, a combination considered a schema. (3) Contention scheduling, a more complex activity that entails a selection of schemas for relatively rapid, routine tasks. Thus, if the trip from work to home was interrupted by a stop to pick up groceries, this would demand contention scheduling, the ordering of separate schemas to complete an already known activity. (4) Supervisory attentional system, a distinctly superordinate function by means of which nonroutine goal achievement could be acquired. The supervisory attentional system is only brought into operation when contention scheduling fails or when there is no known solution for a problem. Once a satisfactory solution has been derived and overlearned, the activity would be continued as a schema or other more basic mental unit. While most of the routine activities, the schemas and much of contention scheduling can be handled by posterior brain activity, the supervisory attentional system is a frontal function.

Luria [1966, 1970]. Based on many years of clinical observations, neuropsychological testing and anatomical studies, the Russian psychologist Luria developed an extensive theory of brain function. A number of crucial features can be extracted from the large volume of his writings to produce a comprehensive theory. Luria suggests three important cerebral zones. The first is basal (brainstem and diencephalon) and primarily operates to maintain cortical tone. The second is the posterior cortex that deals with basic sensorimotor functions. The third, the frontal cortex, regulates brain functions. Luria emphasizes the control functions performed by the frontal lobes through much of his writings. He particularly notes that the prefrontal cortex has reciprocal connections with, and therefore control of, the basal functions; the tone of all mental activity is dependent upon intact basal-prefrontal activity. In addition, he emphasized the feedback/feedforward influence of the prefrontal cortex on sensorimotor functions. Thus, Luria postulated a controlling influence of the prefrontal cortex on basic brain functions. Based on this theory he emphasized that although frontal damage produced a notable decrease in mental tone (alertness, arousal) and posterior brain functions (sensation, perception), most brain activity could still be carried out, just not as efficiently. He also noted that, based on the mental control function, prefrontal damage could produce a separation of thought and action. The frontally damaged individual could express and 'know' the proper or expected response but carry out a totally different action.

Stuss and Benson Theory

Based on clinical studies of both brain-damaged humans and a series of post-leukotomy subjects, experience with neuropsychological testing and review of the world's literature including the theories of brain function mentioned above, we [Stuss and Benson, 1986] proposed a theory of brain function with particular emphasis on the activities of the prefrontal cortex. Our theory is clearly derivative from the theories presented above, both the original clinical/anatomical studies from the turn of the century and the

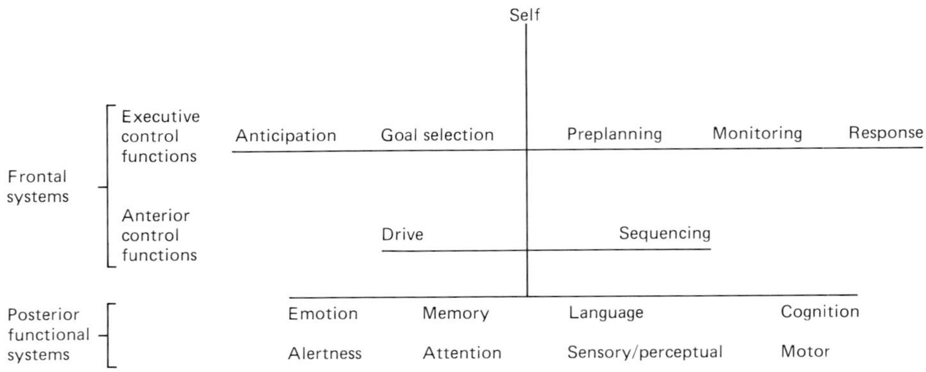

Fig. 3. Schematic illustration of hierarchy of mental functions postulated by Stuss and Benson [1986]. Modified from Stuss and Benson [1986].

more recent theories and anatomical demonstrations. We offer an additional breakdown of frontal lobe activities and propose four separate levels of brain function to illustrate these frontal activities. Figure 3 illustrates the levels of brain activity in a hierarchical pattern.

Posterior Fixed Organized Integrated Functional Systems. Under this heading we have subsumed the major separable behavioral/psychological functions that have been studied over the past century. A great number of terms have been suggested for these systems (e.g. faculties, modules, processes, functions). The eight postulated posterior functional systems, while separable, are not mutually exclusive (in fact, they are integrated). Nonetheless, each has traditionally been studied as a separate entity. The three most basic of the functional systems include alertness (awakeness), attention, and emotion. A middle group represents more cortically directed activity, the basic sensory-perceptual and motor functions. The third group, representing higher human functions includes memory, language, visuospatial skill and cognition. Each of these brain functions has been thoroughly studied by psychologists, each has a fairly well established anatomy and at least some recognized physiological attributes. Each of the eight systems can be specifically disordered by focal brain damage that affects either the posterior or the basal portions of the brain. These functional systems represent the basic building blocks of cerebral activity and are the stuff of both neuropsychology and behavioral neurology.

Frontal Fixed Organized Integrated Functional Systems. Two additional functional systems are posited, both apparently acting in a superordinate fashion to the posterior functional systems and each apparently based on frontal brain activities. The first can be called sequencing, the ability of the brain to handle multiple bits of information in an accurate serial order, the temporal structuring of Fuster [1980]. In addition, the ability to extract relevant information from the sequences and place it into new sequences (sets) of information is a related function. Finally, taking information from sequences and/or sets and integrating it with old, previously learned information is another closely related function. Obviously, these activities are tightly integrated with the posterior functional systems, dependent upon their material, and act exclusively as a superordinate mechanism.

A second, totally different frontal fixed organized integrated functional system concerns drive. One of the most common prefrontal behavioral symptoms is apathy, the lack of initiative. While frontally damaged patients often retain good fund of knowledge and normal motor abilities, they fail to activate these attributes. Drive is closely related to motivation (often defined as more intellectual); both may be seriously deficient in frontally damaged patients. In addition, human will is closely related to (dependent upon) these functions and can also be considered a frontal function. Drive, motivation and will are also superordinate to the posterior functional system and are closely related to important basal functions.

There appears to be an anatomical basis for the two frontal fixed organized integrated functional systems. Sequencing, sets and integration appear to represent lateral prefrontal activity, both the dorsal lateral convexity and the lateral aspects of the orbital surfaces. In contrast, abnormalities of drive and motivation are closely related to medial frontal dysfunction, following damage to the medial orbital as well as the sagittal frontal regions. Both of the frontal fixed systems, however, exert their influence through the posterior/basal systems.

Executive (Cognitive) Control Functions. Apparently superior to all of the fixed organized integrated functional systems outlined above are a number of executive functions. Many terms have been suggested but five activities represent most of these control functions: (a) anticipation; (b) goal selection; (c) pre-planning (means-end establishment); (d) initiation of novel responses; and (e) monitoring (if-then considerations). This control activity, the executive mental functions carried out by human beings, is almost universally recognized as a prefrontal function. Again, while the prefrontal executive activities are truly superordinate and affect (control) all basic brain functions, each of the individual functional systems can operate without this control, the divorce of thought and action stressed by Luria.

Self-Consciousness. Finally, it can be hypothesized that one of the most mysterious of human functions, the recognition of the self, represents another frontal function. Self-consciousness, self-awareness, self-control and so on, all tend to be impaired following frontal damage. The various functions that make up what is called the self include combinations of most or all posterior and frontal functional systems plus the executive control mechanism. This is the level that James [1890] called the 'Me'. Superior to this vast amount of knowledge and action is yet another function, that of knowing the knowledge; this ability to introspect has been called the psyche, the ego, the 'I', the little man in brain, the ghost in the machine, and many other terms. While the knowledge itself can be disturbed by damage to the other systems, disturbance of knowing this knowledge (self-awareness, self-monitoring, etc.) almost invariably indicates frontal lobe malfunction. Konow and Pribram [1970] note that while a frontal lobe patient may recognize his errors, he cannot use this knowledge to correct his behavior.

Conclusion

It must be recognized that all of the theories mentioned here represent hypothetical, imaginary structures set up for test and evaluation. In some, particularly the earlier theories, investigations have confirmed many of the points suggested. Less of the conjecture has been proved for the more recent theories. It can be anticipated that future generations will produce new, more advanced and more comprehensive theories of human brain function. At least some of the theories presented here will be basic to these new theories. It can be confidently anticipated that the functions of the prefrontal cortex will be of increasing importance to future developments of theories of brain activity.

References

Benson, D.F.; Stuss, D.T.; Naeser, M.A.; Weir, W.S.; Kaplan, E.F.; Levine, H.L.: The long term effects of prefrontal leukotomy. Archs Neurol. *38:* 165–169 (1981).

Bianchi, L.: The functions of the frontal lobes. Brain *18:* 497–522 (1895).

Chapman, L.F.; Wolf, H.G.: The cerebral hemispheres and the highest integrative functions of man. Archs Neurol. *1:* 357–424 (1959).

Damasio, A.R.: The frontal lobes; in Heilman, Valenstein, Clinical neuropsychology, pp. 360–412 (Oxford University Press, New York 1979).

Denny-Brown, D.: The frontal lobes and their functions; in Feiling, Modern trends in neurology, pp. 13–89 (Butterworth, London 1951).

Feuchtwanger, E.: Die Funktionen des Stirnhirns, ihre Pathologie und Psychologie. Monogr. Gesamtgebiete Neurol. Psychiat., Berlin *38:* 1–193 (1923).

Flechsig, P.: Gehirn und Seele (Viet, Leipzig, 1896).

Franz, S.I: On the functions of the cerebrum of the frontal lobes (Science Press, New York).

Fulton, J.F.: Frontal lobotomy and affective behavior (Norton, New York 1951).

Fuster, J.M.: The prefrontal cortex: anatomy, physiology and neuropsychology of the frontal lobes (Raven Press, New York 1980).

Goldstein, K.: The significance of the frontal lobes for mental performances. J. Neurol. Psychopathol. *17:* 27–40 (1936).

Goldstein, K.: Mental changes due to frontal lobe damage. J. Psychol. *17:* 187–208 (1944).

Grant, D.A.; Berg, E.A.: A behavioral analysis of reinforcement and ease of shifting to new responses in a Weigl-type card-sorting problem. J. exp. Psychol. *38:* 404–411 (1948).

Harlow, J.: Recovery from the passage of an iron bar through the head. Publ. Mass. med. Soc., Boston *2:* 329–346 (1868).

Hebb, D.O.; Penfield, W.: Human behaviour after extensive bilateral removal from the frontal lobes. Archs Neurol. Psychiat. *44:* 421–438 (1940).

Hécaen, H.: Mental symptoms with tumors of the frontal lobe; in Warren, Akert, The frontal granular cortex and behavior, pp. 335–352 (McGraw-Hill, New York 1964).

Hécaen, H.; Albert, M.L.: Human neuropsychology (Wiley, New York 1978).

James, W.: The principles of psychology (Holt, New York 1890).

Kleist, K.: Kriegsverletzungen des Gehirns in ihrer Bedeutung für Hirnlokalisation und Hirnpathologie (Barth, Leipzig 1934).

Konow, A.; Pribram, K.H.: Error recognition and utilization produced by injury to the frontal cortex in man. Neuropsychologia *8:* 489–491 (1970).

Lashley, K.S.: Brain mechanisms and language (University of Chicago Press, Chicago 1929).

Lishman, W.A.: Psychiatric disability after head injury: the significance of brain damage. Proc. R. Soc. Med. 59: 261–266 (1966).

Luria, A.R.: Two kinds of motor perseveration in massive injuries of the frontal lobes. Brain *88:* 1–10 (1965).

Luria, A.R.: Human brain and psychological processes (transl. by B. Haig) (Harper & Row, New York 1966).

Luria, A.R.: The functional organization of the brain. Sci. Am. *222:* 66–78 (1970).

Marie, P.; Foix, C.: Les aphasies de guerre. Revue neurol. *24:* 53–87 (1917).

McGhie, A.; Chapman, J.: Disorders of attention and perception in early schizophrenia. Br. J. med. Psychol. *34:* 103–116 (1961).

Mettler, F.A. (ed.): Columbia-Greystone Associates: selective partial ablation of the frontal cortex: a correlative study of its effects on human psychotic subjects (Hoeber, New York 1949).

Meynert, T.: Psychiatrie. Klinik der Erkrankungen des Vorderhirns erste Hälfte (Braumuller, Vienna 1884).

Miller, G.A.; Galanter, E.H.; Pribram, K.H.: Plans and the structure of behavior (Holt, Rinehart & Winston, New York 1960).

Milner, B.: Effects of different brain lesions on card sorting. Archs Neurol. *9:* 90–100 (1963).

Monakow, C.V.: Gehirnpathologie; 2nd ed. (Holder, Vienna 1905).

Naeser, M.A.; Levine, H.L.; Benson, D.F.; Stuss, D.T.; Weir, W.S.: Frontal leukotomy size and hemispheric asymmetries on computerized tomographic scans of schizophrenics with variable recovery. Archs Neurol. *38:* 30–37 (1981).

Nauta, W.J.H.: The problem of the frontal lobe: a reinterpretation. J. psychiat. Res. *8:* 167–187 (1971).

Nauta, W.J.H.: Neural associations of the frontal cortex. Acta Neurobiol. exp. *32:* 125–140 (1972).

Pribram, K.H.: The intrinsic systems of the forebrain; in Field, Magoun, Hall, Handbook of physiology, vol. II, pp. 1323–1344 (Am. Physiologic Society, Washington 1960).

Pribram, K.H.: The primate frontal cortex – executive of the brain; in Pribram, Luria, Psychophysiology of the frontal lobes, pp. 293–314 (Academic Press, New York 1973).

Pribram, K.H.; Melges, F.T.: Physiological basis of emotion; in Vinken, Bruyn, Handbook of clinical neurology, vol. III, pp. 316–342 (North-Holland, Amsterdam 1969).

Russell, W.R.: Disability caused by brain wounds. J. Neurol. Neurosurg. Psychiat. *14:* 35–39 (1951).

Salazar, A.M.; Jabbari, B.; Vance, S.C.; Grafman, J.; Amin, D.; Dillon, J.D.: Epilepsy after penetrating head injury. I. Clinical correlates. Neurology *35:* 1406–1414 (1985).

Shallice, T.: The dominant action system: an information processing approach to consciousness; in Pope, Singer, The stream of consciousness, pp. 117–157 (Plenum Press, New York 1978).

Shallice, T.: Specific impairments of planning; in Broadbent, Weiskrantz, The neuropsychology of cognitive function, pp. 199–209 (Royal Society, London 1982).

Stuss, D.T.; Benson, D.F.: Neuropsychological studies of the frontal lobes. Psychol. Bull. *95:* 3–28 (1984).

Stuss, D.T.; Benson, D.F.: The frontal lobes (Raven Press, New York 1986).

Stuss, D.T.; Benson, D.F.; Kaplan, E.F.: Leucotomized and nonleucotomized schizophrenics: comparison on tests of attention. Biol. Psychiat. *16:* 1085–1100 (1981).

Stuss, D.T.; Benson, D.F.; Kaplan, E.F.; Weir, W.S.; Naeser, M.A.; Lieberman, I.; Ferrill, D.: The involvement of orbitofrontal cerebrum in cognitive tasks. Neuropsychologia *21:* 235–248 (1983).

Stuss, D.T.; Kaplan, E.F.; Benson, D.F.: Long-term effects of prefrontal leucotomy: cognitive functions; in Malatesha, Hartlage, Neuropsychology and cognition, vol. II, pp. 252–271 (Nijhoff, The Hague 1982).

Teuber, H.-L.: The riddle of frontal lobe function in man; in Warren, Akert, The frontal granular cortex and behavior, pp. 410–477 (McGraw-Hill, New York 1964).

Teuber, H.-L.: The frontal lobes and their functions: further observations on rodents, carnivores, subhuman primates and man. Int. J. Neurol. *5:* 282–300 (1966).

Teuber, H.-L.: Unity and diversity of frontal lobe functions. Acta Neurobiol. *32:* 615–656 (1972).
Tilney, F.: The brain, from ape to man (Hoeber, New York 1928).
Venables, P.H.: The relationship between level of skin potential and fusion of paired light flashes in schizophrenic and normal subjects. J. psychiat. Res. *1:* 279–287 (1963).
Warren, J.M.; Akert. K. (eds.): The frontal granular cortex and behavior (McGraw-Hill, New York 1964).
Wechsler, D.: Manual for the Wechsler Adult Intelligence Scale (The Psychological Corporation, New York 1955).
Wernicke, C.: Das aphasische Symptomenkompex (Cohn & Weigart, Breslau, 1874).
Worster-Drought, C.: Mental symptoms associated with tumours of the frontal lobes. Proc. R. Soc. Med. *24:* 1007 (1931).

D. Frank Benson, MD, UCLA Department of Neurology, 710 Westwood Plaza, Los Angeles, CA 90024 (USA)

Subject Index